ENTER LAUGHING—

The first ones were left over from the vaudeville
circuit. Then came the nightclub and radio
veterans, followed by those who courageously cracked
their first jokes on live television. Eventually they
all found their way to Hollywood, and stirred up the
laughter that generations of moviegoers and
late-show watchers still break into. . . .

MOVIE COMEDY TEAMS

LEONARD MALTIN is a leading authority on
American films and is the film critic for the
nightly television show "Entertainment
Tonight." His other books include OF MICE AND
MAGIC and THE WHOLE FILM SOURCE BOOK,
both available in Plume editions, and the
bestselling TV MOVIES, available in Plume and
Signet editions.

MOVIE COMEDY TEAMS

Leonard Maltin

With an Introduction by BILLY GILBERT

REVISED AND UPDATED

A PLUME BOOK

NEW AMERICAN LIBRARY

NEW YORK AND SCARBOROUGH, ONTARIO

**Dedicated to my mother and father,
without whom . . .**

NAL BOOKS ARE AVAILABLE AT QUANTITY DISCOUNTS WHEN
USED TO PROMOTE PRODUCTS OR SERVICES. FOR INFORMA-
TION PLEASE WRITE TO PREMIUM MARKETING DIVISION, NEW
AMERICAN LIBRARY, 1633 BROADWAY, NEW YORK, NEW YORK
10019.

PHOTOGRAPH CREDITS AND ACKNOWLEDGMENTS: *Film Fan Monthly,* Abner
Blumenfeld, Ernest D. Burns and Cinemabilia, Carlos Clarens, Doro-
thy Granger, Ron Green, Gary Hough, Al Kilgore, Harold Kinkade,
Jr., Doug McClelland, Jeff Satkin, Lou Valentino, Jerry Vermilye,
Harvey Chertok and Warner Brothers, Hal Roach, RKO Radio Pic-
tures, Metro-Goldwyn-Mayer, Paramount Pictures, Columbia Pictures,
20th Century-Fox, Universal Pictures, Screen Gems, United Artists,
Theatre Collection of the New York Public Library, Independent Inter-
national Pictures, Museum of Modern Art Film Stills Archive, Phil
Johnson. Special thanks to Bernard Maltin for his photographic work.

The chapters on Wheeler and Woolsey and the Three Stooges have been
expanded from articles which originally appeared in *Film Fan Monthly*.

Movie Comedy Teams was published originally in a Signet edition.

SIGNET, SIGNET CLASSIC, MENTOR, PLUME, MERIDIAN AND NAL BOOKS
are published *in the United States* by New American Library,
1633 Broadway, New York, New York 10019,
in Canada by The New American Library of Canada Limited,
81 Mack Avenue, Scarborough, Ontario M1L 1M8

Library of Congress Cataloging in Publication Data

Maltin, Leonard.
  Movie comedy teams.

  Includes index.
  1. Comedy films—United States—History and
criticism. 2. Comedians—United States. I. Title.
PN1995.9.C55M35   1985   791.43′028′0922   85-10449
ISBN 0-452-25694-1

First Signet Printing, December, 1970

First Plume Printing (Revised Edition), August, 1985

1 2 3 4 5 6 7 8 9

PRINTED IN THE UNITED STATES OF AMERICA

CONTENTS

(Complete filmographies follow each of the chapters.)

Preface to the Plume Edition

It's been sixteen years since I wrote *Movie Comedy Teams*. My goal at that time was to chart the careers of movies' greatest comedy partners, and to celebrate some of the teams who'd been neglected. Judging from the mail I received, I did succeed in turning people on to the manic delights of Clark and McCullough, the vaudevillian hokum of Wheeler and Woolsey, and the utter charm of Thelma Todd with ZaSu Pitts and Patsy Kelly. Nothing could have brought me greater satisfaction.

Even today, I think this book will open some eyes—to the delights of the Wiere Brothers, or the evergreen shtick of Smith and Dale. But quite a lot has changed since my book first saw the light.

When I completed the original manuscript in 1969, Groucho Marx was still alive and active. So were the Three Stooges. George Burns had yet to embark on his new acting career. And Cheech and Chong were just starting to light up.

At that time, a Marx Brothers revival was in full swing, and book-length studies of the team were starting to appear. But no book had yet discussed the work of Abbott and Costello or the Three Stooges—or even acknowledged their existence! Research material on these teams, not to mention Wheeler and Woolsey or Clark and McCullough, was virtually nonexistent.

As of this writing, there are now three books in my collection about Abbott and Costello (one of which I edited), eight on the Three Stooges and its individual members (though a full-fledged biography of Shemp has yet to surface), and no less than sixteen on the Marx Brothers! (A magazine called *The Freedonia Gazette* adds still more information to the Marxian mound every year.) But there is still no other book that chronicles the careers of such notable teams as the Ritz Brothers, Burns and Allen, and Olsen and Johnson. And there is no other work that presents the stories of the famous comedy teams—and the forgotten ones—side by side.

So it is that *Movie Comedy Teams* returns, substantially the same as before but with a number of changes and additions. Nearly all the chapters have been updated in some way. Needless to say, Rowan and Martin are not "the country's hottest comedy team" as they were in 1969, and Joey Bishop is no longer welcoming the Three Stooges and the Ritz Brothers to his now long-defunct late-night TV show.

Shortly after the first edition of this book was published, I met and interviewed director H. C. Potter, who revealed some fascinating details about the original version of HELLZAPOP-PIN. A few years later the long-unseen Wheeler and Woolsey version of GIRL CRAZY was given its first public showing in decades. Then, just a few years ago, I got to see the 1925 silent feature TOO MANY KISSES, in which Harpo Marx made his movie debut. These meetings and screenings have enabled me to flesh out certain points in the text. (I recently heard Jerry Lewis name his favorite Martin and Lewis movie; I couldn't resist adding it to the M & L chapter.)

The filmographies reflect additional research "finds." These include some heretofore unpublished credits for Groucho and Chico Marx, Abbott and Costello, Olsen and Johnson, Wheeler and Woolsey, Clark and McCullough, and the Ritz Brothers—most are guest appearances, but interesting footnotes nonetheless. (Finding a new Marx Brothers credit, no matter how obscure, is something of a coup.)

I also couldn't resist replacing some of the stills that appeared in the original volume with newly discovered goodies.

One thing I would *not* think of changing is the introduction to the 1970 edition, which was written by one of my heroes, a delightful comedian named Billy Gilbert. Billy is gone now, and many of the references in his foreword are dated, but his recollections are worth retaining, and his association with the great comedy teams is worth remembering.

I am indebted to Herb Graff, Mary Corliss, Carol Epstein, Eddie Brandt, Alice Cella, Samuel M. Sherman, Douglas Hart, Jim Mulholland, Phil Johnson, Richard Plotkin, the late H. C. Potter, and the late Joe Smith, for helping to make this new edition a reality, with very special thanks, as always, to my wonderful wife, Alice. I am happy to repeat my original list of acknowledgments from 1970 with a sincere thank-you to Gordon Berkow, Joe Bolton, George Burns, Harvey Chertok, David Chierichetti, John Cocchi, Jon Davison, Harvey Deneroff, William K. Everson, Dorothy Granger, Alan Hoffman, the late Moe Howard, the late Al Kilgore, Don Koll, Miles Kreuger, the late Sidney Lanfield, Doug McClelland, Milton Menell, Charles Pavlicek Jr., and Chris Steinbrunner.

And I'm equally happy to repeat my hopes for this book as stated in the original preface: I hope this book fills a gap in film history, however small. I trust it is thorough. But above all, I hope it is fun, for after all, that's what comedy is all about.

LEONARD MALTIN
Los Angeles, California
February 1985

Introduction

I am honored to write the introduction for this new book about comedy teams in motion pictures. I was associated with so many of them in the thirties and forties.

I wrote and acted in nine Laurel and Hardy pictures. I wrote and acted in I don't know how many Thelma Todd and ZaSu Pitts comedies—later when Patsy Kelly joined Thelma I worked with them, too. The Ritz Brothers are good friends of mine, and we appeared together in ON THE AVENUE. The Three Stooges (the original ones) were all friends of mine. Shemp Howard, who formed the act for vaudeville and later did the shorts, was about my dearest friend.

Bud Abbott is an actor today because of me. He was a ticket taker in a theater I played in. When my straight man didn't show up one day I remembered a bright kid out front and sent for him to replace my missing straight man. He was so good I kept him in the show. I was 22 years old and he was 19.

I worked in one of the only feature movies that Olsen and Johnson ever did. I was in A NIGHT AT THE OPERA with the Marx Brothers, and later was guest star on Groucho's radio show many times. We are good friends now. Bert Wheeler was a very dear pal, and I also worked with Clark and McCullough.

I first saw Dean Martin and Jerry Lewis when they had just become a team. They were playing at Bill Miller's Riviera Night Club in New Jersey; I think it was in 1946. After their show they came to my table and introduced themselves and we became friends. Jerry came to our house frequently and I still see him occasionally.

There always seems to be one outstanding comedy team in each era. Rowan and Martin are the current ones. I don't know them but think they are fine.

It is very difficult to be half of a successful comedy team, just as it is difficult to be half of a successful marriage. Some people can't take it—they are simply together too much. They usually protect themselves from each other by having entirely separate private lives. Even so they sometimes break up—Martin and Lewis, and Allen and Rossi are good examples. Laurel and Hardy were never close socially at the peak of their careers. It was only when they were touring in

Britain and Europe and not doing so well in their movie careers that they turned to each other and each found a cherished friend.

I was briefly teamed with Ben Blue, Frank Fay and Shemp Howard, but never cared much for the experience even though I liked all three men. Only one man sticks to my memory who I really enjoyed being teamed with. That was Buster Keaton. We appeared together on a Ken Murray TV show in 1952. *Variety* reviewed our sketch as the funniest scene ever done on television. Ken is my closest friend and he has a print of this scene. We occasionally look at it and I must immodestly say it's wonderfully funny. Buster said to me afterwards, "Isn't it too bad we didn't team up when talkies first started and I took such a beating? I really think we would have made it." You know, I think so, too.

I read not long ago about Elizabeth Taylor and Richard Burton; they were having a discussion about the fact that they had done so many pictures together. Mr. Burton told his wife he wanted to do his next picture without her. He said, "We don't want to become another Laurel and Hardy." Whereupon Miss Taylor cried, "Why? What's so bad about Laurel and Hardy?" And I say "What indeed?"

BILLY GILBERT

[Billy Gilbert, a great comedian and a kind, gentle man, died on September 23, 1971, at the age of 77.]

Billy Gilbert with Laurel and Hardy in THEM THAR HILLS.

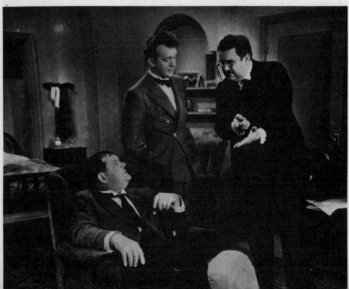

LAUREL and HARDY

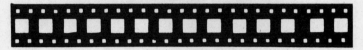

Screen comedy has never been fully appreciated by film students and scholars. Chaplin was the first, and for many years the only comedian to be hailed as an "artist." James Agee was the first one to bring attention to the genius of Buster Keaton, but he did so twenty years after Keaton had passed his prime. Harold Lloyd was always liked, but was seldom considered worthy of analysis.

The comedy teams suffered in particular. Only the Marx Brothers were noticed by the intelligentsia, who also failed to note that the Brothers' films went steadily downhill after A DAY AT THE RACES. Completely lost in the shuffle until very recent years were Laurel and Hardy. Taken for granted, unappreciated by film critics even during their peak years, they suffered at the hands of Hollywood and were forced into premature retirement.

Three things brought Laurel and Hardy back into the spotlight in the 1950's and 60's: First, the constant showing of their films on television: second, the inclusion of L & H footage in Robert Youngson's films like THE GOLDEN AGE OF COMEDY; and third, the publication of a warm, appreciative biography called *Mr. Laurel and Mr. Hardy* by John McCabe. This sudden spurt of interest in L & H made people stop and take a second look at the duo. What they discovered was that Stan Laurel and Oliver Hardy were the greatest comedy team of all time.

The word "great" is overused, mainly by advertisers and press agents, and it has become something of a joke in the entertainment industry, especially when a performer is aware that he is supposed to *be* great. Laurel and Hardy never had any such pretensions; they were simply two very fine clowns who went about their business with love and dedication, and garnered millions of fans in the process. They still have a legion of admirers around the world, and an international club called The Sons of the Desert perpetuates their mem-

1

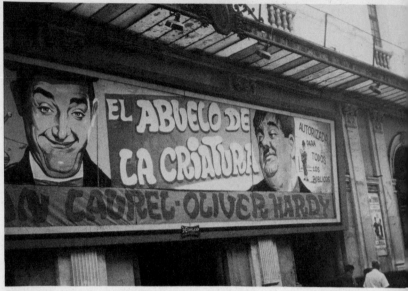

A Laurel and Hardy poster outside a theater in Barcelona.

ory. The members of this group, all dedicated L & H buffs, speak fondly of Stan and Babe (as Hardy was known off screen) as if they were lifelong friends, and to anyone who has seen their films again and again, they are just that. Laurel and Hardy created two very likable, very *believable* characters, and buffs feel they have lived with "the boys" through all their adventures together. No other comedy team, and few other comedians, ever elicited such empathy from an audience, and few ever received such international acclaim. Laurel and Hardy movies are still shown all over the world. A recent visitor to Barcelona, Spain, was amazed to find a local theater advertising, with large, colorful posters, EL ABUELO DE LA CRIATURA, the Spanish name for their 1932 feature PACK UP YOUR TROUBLES. The film's age means nothing to the people who see it; laughter is timeless, and so are Laurel and Hardy.

There is a disturbing tendency to praise Stan Laurel while ignoring Oliver Hardy. The reasons are understandable: Stan was "the brains of the outfit" off screen, working out the gags and supervising the editing of their films. In addition, he outlived Hardy by eight years, living to see the L & H revival in full swing and be lionized by thousands of fans around the world. But Laurel and Hardy were a team in every sense of the word; neither one dominated the other on screen, and off screen their relationship was one of mutual respect and admiration. Ollie's response to any queries about comedy was always "Ask Stan." Comedian Billy Gilbert, who worked with the team for many years, recalled, "There was no rivalry between them. Babe would do anything Stan suggested. To him he was a god, and he had the greatest respect for Stan's genius for thinking up comic situations." Similarly, when John McCabe asked Stan why it appeared that his eyes were always on Hardy when he watched their films, he replied, "I guess it's because the character fascinates me so much. He really is a funny, funny fellow, isn't he?"

They were both funny fellows, from entirely different backgrounds. Stan was born Arthur Stanley Jefferson in Ulverston, Lancashire, England, in 1890. His father, A. J. Jefferson, was a prominent local theatrical entrepreneur.

In one of those stranger-than-fiction coincidences, the actor hired to play a thief in Stan Laurel's 1917 starring comedy LUCKY DOG was none other than Oliver Hardy! The two never worked together until 1926 when they came together under the Hal Roach roof. The film, long thought to be lost, was discovered by Robert Youngson, who used it in his film 30 YEARS OF FUN.

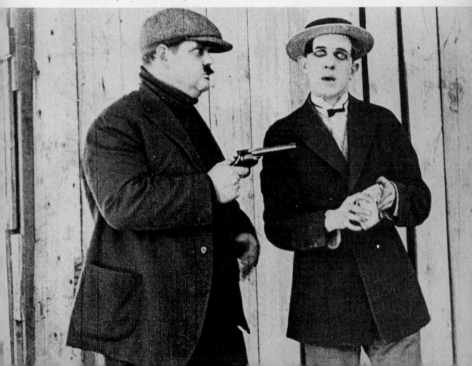

Bitten by the stage bug at an early age, Stan made his debut
at the age of sixteen and, with his parents' reluctant consent,
set out to conquer new worlds. For seven years he toured
England with various theatrical troupes, doing straight plays,
comedies, and sketches. His greatest opportunity came when
he joined the Fred Karno troupe, which included another
comic named Charlie Chaplin. They performed in the classic
sketch *Mumming Birds*, which under the title *A Night in an
English Music Hall* also toured the United States. Stan Laurel (as he was then known) decided to set out on his own, and
became a staple on the various American vaudeville circuits
with a variety of knockabout comedy acts. In 1917 he was
approached to do a one-reel comedy, NUTS IN MAY, which
won him a Universal Pictures contract. At Universal he
starred in a series called HICKORY HIRAM, but before long
his contract lapsed and was not renewed. Stan returned to
vaudeville, but in 1918 was back in films, where he free-
lanced for the next eight years, working on and off for his
future mentor, Hal Roach. At Vitagraph he supported Larry
Semon, and for producer (former cowboy star) "Bronco
Billy" Anderson, he did a now-historic two-reeler, LUCKY
DOG, which featured Oliver Hardy in a minor role as a
crook.

At this point, Stan began to make a name for himself in
films. He did a short series for Anderson, and other producers, which included some first-rate slapstick spoofs of popular feature films of the day. MUD AND SAND parodied
Valentino's BLOOD AND SAND with Stan as "Rhubarb Vaselino." The comedy was frantic, and all the stops were out,
with such scenes as Stan, on horseback, waving good-bye to
his native village as he goes off to the big city, then falling
off the horse into a mud puddle. THE SOILERS poked fun at
Rex Beach's hard-bitten tale of the Yukon, THE SPOILERS,
with all the action stopping periodically to let a local pansy skip
merrily through the scene. DR. PYCKLE AND MR. PRYDE used
trick photography to help Stan make his drastic change from
sedate Dr. Pyckle to lurching Mr. Pryde, whose dastardly
schemes included aiming a pea-shooter at unsuspecting pedestrians in the London streets.

Many of Stan's solo comedies survive today, and most are
quite funny. SMITHY (1925) was a forerunner to the Laurel
and Hardy comedy THE FINISHING TOUCH, with Stan as an
inept construction supervisor who builds a house which, at
the end of the film, collapses entirely. KILL OR CURE (1923)
shows Stan in his most typical role, that of the brash young

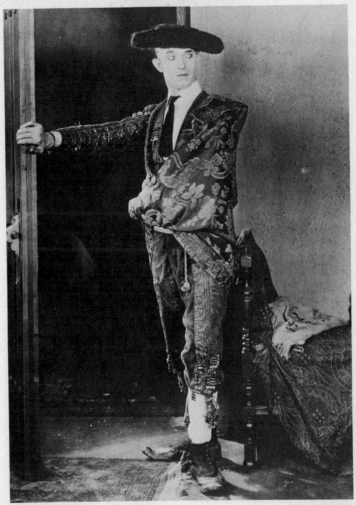

Stan, as Latin lover Rhubarb Vaselino, strikes a pose in MUD AND SAND, his side-splitting spoof of Valentino's BLOOD AND SAND.

man trying to get ahead in the world, as a door-to-door salesman. In 1926 Laurel returned to Hal Roach for good, principally as a gagman and director, not as a comic. Comedy behind-the-scenes fascinated Laurel, and he enjoyed these jobs even more than performing. But fate was to change all that. Fate, and Oliver Hardy.

Oliver Norvell Hardy was born in Harlem, Georgia, in 1892. His mother owned a hotel, and there was no show-business background in the family. Oliver, however, possessed a fine soprano voice and in his early years made the most of it. At the age of eight he was featured in a touring minstrel show, but soon tired of the hectic pace and returned home. He was sent to Georgia Military College, and later studied law at the University of Georgia. Law held no excitement for him, so in 1910 he opened a movie theater, which he operated for three years. Intrigued by what he saw on the screen, Hardy journeyed to Jacksonville, Florida, and joined the Lubin film company as a comedy villain. He remained there for several years, appearing in countless one-and-two-reelers, most of which have disappeared. Two comedies which do exist today are HOP TO IT, BELLHOP, and THE PAPERHANGER'S HELPER, in which Hardy was paired with diminutive Bobby Ray. The "fat and skinny" teaming of these two men often causes people to comment that these were definite ancestors of the Laurel and Hardy films. This is only true on the surface. These two-reelers are typical comedies of the era, with some good slapstick gags, and in some ways they do parallel later L & H work: Hardy is tough and domineering, and makes sure that Ray does all the work. He is arrogant, but always seems to get himself into trouble. Beyond this, however, there is none of the warmth that set Laurel and Hardy apart from other slapstick comedians of the day.

Hardy worked for many studios in the late teens and early 1920's. He supported Billy West, the Charlie Chaplin imitator, in a number of his comedies, and later became a prime fixture in the comedies of Larry Semon. Semon, forgotten today by all but the most avid film buffs, was an extremely popular comedian in the 1920's, with a fine, inventive, comic mind. His gags were among the most elaborate ever staged, and two-reelers like THE SAWMILL bear this out. In Hardy he found an appropriately sinister heavy, and used him in most of his comedies, as well as feature films like THE PERFECT CLOWN and the 1925 version of THE WIZARD OF OZ, in which Hardy played the Tin Woodsman. "Babe" Hardy finally ended up at the Hal Roach studio around 1926. He became part of the stock company Roach had established, which included the double-take master James Finlayson, slow-burn Edgar Kennedy, brawny Noah Young, and comedienne Anita

Garvin. Hardy worked often with Roach star Charley Chase in his two-reelers, and performed with other members of the troupe in the Hal Roach All-Star series.

When asked how they happened to become a team, Laurel and Hardy could never provide a clear-cut answer. Stan's reply was the most accurate: "We just sort of came together—naturally." It happened that the two were appearing in the same Hal Roach comedies in 1926 and 1927, not as a team, but simply as two members of the cast. Thus, in such films as SLIPPING WIVES, LOVE 'EM AND WEEP, and WHY GIRLS LOVE SAILORS, they were part of an ensemble. WITH LOVE AND HISSES, a hilarious Army comedy, had them working together for the first time, as half-witted soldiers at odds with officer James Finlayson. When, after a long hike, the squad decides to go swimming in a nearby lake, Stan is assigned to guard their clothes. Thanks to his alertness and powers of observation, the garments are on fire within minutes, and the soldiers are left in an embarrassing predicament. Their solution forms the film's final, and most inventive, gag—the GIs borrow a nearby billboard sign for the film THE VOLGA BOATMEN, and, poking their heads through those on the advertisement, they shuffle their way back to camp.

Their next film, SAILORS BEWARE, actually did co-star Laurel and Hardy, but not as a team. Each one worked within his own plot in the picture, and their scenes together were few. Nevertheless, the film showed both Stan and Ollie to good advantage, with Stan as a cabdriver who accidentally remains on a ship after it sets sail, and Ollie as the temperamental ship's purser who puts Stan to work as a steward. The film is almost pure slapstick, with Lupe Velez getting early film experience (of sorts) as a haughty young girl whom Stan pushes into the ship's swimming pool. Each successive film after this one made Laurel and Hardy seem more of a team, even though they continued to be featured along with the other Roach comedians in cast listings. DO DETECTIVES THINK? answers its title question by providing us with the boys as bumbling detectives assigned to guard James Finlayson's mansion from a mad killer (Noah Young) who, in actuality, is Finlayson's butler. FLYING ELEPHANTS is a wild caveman comedy with both Stan and Ollie vying for the same girl's hand in marriage. SUGAR DADDIES features Finlayson in the major role, with Stan and Ollie as his lawyer and butler, respectively, who come to his aid when the blackmailing brother (Noah Young) of the girl Fin drunkenly married the night before wants to collect. The best part of the film is a chase through an amusement park with Stan, perched on Fin's shoulders, masquerading as a woman. One memorable gag, the kind indigenous to silent comedy and seldom seen in talkie films, has Finlayson waking "the morning after" with a hangover that makes his head bulge and throb before our eyes!

There has always been some confusion about the first official Laurel and Hardy film. Hal Roach changed distributors in 1927, and films were being released by two different companies at the same time—not always in the same order in which they were made—so it's difficult to determine which film the general public may have seen first. But the order of release is less important than the overall results: within months the Hal Roach staff, led by the resourceful Leo McCarey, helped fashion a team out of two talented comedians, and created for them three memorable comedy vehicles: PUTTING PANTS ON PHILIP, THE BATTLE OF THE CENTURY, and THE SECOND HUNDRED YEARS.

Of the three, only PUTTING PANTS ON PHILIP does not present L & H in their usual character portrayals. In it, Ollie is sent to meet his young Scottish nephew, who has just sailed to America for the first time. A letter from his mother warns Ollie that Philip's (Stan's) one weakness is women—he goes wild any time he sees a pretty girl. One poor girl becomes Stan's victim for the entire film, having the bad fortune to walk past him no matter where the action moves. Stan's reaction is a grin, a mad leap in the air, and a chase after the young lady. All of this is very embarrassing to Ollie, a pillar of respectability in his community. After much trouble he decides the best way to handle the situation is to approach the lady himself, which results in a quick rebuff and one of Ollie's frequent trips into a mud puddle. While not a typical Laurel and Hardy comedy, PUTTING PANTS ON PHILIP is quite funny and was always a special favorite of both Leo McCarey and producer Hal Roach.

THE BATTLE OF THE CENTURY, since its first exposure in many years in Robert Youngson's GOLDEN AGE OF COMEDY and LAUREL AND HARDY'S LAUGHING 20's, has taken on classic status, and deservedly so. Its climax is the greatest pie-throwing battle ever staged for a film and one of the great scenes in all of screen comedy. The episode begins when Ollie drops a banana peel in the path of a pieman loading his goods onto a bakery wagon. The pieman is Charlie Hall, the duo's nemesis in countless later films. He surveys the situation, slowly picks up a pie and throws it into

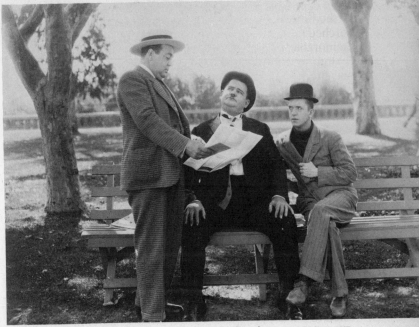

Eugene Pallette sells Ollie an insurance policy for Stan in THE BATTLE OF THE CENTURY. This leads to the now-classic pie fight that climaxed the film.

Ollie's face. In the process of retaliation, one innocent person after another is drawn into the line of fire, from a man in a dentist's chair to a dignified dowager calmly observing the situation from afar. The buildup follows the usual Laurel and Hardy process, labeled "reciprocal destruction" by John McCabe. It consists of the victimized party of some indignity (here, a pie in the face) facing his problem with no outward display of anger, but merely a determined act of revenge. It is this pace that sets even a Laurel and Hardy pie fight apart from imitators; it is precisely the lack of pace that made Blake Edwards' pie fight in THE GREAT RACE (1965) a failure, and an incomplete understanding of slapstick that makes one wish SMASHING TIME (1967) had been handled by someone other than Desmond Davis. Comedy is a definite science, especially slapstick comedy. Few people have mastered it: L & H were among those few.

It's no secret that the basis of slapstick comedy is the puncturing of dignity. Laurel and Hardy knew how to manipulate the formula for maximum results. For instance, one of the notable members of the Hal Roach stock company was a statuesque, dignified, dowager type, Ellinor Van Der Veer. She was with Roach for at least eight years, contributing her imposing presence to everything from THE SECOND HUNDRED YEARS in 1927 to a Hal Roach musical short called APPLES TO YOU in 1934. She seldom spoke a word, or received much of a part, but her contribution was nevertheless quite important. She is the lady who observes the pie fight behind her lorgnette in BATTLE OF THE CENTURY, and suddenly receives a pie in the face; she is the lady who sits on a batch of ice cream cones in A PAIR OF TIGHTS, and registers an unforgettable reaction of astonishment; she is in James Finlayson's party visiting the prison in the L & H comedy THE HOOSEGOW, who receives a parcel of gooey rice in the face; in Charley Chase's GIRL SHOCK she is the target of still *more* pastry. In every case, the scene is uproariously funny. The hearty Miss Van Der Veer was just one of many women who "gave their all" for slapstick comedy in the 1920's and early 30's. Others, like Margaret Dumont in the Marx Brothers films and Symona Boniface in the Three Stooges shorts, performed similar functions. Their stately dignity in the midst of wild situations made the free-for-alls seem that much funnier.

As time went on, screen comedy changed drastically, and slapstick was all but forgotten. Several actors and directors tried to revive it, with varying degrees of success, and in the 1960's there was a short-lived attempt to bring back slapstick on a grand scale. Such films as IT'S A MAD MAD MAD MAD WORLD, THOSE MAGNIFICENT MEN IN THEIR FLYING MACHINES, and THE GREAT RACE resulted. None of them really hit the bull's-eye, although audiences who had never seen anything better enjoyed these films tremendously. To show up these halfhearted Hollywood endeavors, Robert Youngson included the climactic sequence from THE BATTLE OF THE CENTURY in his feature film LAUREL AND HARDY'S LAUGHING 20's (it had previously been used in THE GOLDEN AGE OF COMEDY). The result was solid acclaim from every theater that booked the film, and cries of joy from most of the critics, proof that Laurel and Hardy were still the masters of slapstick comedy.

In 1928 and 1929, Hal Roach's now-starring comedy team turned out an incredible output of 23 two-reel shorts. Not since Chaplin made his "golden dozen" comedies for Mutual in 1916–17 had anyone produced such an outpouring of first-rate two-reelers in rapid succession. Admittedly there are some mediocre entries in this series of shorts, but they

are few, and for the most part these 23 shorts represent
Laurel and Hardy at the height of their powers. LEAVE 'EM
LAUGHING is a perfect example of how L & H could do a
great deal with very little material. The first half centers
around a dentist's office, where Stan goes to have an aching
tooth pulled, but Ollie ends up the unwitting patient. They
receive an overdose of laughing gas, and the remainder of
the film has them creating a mammoth traffic jam and upset-
ting traffic cop Edgar Kennedy, while in hysterics every moment. Laughing scenes were always highlights of L & H
films, including talkies like THE DEVIL'S BROTHER and SCRAM.
THE FINISHING TOUCH is pure visual humor with the boys
trying their best to build a house in the course of an afternoon. One of the best running gags has Ollie swallowing a
handful of nails to work on one section of the house, repeatedly stumbling off a ledge, and swallowing the nails. FROM
SOUP TO NUTS features the boys as waiters-for-hire. Their
business card reads: "Laurel and Hardy—Waiters—All we
ask is a Chance." It is a plotless two-reeler which contains a

Anita Garvin is trying to move into high society by giving a dinner party in
FROM SOUP TO NUTS; the boys look skeptical.

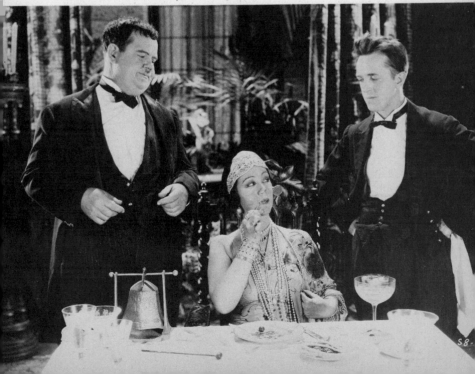

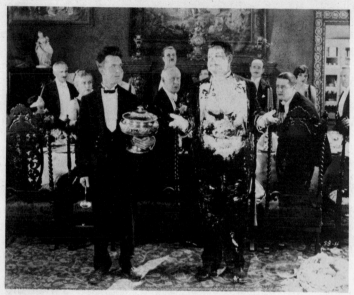

The immediate aftermath of one of Ollie's attempts to serve a cake in FROM SOUP TO NUTS.

tremendous procession of slapstick gags, highlighted by Ollie's continual attempt to serve a huge cake to some dinner guests, and three times ending up face-first in the confection. FROM SOUP TO NUTS features one of the screen's finest, and unjustly forgotten, comediennes, Anita Garvin, a beautiful woman with a mobile and expressive face, and timing that could put many experienced comedians to shame. Although she appeared in many L & H films, this one put her in the spotlight, as a lady trying to crash high society, by giving a swanky dinner party and attempting to adopt the manners and demeanor of a society hostess. *Her* running gag involves a tiara that falls down over her face at periodic crucial moments. The film, incidentally, was directed by Edgar Kennedy, using the name E. Livingston Kennedy. Kennedy was a fine comedian in his own right who often supported L & H before leaving Roach to start his own two-reel series; FROM SOUP TO NUTS and YOU'RE DARN TOOTIN' were among his few directorial efforts.

YOU'RE DARN TOOTIN' features the famous shin-kicking, pants-ripping episode, a parallel to the pie fight in BATTLE

OF THE CENTURY; before it is over, a score of innocent bystanders become involved in the melee. It is not quite as funny as BATTLE, simply because shin kicking, unlike pie throwing, involves physical pain. THEIR PURPLE MOMENT is L & H's first venture into the realm of marital comedy, the wives being, of course, suspicious shrews. The basis of this film was reused many times in later comedies, but no other film ever duplicated PURPLE MOMENT's key sight gag: Stan hiding his secret reserve of money from his wife in a portrait which hangs in their foyer. Before Ollie's disbelieving eyes, Stan actually opens the coat of the man in the picture to reveal a compartment inside his lapel! SHOULD MARRIED MEN GO HOME? spends most of its time on the golf course, where Stan and Ollie join Edgar Kennedy for a succession of inventive sight gags. The film ends in a battle royal with mud as the prime ingredient; no one is spared this indignity, not even the two young girls the boys have taken along, played by two of Hal Roach's loveliest comediennes, Viola Richard and Edna Marian.

EARLY TO BED, another 1928 release, is the oddest film Laurel and Hardy ever made. It does not use any of the typical plot devices of the L & H silents, it takes both Stan and Ollie out of character, and its effect, for a good part of the film, is decidedly melancholy. EARLY TO BED affects different people in different ways. Critic Stanley Kauffman found the film's opening scene brilliant: Ollie opens a letter, passes the envelope to Stan, who in turns passes it to a dog, who deposits it in a trash barrel (for L & H a scene like that was a throwaway). At one New York showing of the film, to *non*buffs, it was greeted with a feeling of bewilderment, and very few laughs. When excerpted in Robert Youngson's THE FURTHER PERILS OF LAUREL AND HARDY, it seemed much funnier than it did in complete form. Charles Barr, author of *Laurel and Hardy*, finds it a superb work, and concludes that the whole essence of the film can be found in its final scene, where after two reels of battling, Ollie smiles and makes up with Stan, affirming their often shaky but eternal friendship. Barr's point on the last scene is well taken, but the action that precedes that sequence remains the most unusual the team ever produced.

The film begins as Ollie discovers he has inherited a fortune, and prepares to move into his late relative's mansion. Stan begins to cry, and asks "What will become of me?" Ollie thinks for a moment, then smiles as he tells Stan that he can be the butler! Stan is content, but not for long.

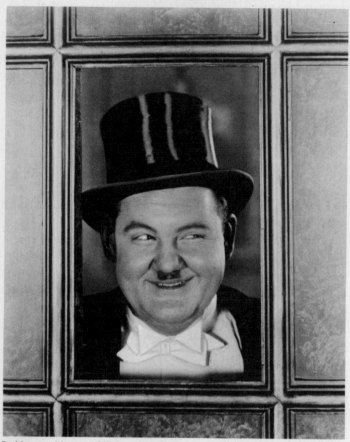

Sudden wealth turns Ollie into a roguish man-about-town in EARLY TO BED.

With his newly acquired standing in society, Ollie becomes an imbibing man-about-town, and one particular night, he returns home very late, in a roguishly playful mood brought on by intoxication. He determines that he's going to give Stan a hard time, starting with some byplay at the front door as Ollie rings the bell and disappears, finally succeeding in locking Stan out. He tortures him in every possible way, sneaking into his room after Stan has fallen asleep and dousing him with water. Stan is not amused by all of this, and finally tells Ollie that he's quitting. Ollie's playful face suddenly turns serious. "You can't quit," he says. "I won't let you." In order to convince Ollie, Stan hits upon the idea of making a shambles of his mansion. He proceeds to find every breakable item in the house and toss each one onto the floor. During the commotion, Stan trips and his face falls into a white cake. Ollie sees him shortly afterward and believes Stan is foaming at the mouth! Stan picks up the cue and begins to chase after Ollie with a wild glint in his eye. Ollie's escape is in a fountain outside the house which has a circular row of gargoyles which bear a strong resemblance to him. He fills his mouth with water and imitates the stone figures beside him until Stan finally catches on and all is forgiven.

There are moments in EARLY TO BED when it seems that the Laurel and Hardy friendship is really at an end. Ollie begins to take great pleasure in torturing Stan, not out of anger or revenge (which usually justify the actions of both Stan and Ollie in their films), but simply for the fun of it. Stan, on the other hand, cannot retaliate at first because he is the servant in this situation, and Ollie his boss. His expressions of annoyance and irritation at Ollie's actions in this film are not amusing, but sad. One finds experimentation, and occasional departures from the norm, in many L & H silents, but no other Laurel and Hardy film ever strayed so far off the beaten path as EARLY TO BED.

Their next film was not only back in their normal groove, but was one of the best they ever made: TWO TARS. The "reciprocal destruction" device, as described in BATTLE OF THE CENTURY, was one of the most successful devices in Laurel and Hardy's bag of tricks, and it served as the basis of some of their funniest films. TWO TARS was one of the most successful shorts based on this theme because its gags were the most inventive, no two being exactly alike. Stan and Ollie are two sailors on leave who pick up a couple of good-time girls for a day's ride. They encounter a tremendous traffic jam, and as these things will happen, violence flares between the boys and an irate motorist behind them (Edgar Kennedy). Before long the traffic jam turns into a gigantic free-for-all, with endless variations on the destruction of an automobile. At one point Stan and Ollie approach the car of an offending driver, and with a mutual nod they pull the front wheels off the car, in perfect unison. On another auto they bend the fenders upward, again with a delicate touch of simplicity. An antagonistic woman musses

the hair of one of the girls in L & H's car. She is promptly
taken care of: the girl empties an entire oil can on the
woman's face. When the battle is over, the cars attempt to
drive away, and the camera shows a procession of odd
vehicles: one with no floorboard, which the driver is walking
along, one with no front wheels, one distorted completely
out of shape, and so on. Stan and Ollie are being kept
behind for punishment by a cop, but they cannot control
their amusement at the passing show. They finally decide to
escape, riding away over a nearby field. The cop tries to
follow them, but each car he jumps into falls apart. Finally,
the whole entourage of cars goes after the boys, following
them into a darkened railroad tunnel. Seconds later, the
pursuants hurriedly back out of the tunnel, and a train
passes through. The camera cuts to the other side of the
narrow tunnel to reveal Stan and Ollie emerging in their car,
which has been squeezed sideways, but valiantly continues
to roll along.

BIG BUSINESS draws a tie with TWO TARS for their best
destruction film; in many ways it is funnier because it is
more basic and focuses on just the boys and James Finlayson.

James Finlayson unleashes his anger on the boys' car, as they look on. Midway
through the melee in BIG BUSINESS.

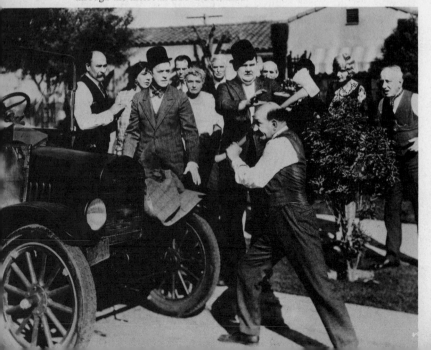

In the film, Stan and Ollie are Christmas tree salesmen in California, trying desperately to sell their wares in the middle of the summer. After several turndowns, they reach the house of Finlayson who, of course, refuses a tree. Walking away, Stan suddenly brightens and tells Ollie, "I have an idea." He returns to Fin's door and asks him if he can take his order for *next* year. From this exchange a small row develops: Fin smashes Ollie's watch. Ollie carves up Fin's doorway. Fin cuts off Ollie's tie. Stan prys the numbers from Fin's front door. The row increases in size and vigor. Soon the battle becomes a true "tit for tat" arrangement. As Ollie breaks a window in Fin's house, Fin smashes the window of the boys' car. When Fin's door is broken through, the angry Scotsman unhinges the car door and violently hurls it to the ground. Before long the boys have torn up all but the foundations of the house, and are working on demolishing its contents (Stan pitches the glassware outside to Ollie, who pulverizes them with a makeshift baseball bat). Meanwhile, Finlayson has exploded their car and is trying to break every piece of machinery in it. Off on the sidelines is the local cop,

When Laurel and Hardy tottered on the skeleton of a skyscraper in LIBERTY, it was for real (although perspective and other tricks helped the illusion along). Tom Kennedy is in pursuit.

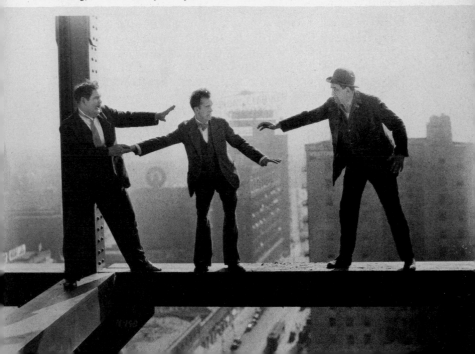

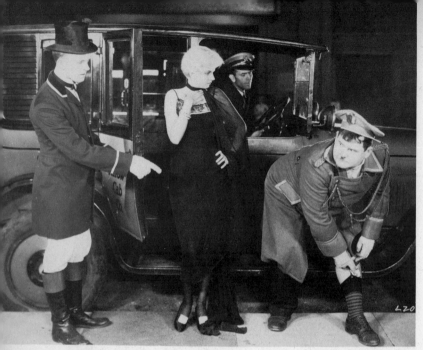

Lovely young Jean Harlow is the focal point of a key gag in DOUBLE WHOOPEE:
Stan closes the taxi door on the train of her dress.

Tiny Sandford, who has been observing the altercation with
a pencil and paper, registering emotions of surprise and
shock at some of the goings-on, but never attempting to
assert his authority. Finally he feels it is time to intervene.
As he tries to get to the cause of the situation, Stan and Ollie,
obviously sorry for what they have done, begin to whimper.
Finlayson also breaks down and expresses regret for his actions. The cop joins in and all four begin to bawl in shame.
Stan hands Fin a cigar as a peace offering. Then Stan and
Ollie glance at each other and sneak in a surreptitious smile.
The cop sees them and gives chase. For a finale, the camera
turns to Finlayson, whose cigar explodes in his face.

Others among their final silents, made in 1929, include
LIBERTY, an excellent two-reeler with the boys as escaped
convicts who, in a desperate attempt to change from prison
garb into their street clothes, end up in an elevator that
takes them to the top of a building under construction. Their
adventures atop the skeletal building are both hair-raising
and hilarious. Like the similar Harold Lloyd comedies,
LIBERTY was filmed just as the audience sees it, without the
aid of process-screens or trick photography. DOUBLE WHOOPEE,
a "simple" film in comparison with these more elaborate

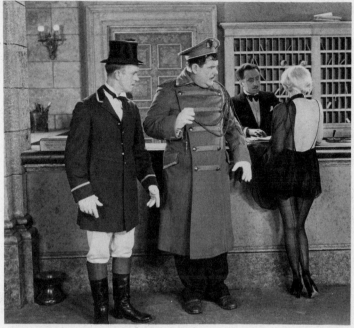

The result of Stan's fumbling: Miss Harlow doesn't realize that most of her dress is missing. Rolfe Sedan is the desk clerk.

endeavors, is a most pleasing comedy with Stan and Ollie as the new doorman and footman at a posh New York hotel (their letter of introduction reads: "These boys were the best we could do on such short notice. There is some reason to believe that they may be competent"). They ruin the visit of an Erich von Stroheim-like prince, and upset the dignity of young Jean Harlow when Stan closes a taxi door on the train of her dress.

Laurel and Hardy's 1929 silent product was for the most part quite good, with pictorial quality and production values that showed the silent film at its zenith. But the silent film was on the way out; by the end of 1929 most of the studios were no longer making silent films, and it looked as if talking pictures were here to stay. Many silent-screen stars' careers came to a sudden and often tragic end with the birth of the microphone. Comedians in particular had trouble, notably Buster Keaton and Harry Langdon, who went from the top of the heap to the very bottom in a few short years.

The luckiest of all silent comics were Laurel and Hardy,

who made the transition to sound with the greatest of ease. Their voices were perfect for their characters, their use of sound and sound effects ingenious, and before long their dialogue as funny as their sight gags. This is not to say that sound did not present some problems at first; for proof of that, one need only look at BERTH MARKS, their first all-talking film (which received simultaneous release in a silent version), probably the worst short they ever made, owing largely to a prolonged sequence of the boys trying to get undressed in an upper berth of a train. The scene seems to go on forever, and to make matters worse, no one bothered to write any dialogue, so Ollie repeats over and over again, "Will you stop *crowding?*"

This handicap was resolved immediately, for the team's next film, MEN O'WAR, contains some of their best dialogue scenes, and remains one of their most enjoyable talkies. It consists of three main sequences. In the first, Stan and Ollie, as sailors out for a day in the park, discover a pair of woman's panties on the ground, and approach two girls to find out if it belongs to one of them. Having lost a pair of gloves, one girl carries on a long dialogue with Ollie consisting of one misunderstanding after another. Ollie is too em-

The boys introduce themselves to a pair of cuties in MEN O'WAR. Later, they wind up in a sinking rowboat.

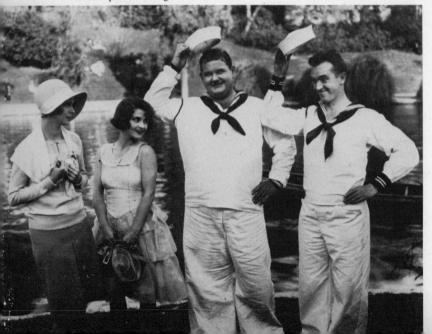

barrassed to say what it is he's found, and the girl assumes
he is talking about her gloves. "Can you describe them?" he
asks sheepishly. "Well, they button on the side," she replies.
Stan and Ollie reexamine the garment to see if they've
missed something "I'll bet you miss them," Ollie continues.
"Well, you can just *imagine*," giggles the girl. "Good thing
we're having warm weather," laughs Ollie. The episode
comes to an abrupt end when a policeman approaches and
returns the girl's gloves. From there, the party of four goes
to James Finlayson's ice cream parlor where Stan and Ollie
try to treat the girls to a soda on a budget of fifteen cents.
Ollie goes through an agonizing series of instructions with
Stan, telling him to refuse a soda so they will be able to pay
the tab for three. When he finally gets the idea, and three
sodas are ordered, Ollie tells Stan to drink his half first. Stan
turns around and gulps down the whole glass. Ollie, smiling,
takes the glass in hand to have his drink, suddenly realizes it
is empty, and turns his smile into a solemn frown. Turning
to Stan, he asks quietly, "Do you know what you've done?"
Stan nods sheepishly. Ollie continues, "Why did you do it?"
Stan breaks down and cries, "I couldn't help it—my half was
on the bottom!" The final episode takes place as the boys
decide to rent a rowboat for an afternoon on the lake. A
run-in with Charlie Hall, in another boat, soon amplifies
into another melee, with half-a-dozen boats going under as
all the refugees clamber aboard the L & H vessel. With
fifteen people aboard, including Finlayson and a cop, the
ship slowly sinks into the lake for the final fade-out.

Although they were to do two more silent and part-talkie
films, MEN O'WAR eliminated most of the clumsiness of their
first talkie effort, and from that point on the team that had
mastered the art of silent comedy had no problem in con-
quering the talkie field as well. Laurel and Hardy were
among the few people in Hollywood who instinctively knew
how to use the medium of sound. They realized that their
appeal was mainly visual, and that their forte was in the
realm of the sight gag. In talkies, they continued to do the
same kind of films they were doing as silents, with sound
added *naturally*. Films like MEN O'WAR utilized a perfect
blend of visual and verbal humor, with fine dialogue sequences like the soda routine, and inventive sight-gag scenes
like the final melee on the lake. It was a formula L & H
were to perfect and use for the next decade at the Hal
Roach studios.

Another early talkie produced hilarity with the artful rep-

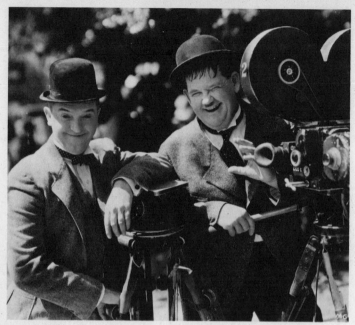

Stan and Ollie at their peak: an off-screen pose from the early 1930's.

etition of the word "good-bye." It was THE PERFECT DAY, an adventure in frustration with the boys, their wives, and grouchy uncle Edgar Kennedy (replete with gouty foot) valiantly trying to take the car for a Sunday picnic. The team's knowledge of how to build a gag provided the inspiration for this film, which has everything imaginable going wrong with their car as they attempt to leave for their outing. Every time they seem ready to go, friendly neighbors on all sides wave and shout, "Good-bye, good-bye!" and the family group answers, "Good-bye, good-bye!" Invariably, as the car is about to go, something goes wrong, causing the boys to stop and investigate. After several attempts, in the midst of "good-byes" Stan adds confidently, "We're going now!"—to no avail. The film ends as the car finally circles the corner and plunges into a deep pit full of water.

The Laurel and Hardy comedies varied sharply over the next few years, with little or no rhyme or reason. It is impossible to pinpoint a "winning streak" or period of consistently good output, for in the middle of a fine group of shorts there is always at least one misfire. It should be said that most of the L & H two-reelers of the 1930's were quite good, and even the weaker ones had their moments, but many could only be called run-of-the-mill. Run-of-the-mill Laurel and Hardy was far better than the top-grade product of certain other studios, and on a comparative basis, L & H fared quite well during their talkie years.

One of their better talkie shorts was THE HOOSEGOW, an extremely funny slapstick comedy with a memorable introductory title: "Neither Mr. Laurel nor Mr. Hardy had any thoughts of doing wrong. As a matter of fact, they had no thoughts of any kind." The film takes place in a prison camp where the boys have run-ins with burly guard Tiny Sandford and visiting governor James Finlayson, climaxing in a battle with a gooey rice mixture for ammunition. BELOW ZERO starts with the boys as sidewalk musicians, serenading the populace with "In the Good Old Summertime"—in the middle of the winter. One party in a second-story apartment asks them how much they make on one block. They tell him their net is usually 25 cents. He tosses down a half-dollar and tells them to move down two blocks. The film ends with one of the strangest gags L & H ever devised: Stan hides from a pursuing policeman in a barrel of water. When Ollie goes to get him, he looks inside and asks what happened to all the water. Stan gulps and cries, "I drank it!" When he

Nothing goes right when Stan and Ollie try to install an antenna on Ollie's roof. A scene from HOG WILD.

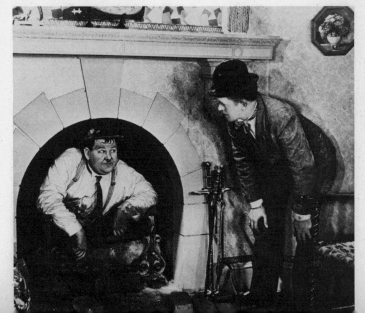

emerges from the barrel he has taken on the gigantic proportions of the container! HOG WILD has Stan and Ollie trying to
put up a radio antenna on Ollie's roof, with predictable but
very funny results, including Ollie repeatedly sliding down
the roof into a lily pond below. As he is climbing the ladder
back up to the top again, Stan accidentally starts his car, and
the ladder, perched in the back seat, goes with it. The car,
with Ollie holding onto the ladder for dear life, careens
down the city streets, sideswipes a streetcar, and finally crashes
to a halt as Ollie is deposited on the ground. It is essential to
Laurel and Hardy logic that during this sequence, Ollie
never tries to climb down the ladder, and Stan never tries to
stop the car.

CHICKENS COME HOME is a fine short helped in no small
way by the supporting cast: Thelma Todd as Ollie's wife,
Mae Busch as his old flame and James Finlayson as his
butler (!). The story has Mae trying to blackmail Ollie, who
is (incredibly) running for mayor, with the boast of a spot-
less reputation. Fin plays Ollie's suspicious butler, and in
one scene gives out with a fantastic triple-take that surely
rates as one of Fin's greatest moments on film. COME CLEAN
is one of the funniest L & H shorts, with Stan and Ollie

Ollie is happily married to Thelma Todd in CHICKENS COME HOME, and he's
running for mayor. But an indiscreet old flame (Mae Busch) tries to blackmail him.

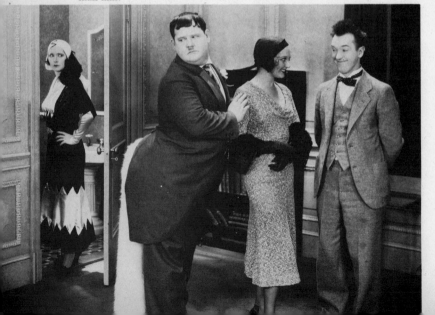

saving Mae Busch from a watery suicide, only to find her decidedly ungrateful, and a blackmailer to boot!

HELPMATES, made in 1931, is one of the team's classic films, with a perfect blend of nonsense dialogue and slapstick sight gags, as Ollie recruits Stan to help him straighten out his house after a wild party. He's just gotten word that his wife is coming home at noon and the house is a mess. Stan comes over immediately, and Ollie asks, "You never met my wife, did you?" "Yes, I never did," Stan replies. Ollie shows him their wedding portrait; Amazonian Blanche Payson is the "bride," with a fierce scowl on her face. As Ollie gets dressed to meet her at the train station, Stan miraculously manages to gather all the dishes, wash them, and stack them neatly in the kitchen. This is too good to last. Ollie approaches, trips on a stray carpet sweeper, and flies head first into the kitchen. From the ensuing racket, we know what has happened. From that point on, *everything* goes wrong, with Ollie ruining three suits of clothes and finally being forced to go out in an old Napoleon costume left over from a party. After Ollie barks a long complaint to Stan, Stan gets angry and protests, "Say, who do you think I am, Cinderella? You know, if I had any sense I'd leave." "Well," shouts Ollie, "it's a good thing you haven't!" "It certainly is!" returns Stan, after which he stands perplexed, trying to figure out what he has just said. Among the many

Ollie demonstrates to Stan how easy it is to prop open a window in HELPMATES In a moment, Ollie will be doused with dishwater.

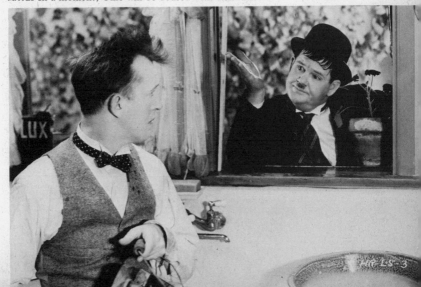

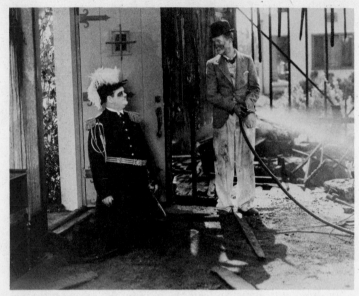

The end of a perfect day. Ollie returns from meeting his wife (note the black eye) only to find his house demolished, in HELPMATES.

calamities that befall Ollie before he manages to leave the house are a tin of flour falling on his head, a sooty stove pipe depositing dirt all over him, and a garden hose positioned outside so that he is in its range when he walks into his bedroom.

Finally, everything somehow straightened out, Ollie, in his Napoleon suit, goes to meet his wife, leaving Stan to put the finishing touches on the house. As a parting gesture, Stan decides to light a fire for the returning couple, and douses the logs in the fireplace with a can of gasoline. We are spared the results by a convenient fade-out, after which we see Ollie driving up to the house *without* his wife, and sporting a black eye. He turns to his home and sees only the skeleton of a smoldering house, with Stan in the middle, using a water-hose on the rubble. Incredulous, Ollie tries to find out what happened, and Stan gulps out a simple explanation of how he was trying to help by lighting a nice fire. Calming down, Stan looks around aimlessly and says, "Well, I think I'll be going. Is there something else I can do?" "No," says Ollie calmly, "You've done quite enough already." Sinking into a remaining easy chair, Ollie calls after Stan. "Hey!" he shouts,

"Would you mind closing the door? I'd like to be alone."
Stan closes the front door of the house (the doorframe is still
standing), and leaves. As Ollie stares at the camera, it
begins to rain, and with a rueful sigh, he picks a speck of lint
from his sleeve as the picture fades out.

A short two films later, another L & H classic was produced, the only film of theirs to win an Academy Award:
THE MUSIC BOX. Without going into detail, the three-reel
comedy is a superb series of variations on one theme: Laurel
and Hardy delivering a piano to a hilltop home. There is very
little dialogue, most of it coming from antagonistic Billy Gilbert, in one of his funniest roles as a bombastic intruder who
is trying to come down the narrow steps occupied by Stan,
Ollie and their piano. "Well?" he asks impatiently. "Well,
what?" pants Ollie. "Well, aren't you going to move it?" he
asks. "Why don't you walk around?" suggests Stan. "What?"
explodes Gilbert. "Walk around! Me, Professor Theodore
von Schwarzenhoffen, M.D., A.D., D.D.S., F.L.D., F.F.F.
and F., should walk around?" He tangles with the boys, who
send his top hat flying down to the street below, where it is
demolished by a passing truck. With a shake of the fist,
Gilbert follows his hat, and is not seen again until the end of
the film, when after a full day of exhaustive efforts, Stan and
Ollie finally get their piano into the home of the new owner—
none other than the ungrateful Gilbert. HELPMATES is too
slapsticky for some audiences, and some of the silent L & H
films are seemingly too subtle, but THE MUSIC BOX has wide
and instant appeal. It is one of the team's most famous
shorts, and one of the best-loved. In addition, it is the only
one of the three-reel shorts they made that does not show
padding (Hal Roach experimented with the three-reel format for several years with most of his stars, but the extra
length was unnecessary and only resulted in weak and drawn-
out shorts). It is also one of the only times Laurel and Hardy
were ever recognized with some sort of honor, such as the
Academy Award. While the team was always popular with
audiences, and Hal Roach profited quite well from their
films, critics were generally cool in responding to their efforts. THE MUSIC BOX was a notable, and deserved, exception.

A long-ignored short called THEIR FIRST MISTAKE, made in
1932, is a screamingly funny film that in recent years has
taken on almost classic status. It holds up better than many
other L & H talkies, and contains some of the funniest
dialogue the team ever had. Mae Busch chases husband
Ollie out of their apartment, because he's been spending all

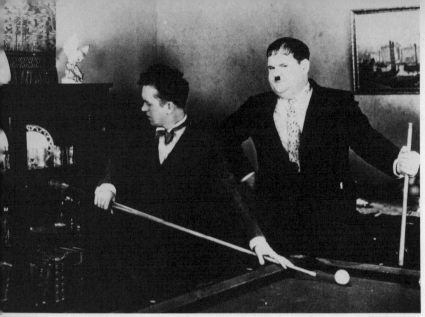

Laurel and Hardy stills are often just as funny as their films. Case in point: this shot from BRATS.

Stan disrupts a quiet domestic scene in the Oliver Hardy household. Mae Busch is the wife who sues Stan for the alienation of her husband's affections in THEIR FIRST MISTAKE.

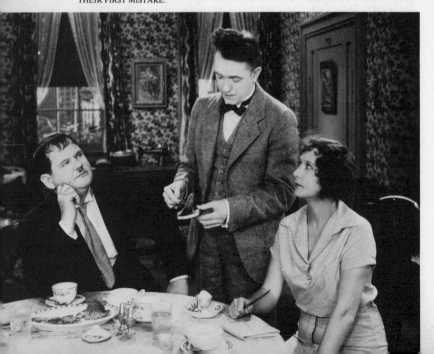

his time with Stan. Stan suggests to Ollie that what he needs in his house is a baby; after all, he reasons, if the wife is kept occupied at nights with the baby, she won't mind Ollie going out with him. Ollie agrees, and the two go out to adopt a child. When they return they discover that Mae has walked out, and soon afterward, process server Billy Gilbert presents Ollie with her divorce papers. "Gee, that's tough," says Stan. "Your name Laurel?" asks Gilbert. "Yes, ma'am," Stan answers blankly. "This is tougher," snaps Gilbert. "She's suing *you* for the alienation of Mr. Hardy's affections. And she's going to take you hook, line and sinker."

After the two digest all of this, Stan hands the baby to Ollie and mumbles something about leaving. Ollie is aghast; "You can't leave me here with this child," he says. "What have I got to do with it?" asks Stan. Ollie turns to him and says, "What have you got to do with it?" He steps closer to the camera and repeats, with real concern, "What have *you* got to do with it?" Then, looking sadly at the child, "Why, you were the one that wanted me to have a baby. And now that you've gotten me into this trouble, you want to walk out and leave me flat." "Well, I don't know anything about babies," Stan protests. "You should have thought of that before we got it," Ollie replies sorrowfully. "I don't want to get mixed up in this thing," Stan says. "I have my *future*, my *career* to think of." "Your career," mutters Ollie. "What about me? What will my friends say? Why, I'll be *ostracized!*" The scene is one of their most hilarious, with Ollie playing his part to the hilt. He finally convinces Stan to stay, and the rest of the film concerns their trouble in getting the baby to stop crying and go to sleep.

Disaster reigns through the night as the boys meet one catastrophe after another, succeeding in waking the baby every time they get him quiet. At one point, Stan turns out the lights in the room, then goes back, strikes a match, and looks at the switch. "Why did you strike that match?" Ollie asks. "Well, I wanted to see if the light switch was off," Stan replies. "Oh," says Ollie, comprehending at first, then registering a beautiful double-take. Then, perfectly illustrating the idea that Ollie is even dumber than Stan but doesn't know it (Hardy's own analysis of his character), he tells Stan, "Go get that lamp and bring it here. We can't have you striking matches all night!" The film ends as Ollie, half-asleep in bed, tries to quiet the baby by giving him his bottle, but accidentally puts the nipple into Stan's mouth instead. Stan likes it very much, and devours two bottles before Ollie wakes up and sees what is going on.

Many of their later shorts have great possibilities, like THE MIDNIGHT PATROL, which casts them as policemen on their first night on the job, but this, and others, never reach their full potential. BUSY BODIES is top-grade slapstick set in a construction firm where the boys work, where absolutely everything goes haywire. Its final gag is one of the most ingenious ever devised: escaping from their angry boss, they jump in their car and unwittingly drive head-on into a buzz saw which splits the car in half! GOING BYE BYE has some unforgettable moments, particularly at the beginning when Stan and Ollie, as prime witnesses in sending villainous Walter Long to prison for life, receive Long's promise that if he ever sees them again he's going to take their legs and tie them around their necks. This was brought on when the judge sentenced Long to life imprisonment and Stan exclaimed, "Aren't you going to hang him?" Outside in their car, Ollie reprimands Stan for his stupidity and asks, "Couldn't you see that he was *annoyed?*" A later episode is also a classic, with Ollie taking the phone from Stan, accidentally picking up instead a can of evaporated milk,

Sultan Maurice Black invites the boys to do away with themselves in a tense moment from BONNIE SCOTLAND. A heavily made-up Charlie Hall is offering the weapons; Leo Willis is directly over Stan's right shoulder.

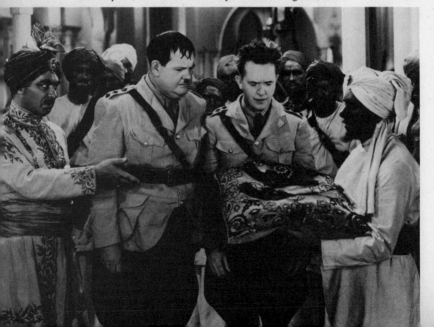

and hastily telling his caller, "Pardon me, but my ear is full of milk."

THEM THAR HILLS starts as Doctor Billy Gilbert orders Ollie to get some relaxation by taking a trip to the mountains with Stan. They drive up to a spot recently deserted by moonshiners, "in the high multitudes," as Stan says. Unbeknownst to them, the moonshiners had just dumped their product into the well before leaving. When Stan asks what makes the water taste so funny, Ollie explains that it's the iron in it. Charlie Hall and Mae Busch, stranded nearby, come to ask for help. While Hall goes to get gasoline, Mae stays with the boys and partakes of the well water. When Charlie returns he finds all three completely soused, and engages in a tit-for-tat battle with Stan and Ollie which starts with Hall tweaking Ollie's nose, proceeds as the boys pour molasses and feathers all over Hall, and climaxes with Ollie's pants being set on fire. Running around ablaze, Stan suggests that Ollie jump in the well, which he does, only to be blasted high into the air and dropped head-first into the ground for the final fade-out. In an unusual move, a follow-up film, TIT FOR TAT, was made the following year with the same cast meeting again as neighboring storekeepers, in a small town. It is enjoyable, but contrived, and not nearly as good as THEM THAR HILLS.

THEM THAR HILLS was Laurel and Hardy's last really good short. THE LIVE GHOST, TIT FOR TAT, FIXER UPPERS, and especially THICKER THAN WATER all have their moments, but none really come up to L & H's highest standard. By 1935 they were out of the short-subject field and devoting themselves entirely to feature films.

The debate continues, after all these years, about Laurel and Hardy's entry into the field of feature films. Stan Laurel himself had no doubt about it: he felt it was a mistake. So did many others, including critics who complained that Stan and Ollie could not sustain a 60- or 70-minute film. Of all their features, the ones that received widest acceptance were those which combined L & H comedy with musical subplots. To say that Laurel and Hardy could not support a feature-length film is ridiculous. They could, and *did*, in SONS OF THE DESERT and WAY OUT WEST. But it took a lot of additional effort behind the scenes to make an L & H feature work, and the Roach team missed the mark as often as they hit. None of the Roach features, with the possible exception

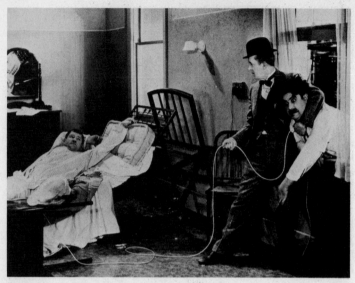

Everything is fine until Stan comes to visit Ollie in COUNTY HOSPITAL. Billy Gilbert is the doctor in distress.

of SWISS MISS, is really *bad*, but several of them fail to sustain a constant level of comedy, mostly due to interference by subplots, musical numbers and the like. Padding shows in many cases, and many feature films that come off as fair might have been excellent as two- or three-reel shorts.

PARDON US was not a bad start for L & H in the feature-film area; its chief asset was the same charm possessed by their shorts. For a while it was hard to believe that the L & H features and the L & H shorts were being made for the same company. Roach spent quite a bit of money on some of the feature films, and in the process eliminated the rough edges and familiarity of sets, actors and other elements that made the two-reelers so enjoyable. PARDON US avoided this by featuring most of the L & H stock company (Charlie Hall, Tiny Sandford, Jimmy Finlayson, Walter Long, etc.), as well as some newcomers. Wilfred Lucas was so good as the clichéd warden that he remained on the Roach lot for several years; heroine June Marlowe was just getting known as the teacher, "Miss Crabtree," in Roach's Our Gang comedies. If PARDON US has any real flaw, it is its lack of unity. Stan Laurel described it as a "three-story building on a one-story base," referring to the fact that it had originally

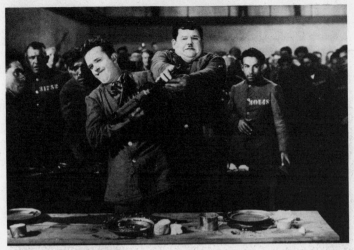

The boys have no intention of causing trouble in prison, but that's just what they do in PARDON US.

been planned as a short but was later expanded into a feature.

Basically, PARDON US is a spoof of the then-current movie THE BIG HOUSE, starring Wallace Beery and Chester Morris. Walter Long takes the Beery role as the tough inmate determined to break out; Stan and Ollie are bootleggers who are sent to prison for selling a case of beer to a policeman. The film has numerous unrelated episodes, including a reprise of the dentist routine from LEAVE 'EM LAUGHING, a musical interlude as the boys escape and disguise in blackface at a cotton plantation, a prison-schoolroom sequence with Finlayson as the harried teacher, and the boys' unintentional involvement with convict Long's prison break. It has some individual hilarious moments, and the musical section, like all those in their films, is a delight. But in the long-run, PARDON US lacks the real hilarity in its individual scenes to overcome its disjointed plot and clumsy construction.

PACK UP YOUR TROUBLES is a smoother-running film than PARDON US, but it isn't as good. The first half is quite funny, with Stan and Ollie drafted into the Army during World War I and waging a continuing battle with the camp cook, played by director George Marshall. After collecting the camp's garbage, they ask Marshall what they are to do with it. "What do you think you do with it?" he replies sarcastically. "Take it to the General!" Stan looks at Ollie and asks,

"What do you suppose the General wants with it?" Ollie sighs and answers, "There you go asking questions again. When will you learn to follow the Army curriculum? If the General wants it, he can have it!" They therefore deliver the cans of refuse to the quarters of the General (James Finlayson, of course), who sputters in disbelief and sends them to the guardhouse. After this promising opening, the film bogs down in a story of the boys trying to locate the family of a little girl who has been orphaned during the war.

THE DEVIL'S BROTHER, also known as FRA DIAVOLO, is considered one of the team's best features, and it received more critical acceptance than any previous L & H film at the time of its release. The reason is simple: FRA DIAVOLO manages to take elements of Auber's operetta, and liberal doses of Laurel and Hardy's comedy, and blend them together in perfect mixture. Stan and Ollie play would-be bandits who go nowhere on their own (their first "victim" is hard of hearing, causing Stan to shout, "We've come to take your money!" When the man hears who they are, he starts to cry and tell them the story of his destitute family. The episode ends with the boys giving *him* some money to take care of his children) but inadvertently become assistants to the notorious Fra Diavolo, well-known bandit and rogue

Director William Seiter talks to Stan and Babe (as Hardy was known off-screen) before shooting a scene for SONS OF THE DESERT.

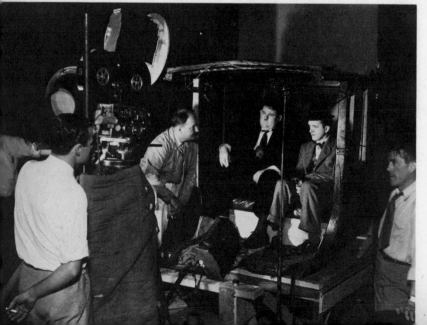

(Dennis King). The rest of the film alternates between Diavolo's attempts to woo lovely Thelma Todd, and steal the fortune owned by her father, Lord Rocburg (James Finlayson), and wonderful comic vignettes with Stan and Ollie. Their routines in this film are quite good, including Stan's famous hand games which never fail to baffle Ollie. A laughing scene, provoked by Stan's overindulgence in the wine cellar, is one of the best they ever did. The idea of blending L & H comedy with a well-known operetta worked so well in FRA DIAVOLO that the formula was repeated several times.

Their next feature, SONS OF THE DESERT, was the best the team ever did. It manages to take the kind of material used in the L & H two-reelers and expand it to feature-length without padding or musical subplots. It remains 100% pure Laurel and Hardy, as the boys try to fool their wives by pretending to go to Hawaii to cure Ollie of a bad cold, when in fact they are attending a convention of the Sons of the Desert in Chicago. The ruse is discovered when the ship they are supposedly taking sinks at sea, and the wives, trying to forget their sorrows at the movies, see Stan and Ollie in a newsreel of the Chicago frolic. The film moves along at a brisk pace, directed by comedy expert William A. Seiter, who, unfortunately, never worked with the boys again. At the convention itself, Stan and Ollie share the spotlight with fellow Roach comedian Charley Chase, seen in the atypical

Stan and Ollie mingle with a fellow conventioneer (Charley Chase) in SONS OF THE DESERT.

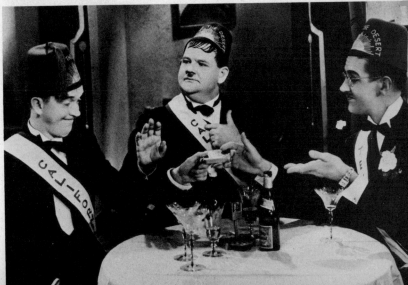

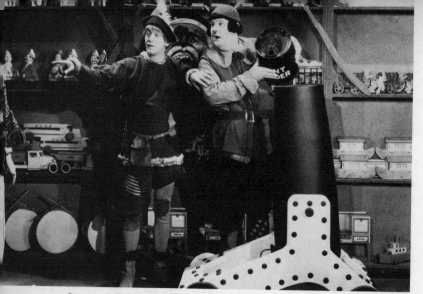

Stan and Ollie as bumbling toymakers in the delightful operetta BABES IN TOYLAND.

role of a loud, obnoxious conventioneer who also happens to be Ollie's brother-in-law. When the boys return home, Ollie tries to talk his way out of their predicament, but Stan breaks down and admits everything. The results: Stan's wife treats him royally, reminding him that honesty is the best policy, while Ollie's wife deposits her entire collection of crockery on Ollie's head.

BABES IN TOYLAND (now known as MARCH OF THE WOODEN SOLDIERS) is a delightful adaptation of Victor Herbert's operetta, with Laurel and Hardy fitting into the proceedings so well it almost seems as if they were written into the original production. Most of the lovely Victor Herbert score remains, with Felix Knight and Charlotte Henry taking the romantic leads and handling the music department, while Stan and Ollie play employees of the Toyland Toymaker. Stan's mix-up on an order from Santa Claus becomes a blessing in disguise; instead of 600 one-foot soldiers, the toymakers have built 100 *six*-foot soldiers, who are pressed into action when the dreaded Bogeymen attack Toytown. The result is a charming fantasy, particularly fine for children, and miles ahead of the 1961 remake by Walt Disney. When Bo-Peep (Charlotte Henry) is forced to marry the villainous Barnaby (Henry Kleinbach—later known as Henry Brandon), Ollie tells her, "Why, Stan is so upset he's not even going to the wedding—are you, Stan?" "Upset?" Stan replies, "Why I'm housebroken!"

Their next features, BONNIE SCOTLAND, THE BOHEMIAN GIRL, and OUR RELATIONS, are enjoyable, but unremarkable, with BOHEMIAN the best of the three. BONNIE SCOTLAND suffers from a stale framework, and too much emphasis on characters other than Laurel and Hardy. OUR RELATIONS, although it is short, is handicapped by repetition and predictability; it picks up tremendously when Stan and Ollie go into Alan Hale's beer garden. With only enough money for one order of beer, they ask for one glass with two straws. The beer arrives, 90% head and 10% liquid. Stan accosts the waiter and asks if he can turn in his straw for a spoon! BOHEMIAN GIRL is an enjoyable, leisurely-paced operetta with Stan and Ollie as vagabond gypsies who have raised an orphan girl from childhood, never dreaming that she is really the daughter of a prominent nobleman. The film's best scenes involve the boys' escapades in the gypsy camp. While Ollie goes to take a zither lesson, Stan is told to transfer their freshly made wine from a large keg to small bottles. To start the flow, he sucks on a piece of rubber tube, but before he can put the end of the tube into a bottle, he realizes that he likes the taste of the wine, and continues to drink it. Before long the keg is empty, and so are the bottles: Stan has devoured the contents single-handedly.

WAY OUT WEST ranks as one of L & H's best features, with our heroes going West to deliver a mine deed to the daughter of a recently departed friend (one wonders who would have trusted them with such a task). Stan makes the mistake

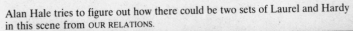

Alan Hale tries to figure out how there could be two sets of Laurel and Hardy in this scene from OUR RELATIONS.

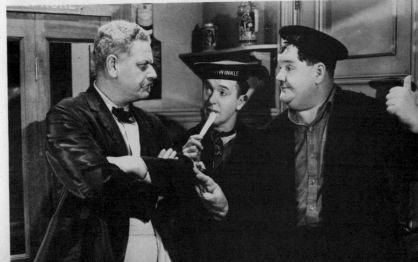

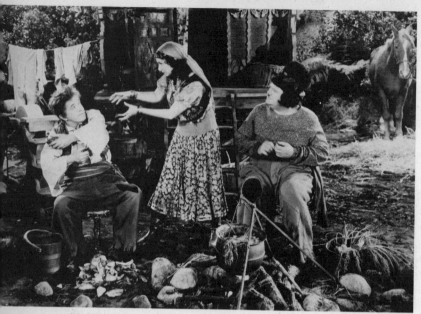

Mae Busch threatens Stan in a gypsy-camp scene from BOHEMIAN GIRL.

James Finlayson laughs triumphantly, but Ollie is about to snatch the valuable mine deed from Sharon Lynne in this scene from WAY OUT WEST.

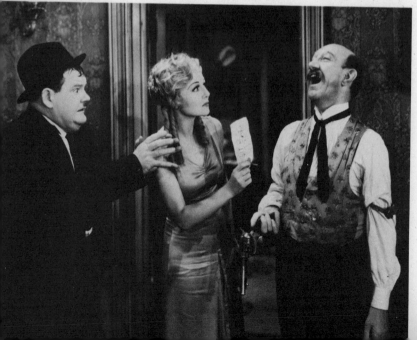

of telling their plans to the town's crooked saloon-keeper (Finlayson), and Fin proceeds to convince them that his girl friend (Sharon Lynne) is the daughter in question, leaving the real girl (Rosina Lawrence) in the dark. The film moves quickly—again it is short, only 65 minutes—and keeps the focus of attention on Stan and Ollie all the way, even allowing them to do two of their always-delightful musical numbers. The film's highlight comes when the boys realize they have been duped, and go to retrieve the deed from Finlayson. There follows a mad chase around Fin's room with Stan, Ollie, Sharon Lynne and Finlayson running around in circles, passing the deed from one to the other. At one point Stan holds the deed triumphantly and proclaims "Ha-Ha!" Fin grabs it and sneers "Ho-Ho!" Then Ollie snatches it, yelling "He-He!" as he runs off with the precious document. Stan deposits it in his shirt, and the determined Lynne goes after it, sending him into a fit of hysteria as she tries to retrieve the deed from the ticklish Laurel. WAY OUT WEST is thoroughly enjoyable, vintage Laurel and Hardy, showing the team at their prime.

Unfortunately, their next starring feature, SWISS MISS, set them back a number of years. The L & H sequences are good, with several—Ollie serenading his sweetheart while Stan plays tuba, Stan trying to outwit a St. Bernard, and so on—among their best, but the film as a whole is dreadful, suffering from an asinine subplot about bickering husband-and-wife musicians, played by Walter Woolf King and Della Lind. The songs include a forgettable ditty called "Crick-Crick-Crick Goes the Cricket," composed by King in his room and immediately taken up by the entire population of the Swiss lodge, who seem to have received the words and music via ESP. One would think that after the success of WAY OUT WEST, the Hal Roach people would have stopped inflicting Laurel and Hardy with unnecessary subplots, but this was not the case in SWISS MISS. Happily, their next film, BLOCKHEADS, returned them to safe ground, the result being another first-rate feature film. It starts with one of the greatest gags ever devised for *any* film: During World War I, the boys' regiment goes "over the top," with the commanding officer leaving Stan to guard the trench, with strict orders not to stop until relieved. A montage shows us the end of the war, the coming of the 1920's and the emergence of the 1930's. In 1938, we return to the same trench to find Stan still marching back and forth in the trench (by now he has dug a sizable hole where he pivots around)—nobody told

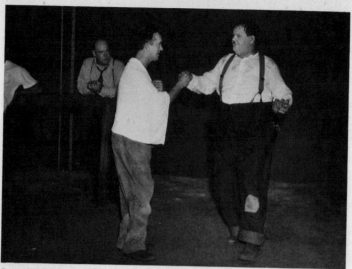

Stan and Babe rehearse their now-classic dance routine for WAY OUT WEST on a bare stage. Supporting player James C. Morton watches.

him the war was over! At noon he sits down to have lunch (a can of beans) and when he's through, he tosses the empty container over to a tremendous stack of cans alongside the trench. Eventually, someone discovers him and takes him back to America, where he stays at an old soldiers' home. Ollie hears he is back, and goes to get him. Stan is seated in a chair designed for amputees, and has one leg tucked under him. Ollie sees this and thinks that Stan must have lost a leg. There is a warm scene when the two friends meet after twenty years' passing. "You remember how dumb I used to be?" Stan asks. "Well, I'm better now." Ollie humors him along, and when they leave for Ollie's home, he insists on carrying Stan, failing to notice that he has full use of both legs. When he makes the discovery, after several trying moments, and asks Stan why he didn't tell him he had two legs, Stan replies innocently, "Well, you didn't ask me!" Then, to himself, he mumbles, "I've always had them." Ollie looks angrily at Stan and repeats sarcastically, "You're better now!" The film goes from there into a series of unrelated gags at Ollie's apartment, with one hilarious scene after another. The climax comes when they are innocently involved with the wife of Ollie's neighbor, temperamental big-game hunter Billy Gilbert (the scene is a reworking of their earlier short UNACCUSTOMED AS WE ARE).

BLOCKHEADS was reported to be, at the time, the team's farewell to the screen, but the very next year they were working again, at RKO, in THE FLYING DEUCES. Producer Boris Morros and director Eddie Sutherland wisely hired the writing team which had been doing L & H's material for Hal Roach, and several of the inimitable stock company from the Laurel and Hardy films—dour Charles Middleton, repeating his role from BEAU HUNKS, sneering Richard Cramer, and forever flustered James Finlayson. The film moves quickly—perhaps too quickly for perfection of the L & H technique—but it manages to pack in more laughs than even some of the Roach endeavors. Highlights include a song-and-dance of "Shine on, Harvest Moon," and a completely insane moment when, in a jail cell awaiting execution the next morning, Stan plays "The World Is Waiting for the Sunrise" on his bedsprings, with all the flair and seriousness of Harpo Marx. In 1940 Laurel and Hardy returned to Hal Roach for two short features, A CHUMP AT OXFORD and SAPS AT SEA. OXFORD, while disjointed, is a very pleasing film, mainly because of Stan's unique role. By foiling a gang of bank robbers, the boys are given the chance to get the education they have always wanted, at Oxford University in England. They are the butt of endless practical jokes played by other

Ollie plays it straight in his role as a doctor in ZENOBIA. his first film without Stan since their teaming. With him are Jean Parker, James Ellison and Billie Burke.

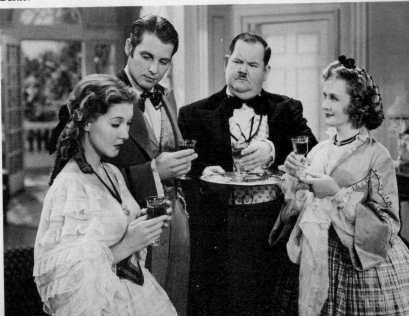

students (led by later British star Peter Cushing) until a window falls on Stan's head and transforms him into a totally different personality, a brilliant scholar who had gone to Oxford years before and remained a legendary figure there. The metamorphosis is complete: Stan becomes vain, aristocratic, and has no recollection of Ollie at all. He keeps him as valet, calling him "Fatty, old thing," and tries to make a decent servant of him. "Lift up your chin," he instructs as he trains Ollie in carrying a tray. "No, no, no," he reprimands, "both of them, both of them!" Finally, Ollie can stand no more. He bursts into a fit of anger, shouting insults at Stan as he packs his bags and gets ready to leave, suddenly coming back to add, "And I didn't like that double-chin crack!" At this point Stan leans out his window again, and the slippery pane crashes down, returning him to his old self. He meekly asks Ollie what is going on, and seeing that he's back to normal, Ollie bursts into laughter and embraces his old friend. This part of OXFORD is so good it seems a shame there is so much mediocre footage preceding it. The film might have worked much better as a three- or four-reeler than as a short feature film. Still, the opening sequences are not all that bad (just unnecessary), and A CHUMP AT OXFORD remains a most enjoyable little film.

SAPS AT SEA, like OXFORD, has little unity, but it does have many amusing sequences, most of them in the first half of the film. The boys work at the Sharp and Pierce horn factory, where one day Ollie goes crazy. "Horns!" he screams, "Horns! Nothing but horns!" Doctor James Finlayson orders him to take a rest, so he and Stan rent a boat, which they plan to keep tied to the dock. Unbeknownst to them, a fleeing criminal (Richard Cramer) stows aboard, sets them adrift, and the next morning makes all sorts of trouble for the boys. They try to put one over on the crook by serving him an "artificial meal" (string representing spaghetti, etc.) but Cramer catches on and makes the boys eat it instead. After this feature, Laurel and Hardy ended their long and fruitful association with Hal Roach.

There was no love lost between Roach and his breadwinning stars; he and Stan Laurel had clashed many times over the years over creative control of the films. Moreover, Roach insisted on keeping each performer under separate contract, making it impossible for them to negotiate as a team. (It was the staggered completion of Hardy's agreement in 1939 that obliged him to make a feature without Stan—a bucolic comedy called ZENOBIA in which he costarred with Harry Langdon).

But Hal Roach's studio was the very best place for Laurel and Hardy to have functioned. With Mack Sennett's decline in the late 1920s, the Roach lot in Culver City became the comedy capital of the world. It was a happy shop, full of comics and craftsmen whose sole ambition was to make good, funny movies. There was a genuine family feeling at the Hal Roach studio, and an important sense of continuity over the years on both sides of the camera. The stars, the supporting players, the directors, gagmen, and technicians worked in great harmony because they knew and understood each other so well. For audiences, there was a similar (and welcome) continuity in the familiar faces, settings, and music scores of those Hal Roach comedies. When Laurel and Hardy left Roach after SAPS AT SEA, they did not appreciate how unique their working conditions had been and had no idea of what was in store for them. (Ironically, Hal Roach's fortunes fell almost as precipitously as Laurel and Hardy's during the 1940s.)

The team signed contracts with 20th Century-Fox and MGM for feature-film comedies, assuming that they would be made the same way their films had been done for the past fifteen years. Unfortunately, Laurel and Hardy were coming

Their first day at Army camp, two tough guys (Max Wagner and Jimmy Dundee) swipe the boys' lunch. A scene from GREAT GUNS.

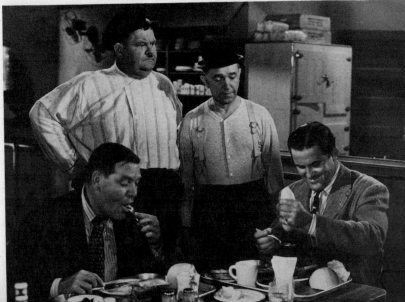

face to face with the Hollywood studio system at the peak of
its powers. The System was a mass-assembly process, and its
foremen (the studio heads) asked only that their films be
made professionally, as quickly as possible. Directors or
stars with big enough box-office returns, and plenty of nerve,
could battle the system in order to turn out films of an
unusual or uncommercial nature, but in 1941 Laurel and
Hardy did not have this stature. Fox intended to treat them
as they would any other actors: give them a script and expect
them to perform. Laurel and Hardy were *not* actors, however; they were comedians who liked to "feel" their way
through a film, relying on instinct and interplay as much as
possible. And in Stan's case, he enjoyed nothing more than
working out the various gags himself with the writers and the
director. Fox did not see it this way at all, and forced L & H
into a confining situation with tired scripts turned out by
writers who had had no previous association with the boys.
Missing, too, were the wonderful comedians who supported
them during their years at Roach—James Finlayson, Edgar
Kennedy, Charlie Hall, Mae Busch and all the others. Laurel and Hardy found themselves trapped, like little fish in a
big pond.

Some of the films that resulted were not bad by normal
standards, but for Laurel and Hardy they were great let-
downs. Others in the Fox series were abominable by *any*
standards. All of them lacked the charm that had made the

Stan disguises as Vivian Blaine's aunt, and Ollie pretends to be a Southern
colonel, in JITTERBUGS.

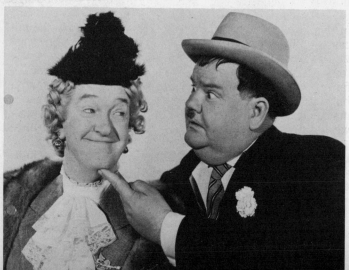

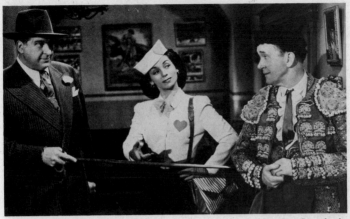

Ralph Sanford and Margo Woode seem sure of themselves, but Stan looks nervous in this shot from THE BULLFIGHTERS.

team great, and in four short years they brought an end to the team's career in Hollywood.

Of the six films made for Fox, only two are worth discussing: JITTERBUGS and THE BULLFIGHTERS. JITTERBUGS is rather pleasant, with Stan and Ollie as traveling sideshow men who, along with hero Bob Bailey, decide to come to the aid of young Vivian Blaine, who is being swindled by crooked Douglas Fowley. One scene in particular, with Ollie trying to win over shady Lee Patrick (who in turn is trying to woo Ollie) is delightful. She pretends to be a Southern belle, and Ollie rises to the occasion as a Southern colonel full of flowery compliments. The film's climax involves a good sight gag as the boys use their invention, "gas pills," to put some of their abductors out of the way. When swallowed, the pills cause their victims to inflate and float to the ceiling. THE BULLFIGHTERS lacks this inventiveness, relying on strictly formula material, but it is tried-and-true stuff, and comes off fairly well. Stan bears an amazing resemblance to a famous bullfighter, and this gets the boys mixed up with gangsters, including one who threatens to skin them alive. One scene with Margo Woode reprises the egg-breaking routine introduced in HOLLYWOOD PARTY (1934) with Lupe Velez, and the final scene, as expected, has Stan and Ollie "skinned alive," their skeletal bodies, with heads intact, walking toward the camera as Ollie mutters, "Well, here's another nice mess you've gotten us into!"

The other Fox films, THE BIG NOISE in particular, are not

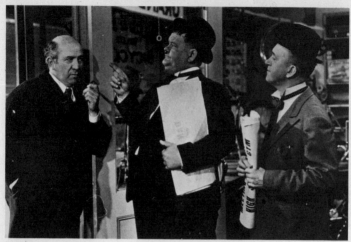

Guess who? The boys are reunited with Edgar Kennedy, an old Hal Roach colleague, in AIR RAID WARDENS.

only unfunny, but for anyone who loves Laurel and Hardy, very sad. A-HAUNTING WE WILL GO has no laughs at all, GREAT GUNS very few, and DANCING MASTERS about the same. The two MGM films aren't quite as bad, but like the Fox efforts, they spend too much time on plot and not enough on gags. AIR RAID WARDENS reunites them with Edgar Kennedy in one scene, but the encounter lacks the sparkle it would have had ten years earlier at the Roach

Stan and Ollie in a sad farewell to the screen: ATOLL K, with Max Elloy and Adriano Rimoldi.

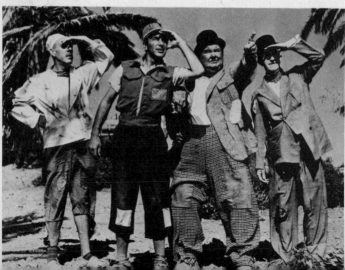

studio. NOTHING BUT TROUBLE benefits from the comedy expertise of Mary Boland as an unsuspecting matron who hires Stan and Ollie as servants. A chief fault of these films is that the writers obviously did not understand the characters of Stan and Ollie; instead of making them likably dumb, they created characters so incredibly stupid one would have no sympathy for them at all. Any warmth the films generated was due to feelings viewers had already formed by watching earlier, better L & H films.

After BULLFIGHTERS, Laurel and Hardy left Hollywood, two men who were still willing and able to make people laugh. They spent much time here and abroad doing live shows, both for the U.S.O. and in commercial theaters. While in Europe, they received a film offer from a French production company to star in a feature film; they accepted, never dreaming the production would turn into a disaster. Stan Laurel had nightmarish recollections of the film, and looked rather nightmarish *in* the film, due to a severe stroke he had suffered during shooting. There were times when one couldn't get involved in the story for fear that poor Stan was going to collapse any minute. The film, like so many they made over the years, has an intriguing premise, and individual scenes that are funny and fond throwbacks to their great years, but as a whole it is disappointing, to say the least. Financially it was a bust, and when it finally was imported to this country its stay was short, and its release erratic. The film, best known as ATOLL K, was also released as ROBINSON CRUSOELAND and UTOPIA. It was Laurel and Hardy's last film.

During the 1950's there were more tours, and occasional oddities such as Ralph Edwards' *This Is Your Life* television show. British producer Bernard Delfont invited the boys to his suite in a Hollywood hotel as part of the plan to surprise them on the show. They were surprised indeed; and after a nervous host (Edwards) ad-libbed for several minutes longer than planned, Stan and Babe walked onto the NBC stage to be honored by Edwards' program. The reason for their delay was that Stan was angered by the "surprise," and did not want to go on. Some fast talking convinced him to go along with the show, and he reluctantly agreed. Once on stage, Laurel and Hardy were perfect showmen, laughing at their host's feeble jokes, looking sad when they were supposed to, and pretending to remember people from their past they probably preferred to forget. The show actually did locate Hardy's childhood sweetheart, and Oliver, oblivi-

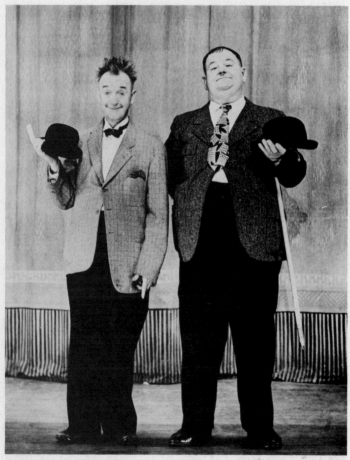

Still clowning in the 1950's, on stage in England.

ous of Edwards' rush to move on to other things, couldn't
hide the fact that he was a gentleman by saying some kind
words about the woman after she left. The show-business people who came on to greet the boys included Hal Roach, Jr.,
who announced that a pond at the studio was being named
Laurel and Hardy Lake in their honor, and Vivian Blaine,
who recalled how kind the two were to her during the

filming of JITTERBUGS. Edwards reminded viewers that Laurel and Hardy had made three hundred films together (sic), and in one of the show's few honest moments, called them two of the greatest funnymen of all time.

"Laurel and Hardy Lake" didn't see much action, except

Laurel and Hardy welcome fellow Hal Roach players Spanky McFarland and Darla Hood on the set of OUR RELATIONS. Looks like Spanky and Babe are trying to outmug each other!

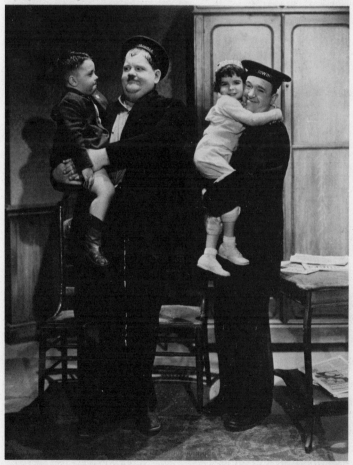

for a moment in an episode of *The Gale Storm Show*, a TV comedy series filmed on the Roach lot. In one episode Miss Storm and ZaSu Pitts were shown prowling around the Roach studios, and noted the sign that bore the name "Laurel and Hardy Lake." Stan and Babe didn't see much action themselves in the 1950's, until Hal Roach, Jr., proposed a series of television specials for the team, filmed shows that would be done in the style of their old two-reel comedies. What might have come of this plan is open to vast speculation, but unfortunately the films were never made. Just before shooting was to start, Stan suffered a stroke that temporarily put him out of commission. As he recovered, Babe Hardy fell ill, and died in August 1957.

Stan lived long enough to become the idol of a new generation of Laurel and Hardy fans, mostly youngsters who came to know the team through television showings of their films. He kept up a steady correspondence with many, and his home in Santa Monica was a shrine for such admirers as Dick Van Dyke, Jerry Lewis and pantomimist Marcel Marceau. Stan had many offers to appear on television, but he always turned them down, preferring to stay home with his wife, Eda. In February 1964, after a brief stay in a hospital, he died.

The men are dead, but their films keep them alive year after year. The Sons' of the Desert organization features showings of the films at every meeting, so that people can enjoy Laurel and Hardy the way they were supposed to— surrounded by an audience that enjoys laughing out loud.

Even Laurel and Hardy *imitators* are thriving—in television commercials, for the most part—which says something about the enduring appeal, and uniqueness, of Stan and Ollie.

The debates will always continue, but most aficionados agree: Stan Laurel and Oliver Hardy were the greatest comedy team of all time.

The Films of Laurel and Hardy

Stan Laurel and Oliver Hardy had extensive solo screen careers: this index details their work as a team, including guest appearances in the films of fellow Hal Roach–studio stars Charley Chase, Thelma Todd and ZaSu Pitts, and

Our Gang. All films are two reels (approximately 20 minutes) in length unless otherwise stated. Director's name follows year.

1. **Lucky Dog**—G. M. Anderson/Metro 1917—Jess Robbins—Florence Gillet.
2. **Forty Five Minutes from Hollywood**—Hall Roach/Pathe 1926—Fred L. Guiol—Glenn Tryon, Charlotte Mineau, Rube Clifford, Sue O'Neil, Edna Murphy, Jerry Mandy, Stanley "Tiny" Sandford, guest stars Theda Bara, Our Gang.
3. **Duck Soup**—Hal Roach/Pathe 1927—Fred L. Guiol—Madeleine Hurlock, William Austin, Robert Kortman.
4. **Slipping Wives**—Hal Roach/Pathe 1927—Fred L. Guiol—Priscilla Dean, Herbert Rawlinson, Albert Conti.
5. **Love 'em and Weep**—Hal Roach/Pathe 1927—Fred L. Guiol—Mae Busch, James Finlayson, Charlotte Mineau, Vivien Oakland, Charlie Hall, May Wallace, Gale Henry, Ed Brandenberg.
6. **Why Girls Love Sailors**—Hal Roach/Pathe 1927—Fred L. Guiol—Anna May Wong, Sojin, Eric Mayne, Bobby Dunn.
7. **With Love and Hisses**—Hal Roach/Pathe 1927—Fred L. Guiol—James Finlayson, Frank Brownlee, Chet Brandenberg, Anita Garvin, Eve Southern, Josephine Dunn, Jerry Mandy.
8. **Sugar Daddies**—Hal Roach/MGM 1927—Fred L. Guiol—James Finlayson, Noah Young, Edna Marian, Eugene Pallette, Dorothy Coburn.
9. **Sailors, Beware!**—Hal Roach/Pathe 1927—Anita Garvin, Stanley "Tiny" Sandford, Viola Richard, May Wallace, Connie Evans, Barbara Pierce, Lupe Velez, Will Stanton, Ed Brandenberg, Dorothy Coburn, Frank Brownlee, Harry Earles.
10. **The Second Hundred Years**—Hal Roach/MGM 1927—Fred L. Guiol—James Finlayson, Eugene Pallette, Stanley "Tiny" Sandford, Ellinor Van Der Veer, Edgar Dearing, Otto Fries, Frank Brownlee, Dorothy Coburn, Charlie Hall, Rosemary Theby, Bob O'Conor.
11. **Call of the Cuckoos**—Hal Roach/MGM 1927—Clyde A. Bruckman—Max Davidson, Lillian Elliott, Spec O'Donnell, Frank Brownlee, Charlie Hall, Leo Willis, Lyle Tayo, Edgar Dearing, Fay Holderness, Otto Fries, Charles Meakin; gag appearances by Charley Chase, James Finlayson, Laurel & Hardy.

12. **Hats Off**—Hal Roach/MGM 1927—Hal Yates—James Finlayson, Anita Garvin, Dorothy Coburn, Ham Kinsey, Sam Lufkin, Chet Brandenberg.
13. **Do Detectives Think?**—Hal Roach/Pathe 1927—Fred L. Guiol—James Finlayson, Viola Richard, Noah Young, Frank Brownlee, Will Stanton, Charley Young, Charles Bachman.
14. **Putting Pants on Philip**—Hal Roach/MGM 1927—Sam Lufkin, Harvey Clark, Lee Phelps, Ed Brandenberg, Dorothy Coburn, Chet Brandenberg, Bob O'Conor, Charles Bachman, Retta Palmer.
15. **The Battle of the Century**—Hal Roach/MGM 1927—Clyde A. Bruckman—Eugene Pallette, Noah Young, Anita Garvin, Charlie Hall, Dorothy Coburn, Sam Lufkin, Gene Morgan, George K. French, Dick Sutherland, Dick Gilbert, Lyle Tayo, Ham Kinsey, Bob O'Conor, Ed Brandenberg, Charley Young, Ellinor Van Der Veer.
16. **Leave 'em Laughing**—Hal Roach/MGM 1928—Clyde A. Bruckman—Edgar Kennedy, Viola Richard, Dorothy Coburn, Charlie Hall, Stanley "Tiny" Sandford, Sam Lufkin, Edgar Dearing, Otto Fries, Jack V. Lloyd, Al Hallet, Jack Hill.
17. **Flying Elephants**—Hal Roach/MGM 1928—Frank Butler—Dorothy Coburn, Leo Willis, Stanley "Tiny" Sandford, Bud Fine.
18. **The Finishing Touch**—Hal Roach/MGM 1928—Clyde A. Bruckman—Edgar Kennedy, Dorothy Coburn, Sam Lufkin.
19. **From Soup to Nuts**—Hal Roach/MGM 1928—E. Livingston (Edgar) Kennedy—Anita Garvin, Stanley "Tiny" Sandford, Edna Marian, Otto Fries, Ellinor Van Der Veer, Dorothy Coburn, Sam Lufkin, Gene Morgan.
20. **You're Darn Tootin'**—Hal Roach/MGM 1928—E. Livingston (Edgar) Kennedy—Otto Lederer, George Rowe, Agnes Steele, Sam Lufkin, Chet Brandenberg, Christian Frank, Rolfe Sedan, Ham Kinsey, Charlie Hall, William Irving, Dick Gilbert, Frank Saputo.
21. **Their Purple Moment**—Hal Roach/MGM 1928—James Parrott—Fay Holderness, Lyle Tayo, Anita Garvin, Kay Deslys, Jimmy Aubrey, Leo Willis, Stanley "Tiny" Sandford, Sam Lufkin, Ed Brandenberg, Patsy O'Byrne, Jack Hill, Retta Palmer.
22. **Should Married Men Go Home?**—Hal Roach/MGM 1928—James Parrott—Edgar Kennedy, Kay Deslys, Edna Marian, Viola Richard, Dorothy Coburn, Jack

Hill, John Aassen, Lyle Tayo, Chet Brandenberg, Sam Lufkin, Charlie Hall.

23. **Early to Bed**—Hal Roach/MGM 1928—Emmett Flynn—no supporting cast.

24. **Two Tars**—Hal Roach/MGM 1928—James Parrott—Thelma Hill, Ruby Blaine, Edgar Kennedy, Edgar Dearing, Charley Rogers, Clara Guiol, Jack Hill, Charlie Hall, Harry Bernard, Sam Lufkin, Baldwin Cooke, Charles McMurphy, Ham Kinsey, Lyle Tayo, Lon Poff, Retta Palmer, George Rowe, Chet Brandenberg, Dorothy Walbert, Frank Ellis, Helen Gilmore, Fred Holmes.

25. **Habeas Corpus**—Hal Roach/MGM 1928—James Parrott—Richard Carle, Charles Bachman, Charley Rogers.

26. **We Faw Down**—Hal Roach/MGM 1928—Leo McCarey—Vivien Oakland, Bess Flowers, Kay Deslys, Vera White, George Kotsonaros, Allen Cavan.

27. **Liberty**—Hal Roach/MGM 1929—Leo McCarey—James Finlayson, Tom Kennedy, Jean Harlow, Harry Bernard, Ed Brandenberg, Sam Lufkin, Jack Raymond, Jack Hill.

28. **Wrong Again**—Hal Roach/MGM 1929—Leo McCarey—Del Henderson, Harry Bernard, Charlie Hall, William Gillespie, Jack Hill, Sam Lufkin, Josephine Crowell, Fred Holmes.

29. **That's My Wife**—Hal Roach/MGM 1929—Lloyd French—Vivien Oakland, Charlie Hall, Jimmy Aubrey, William Courtwright, Sam Lufkin, Harry Bernard.

30. **Big Business**—Hal Roach/MGM 1929—James W. Horne—James Finlayson, Stanley "Tiny" Sandford, Lyle Tayo, Retta Palmer, Charlie Hall.

31. **Unaccustomed as We Are**—Hal Roach/MGM 1929—Lewis R. Foster—Mae Busch, Thelma Todd, Edgar Kennedy. The team's first talking picture.

32. **Double Whoopee**—Hal Roach/MGM 1929—Lewis R. Foster—Jean Harlow, Charlie Hall, Ham Kinsey, Stanley "Tiny" Sandford, Rolfe Sedan, Sam Lufkin, William Gillespie, Charley Rogers, Ed Brandenberg.

33. **Berth Marks**—Hal Roach/MGM 1929—Lewis R. Foster—Harry Bernard, Baldwin Cooke, Charlie Hall, Pat Harmon, Silas D. Wilcox.

34. **Men O'War**—Hal Roach/MGM 1929—Lewis R. Foster—James Finlayson, Anne Cornwall, Gloria Greer, Harry Bernard, Peter Gordon, Charlie Hall, Baldwin Cooke.

35. **Perfect Day**—Hal Roach/MGM 1929—James Parrott—Edgar Kennedy, Kay Deslys, Isabelle Keith, Harry

Bernard, Clara Guiol, Baldwin Cooke, Lyle Tayo, Charley Rogers.

36. **They Go Boom**—Hal Roach/MGM 1929—James Parrott—Charlie Hall, Sam Lufkin.

37. **Bacon Grabbers**—Hal Roach/MGM 1929—Lewis R. Foster—Edgar Kennedy, Jean Harlow, Charlie Hall, Bobby Dunn, Eddie Baker, Sam Lufkin, Harry Bernard.

38. **The Hoose-Gow**—Hal Roach/MGM 1929—James Parrott—James Finlayson, Stanley "Tiny" Sandford, Leo Willis, Dick Sutherland, Ellinor Van Der Veer, Retta Palmer, Sam Lufkin, Eddie Dunn, Baldwin Cooke, Jack "Tiny" Ward, Ham Kinsey, Blackie Whiteford, Ed Brandenberg, Chet Brandenberg, Charles Dorety, Charlie Hall.

39. **The Hollywood Revue of 1929**—MGM 1929—Charles F. Riesner—Conrad Nagel, Jack Benny, Norma Shearer, John Gilbert, Bessie Love, Joan Crawford, William Haines, Buster Keaton, Anita Page, Karl Dane, George K. Arthur, Gwen Lee, Marie Dressler, Marion Davies, Cliff Edwards, Charles King, Polly Moran, Gus Edwards, Lionel Barrymore, Nils Asther, the Brox Sisters, John Gilbert, Ann Dvorak (chorus girl), Ernest Belcher's Dancing Tots, the Albertina Rasch Ballet, Natacha Nattova and Company, the Rounders, the Biltmore Quartet. Partly filmed in Technicolor. 120 minutes.

40. **Angora Love**—Hal Roach/MGM 1930—Lewis R. Foster—Edgar Kennedy, Charlie Hall, Harry Bernard, Charley Young.

41. **Night Owls**—Hal Roach/MGM 1930—James Parrott—Edgar Kennedy, James Finlayson, Anders Randolph, Harry Bernard, Charles McMurphy, Baldwin Cooke.

42. **Blotto**—Hal Roach/MGM 1930—James Parrott—Anita Garvin, Stanley "Tiny" Sandford, Baldwin Cooke, Charlie Hall, Frank Holliday, Dick Gilbert, Jack Hill.

43. **Brats**—Hal Roach/MGM 1930—James Parrott—L & H play themselves as children.

44. **Below Zero**—Hal Roach/MGM 1930—James Parrott—Stanley "Tiny" Sandford, Leo Willis, Frank Holliday, Charlie Hall, Kay Deslys, Blanche Payson, Lyle Tayo, Retta Palmer, Baldwin Cooke, Robert "Bobby" Burns, Jack Hill, Charley Sullivan, Charles McMurphy, Bob O'Conor.

45. **The Rogue Song**—MGM 1930—Lionel Barrymore—Lawrence Tibbett, Catherine Dale Owen, Judith Voselli,

Nance O'Neil, Florence Lake, Lionel Belmore, Ullrich Haupt, Kate Price, Wallace McDonald, Burr McIntosh, James Bradbury, Jr., H. A. Morgan, Elsa Alsen, the Albertina Rasch Ballet, Harry Bernard. Color—115 minutes.

46. **Hog Wild**—Hal Roach/MGM 1930—James Parrott—Fay Holderness, Dorothy Granger, Charles McMurphy.

47. **The Laurel-Hardy Murder Case**—Hal Roach/MGM 1930—James Parrott—Fred Kelsey, Stanley "Tiny" Sandford, Del Henderson, Robert "Bobby" Burns, Dorothy Granger, Frank Austin, Lon Poff, Rosa Gore, Stanley Blystone, Art Rowlands. Three reels.

48. **Another Fine Mess**—Hal Roach/MGM 1930—James Parrott—Thelma Todd, James Finlayson, Eddie Dunn, Charles Gerrard, Gertrude Sutton, Harry Bernard, Robert "Bobby" Burns. Three reels.

49. **Be Big**—Hal Roach/MGM 1931—James Parrott—Anita Garvin, Isabelle Keith, Charlie Hall, Baldwin Cooke, Jack Hill, Ham Kinsey, Chet Brandenberg. Three reels.

50. **Chickens Come Home**—Hal Roach/MGM 1931—James W. Horne—Thelma Todd, Mae Busch, James Finlayson, Frank Holliday, Elizabeth Forrester, Norma Drew, Patsy O'Byrne, Charles French, Gertrude Pedlar, Frank Rice, Gordon Douglas, Ham Kinsey, Baldwin Cooke, Dorothy Layton. Three reels.

51. **The Stolen Jools**—National Variety Artists 1931—William McGann—A fund-raising short, featuring Eddie Kane and cameo appearances by Norma Shearer, Wallace Beery, Buster Keaton, Edward G. Robinson, George E. Stone, Our Gang, Polly Moran, Hedda Hopper, Joan Crawford, William Haines, Dorothy Lee, Edmund Lowe, Victor McLaglen, Joyce Compton, El Brendel, Charlie Murray, George Sidney, Willie Lightner, Fifi D'Orsay, Warner Baxter, Irene Dunne, Bert Wheeler, Robert Woolsey, Richard Dix, Claudia Dell, Lowell Sherman, Stuart Erwin, Eugene Pallette, Skeets Gallagher, Gary Cooper, Wynne Gibson, Charles "Buddy" Rogers, Maurice Chevalier, Loretta Young, Douglas Fairbanks, Jr., Richard Barthelmess, Louise Fazenda, Charles Butterworth, Bebe Daniels, Ben Lyon, Barbara Stanwyck, Frank Fay, Jack Oakie, Fay Wray, Joe E. Brown, Little Billy, Mitzi Green, George "Gabby" Hayes.

52. **Laughing Gravy**—Hal Roach/MGM 1931—James W. Horne—Charlie Hall, Harry Bernard, Charles Dorety.

53. **Our Wife**—Hal Roach/MGM 1931—James W. Horne—Babe London, James Finlayson, Ben Turpin, Charley Rogers, Blanche Payson.

54. **Pardon Us**—Hal Roach/MGM 1931—James Parrott—Walter Long, James Finlayson, June Marlowe, Charlie Hall, Wilfred Lucas, Frank Holliday, Harry Bernard, Sam Lufkin, Silas D. Wilcox, George Miller, Stanley "Tiny" Sandford, Robert "Bobby" Burns, Frank Austin, Otto Fries, Robert Kortman, Leo Willis, Jerry Mandy, Bobby Dunn, Eddie Dunn, Baldwin Cooke, Charles Dorety, Dick Gilbert, Will Stanton, Jack Herrick, Jack Hill, Gene Morgan, Charles Bachman, Blackie Whiteford, Charley Rogers, Gordon Douglas, James Parrott, Hal Roach, Eddie Baker, the Etude Ethiopian Chorus. 55 minutes.

55. **Come Clean**—Hal Roach/MGM 1931—James W. Horne—Gertrude Astor, Linda Loredo, Mae Busch, Charlie Hall, Eddie Baker, Stanley "Tiny" Sandford, Gordon Douglas.

56. **One Good Turn**—Hal Roach/MGM 1931—James W. Horne—Mary Carr, Billy Gilbert, Lyle Tayo, Dorothy Granger, Snub Pollard, Gordon Douglas, Dick Gilbert, George Miller, Baldwin Cooke, Ham Kinsey, Retta Palmer, William Gillespie, Charley Young.

57. **Beau Hunks**—Hal Roach/MGM 1931—James W. Horne—Charles Middleton, Charlie Hall, Stanley "Tiny" Sandford, Harry Schultz, Gordon Douglas, Sam Lufkin, Marvin Hatley, Jack Hill, Leo Willis, Robert Kortman, Baldwin Cooke, Dick Gilbert, Oscar Morgan, Ham Kinsey, Broderick O'Farrell, James W. Horne (billed as Abdul Kasim K'Horne). Four reels.

58. **On the Loose**—Hal Roach/MGM 1931—Hal Roach—Thelma Todd, ZaSu Pitts, John Loder, Claud Allister, Billy Gilbert, Charlie Hall, Gordon Douglas, Jack Hill, Buddy MacDonald, Otto Fries, gag appearance by Laurel & Hardy.

59. **Helpmates**—Hal Roach/MGM 1932—James Parrott—Blanche Payson, Robert "Bobby" Burns, Robert Callahan.

60. **Any Old Port**—Hal Roach/MGM 1932—James W. Horne—Walter Long, Jacqueline Wells (Julie Bishop), Harry Bernard, Charlie Hall, Robert "Bobby" Burns, Sam Lufkin, Dick Gilbert, Eddie Baker, Will Stanton, Jack Hill, Baldwin Cooke, Ed Brandenberg.

61. **The Music Box**—Hal Roach/MGM 1932—James Par-
    rott—Billy Gilbert, William Gillespie, Charlie Hall,
    Gladys Gale, Sam Lufkin, Lilyan Irene. Academy
    Award winner. Three reels.
62. **The Chimp**—Hal Roach/MGM 1932—James Parrott—
    Billy Gilbert, James Finlayson, Stanley "Tiny" Sandford,
    Charles Gamora, Jack Hill, Robert "Bobby" Burns,
    George Miller, Baldwin Cooke, Dorothy Layton, Belle
    Hare, Martha Sleeper. Three reels.
63. **County Hospital**—Hal Roach/MGM 1932—James Par-
    rott—Billy Gilbert, Sam Lufkin, Baldwin Cooke, Ham
    Kinsey, May Wallace, Frank Holliday, Lilyan Irene,
    Belle Hare, Dorothy Layton, William Austin.
64. **Scram!**—Hal Roach/MGM 1932—Raymond McCarey—
    Arthur Housman, Richard Cramer, Vivien Oakland, Sam
    Lufkin, Charles McMurphy, Baldwin Cooke, Charles
    Dorety.
65. **Pack Up Your Troubles**—Hal Roach/MGM 1932—
    George Marshall and Raymond McCarey—Donald
    Dillaway, Mary Carr, Charles Middleton, Richard
    Cramer, Tom Kennedy, Billy Gilbert, Grady Sutton,
    Jacquie Lyn, James Finlayson, Richard Tucker, George
    Marshall, Frank Brownlee, John Rogers, Ben Hen-
    dricks, Jr., James C. Morton, Bill O'Brien, C. Montague
    Shaw, Nora Cecil, Muriel Evans, Mary Gordon, Lew
    Kelly, Robert E. Homans, Adele Watson, Al Hallet,
    Frank Rice, Gene Morgan, James Mason, Charles
    Dorety, Dorothy Layton, Charley Young, Marvin
    Hatley, Bud Fine, Pat Harmon, Frank Hagney, Bob
    O'Conor, Pete Gordon, Henry Hall, Ellinor Van Der
    Veer, Chet Brandenberg. 68 minutes.
66. **Their First Mistake**—Hal Roach/MGM 1932—George
    Marshall—Mae Busch, Billy Gilbert, George Marshall.
67. **Towed in a Hole**—Hal Roach/MGM 1932—George Mar-
    shall—Billy Gilbert.
68. **Twice Two**—Hal Roach/MGM 1933—James Parrott—
    Baldwin Cooke, Charlie Hall, Ham Kinsey, voices of
    Carol Tevis and May Wallace.
69. **Me and My Pal**—Hal Roach/MGM 1933—Charles Rog-
    ers and Lloyd French—James Finlayson, James C. Mor-
    ton, Eddie Dunn, Charlie Hall, Bobby Dunn, Carol
    Borland, Mary Kornman, Charles McMurphy, Eddie
    Baker, Marion Bardell, Charley Young, Walter Plinge.
70. **The Devil's Brother (Fra Diavolo)**—Hal Roach/MGM
    1933—Hal Roach and Charles Rogers—Dennis King,

Thelma Todd, James Finlayson, Henry Armetta, Lane Chandler, Arthur Pierson, Lucile Browne, George Miller, Stanley "Tiny" Sandford, Harry Bernard, James C. Morton, Nina Quartaro, Jack Hill, Dick Gilbert, Arthur Stone, John Qualen, Edith Fellows, Jackie Lynn Taylor, Rolfe Sedan, Kay Deslys, Leo White, Lillian Moore, Walter Shumway, Louise Carver, Matt McHugh. 90 minutes.

71. **The Midnight Patrol**—Hal Roach/MGM 1933—Lloyd French—Walter Plinge, Robert Kortman, Charlie Hall, Harry Bernard, Frank Brownlee, James C. Morton, Stanley "Tiny" Sandford, Edgar Dearing, Eddie Dunn, Billy Bletcher.

72. **Busy Bodies**—Hal Roach/MGM 1933—Lloyd French— Charlie Hall, Stanley "Tiny" Sandford, Jack Hill, Dick Gilbert, Charley Young.

73. **Wild Poses**—Hal Roach/MGM 1933—Robert F. McGowan—Our Gang (Spanky McFarland, Stymie Beard, Tommy Bond, George Billings, Jerry Tucker), Franklin Pangborn, Emerson Treacy, Gay Seabrook, gag appearance by Laurel & Hardy.

74. **Dirty Work**—Hal Roach/MGM 1933—Lloyd French— Lucien Littlefield, Sam Adams.

75. **Sons of the Desert**—Hal Roach/MGM 1933—William A. Seiter— Charley Chase, Mae Busch, Dorothy Christy, Lucien Littlefield, John Elliott, Philo McCullough, Charita, Ty Parvis, Charley Young, John Merton, William Gillespie, Charles McAvoy, Robert "Bobby" Burns, Al Thompson, Eddie Baker, Jimmy Aubrey, Chet Brandenberg, Don Brodie, Harry Bernard, Sam Lufkin, Ernie Alexander, Baldwin Cooke, Charlie Hall, Stanley Blystone, Max Wagner, Pat Harmon, Nina Quartaro, Lillian Moore, Brooks Benedict, voice of Billy Gilbert. 68 minutes.

76. **Oliver the Eighth**—Hal Roach/MGM 1934—Lloyd French—Mae Busch, Jack Barty.

77. **Hollywood Party**—MGM 1934—Richard Boleslawski, Allan Dwan, Roy Rowland—Jimmy Durante, Lupe Velez, Charles Butterworth, Eddie Quillan, Ted Healy and his Stooges, Polly Moran, Jack Pearl, Mickey Mouse, George Givot, June Clyde, Frances Williams, Art Jarrett, Robert Young, Tom Kennedy, Ben Bard, Richard Carle, Leonid Kinskey, Tom Herbert, Tom London, Jed Prouty, Harry Barris, the Shirley Ross Quartet, Edwin Maxwell, Richard Cramer, Clarence

Wilson, Nora Cecil, Baldwin Cooke, Bess Flowers, Muriel Evans, Sidney Bracy, Arthur Treacher, Irene Hervey, Frank Austin, Ray Cooke, Ernie Alexander, Mrs. Jimmy Durante. Animated sequence in Technicolor by Walt Disney. 68 minutes.

78. **Going Bye Bye!**—Hal Roach/MGM 1934—Charles Rogers—Walter Long, Mae Busch, Sam Lufkin, Harry Dunkinson, Ellinor van Der Veer, Baldwin Cooke, Fred Holmes, Jack "Tiny" Lipson, Lester Dorr, Charles Dorety.

79. **Them Thar Hills**—Hal Roach/MGM 1934—Charles Rogers—Mae Busch, Charlie Hall, Billy Gilbert, Bobby Dunn, Sam Lufkin, Dick Alexander, Eddie Baker, Baldwin Cooke, Robert "Bobby" Burns.

80. **Babes in Toyland1 (March of the Wooden Soldiers)** —Hal Roach/MGM 1934—Charles Rogers and Gus Meins—Charlotte Henry, Felix Knight, Henry Kleinbach (Brandon), Johnny Downs, Jean Darling, Marie Wilson, Virginia Karns, Florence Roberts, William Burress, Ferdinand Munier, Frank Austin, Gus Leonard, John George, Scotty Beckett, Marianne Edwards, Tommy Bupp, Georgia Billings, Jerry Tucker, Jackie Lynn Taylor, Dickie Jones, Alice Dahl, Pete Gordon, Sumner Getchell, Billy Bletcher, Alice Moore, Alice Cooke, Kewpie Morgan, Stanley "Tiny" Sandford, Eddie Baker, Dick Alexander, Richard Powell, Scott Mattraw, Fred Holmes, Jack Raymond, Eddie Borden, Sam Lufkin, Jack Hill, Baldwin Cooke, Charlie Hall, Payne Johnson, Angelo Rossitto. 79 minutes.

81. **The Live Ghost**—Hal Roach/MGM 1934—Charles Rogers—Walter Long, Mae Busch, Arthur Housman, Harry Bernard, Pete Gordon, Leo Willis, Charlie Hall, Sam Lufkin, Charlie Sullivan, Jack "Tiny" Lipson, Dick Gilbert, Baldwin Cooke, Arthur Rowlands, Hubert Diltz.

82. **Tit for Tat**—Hal Roach/MGM 1935—Charles Rogers—Charlie Hall, Mae Busch, James C. Morton, Bobby Dunn, Baldwin Cooke, Jack Hill, Pete Gordon, Elsie MacKaye, Dick Gilbert, Lester Dorr, Viola Richard.

83. **The Fixer-Uppers**—Hal Roach/MGM 1935—Charles Rogers—Mae Busch, Arthur Housman, Charles Middleton, Bobby Dunn, Noah Young, Dick Gilbert, Jack Hill, James C. Morton, Bob O'Conor.

84. **Thicker Than Water**—Hal Roach/MGM 1935—James W. Horne—Daphne Pollard, James Finlayson, Harry

Bowen, Ed Brandenberg, Charlie Hall, Grace Goodall, Bess Flowers, Lester Dorr, Gladys Gale, Allen Cavan, Baldwin Cooke.

85. **Bonnie Scotland**—Hal Roach/MGM 1935—James W. Horne—William Janney, June Lang, David Torrence, Anne Grey, James Finlayson, Mary Gordon, James Mack, May Beatty, Daphne Pollard, James May, Jack Hill, Kathryn Sheldon, Minerva Urecal, Claire Verdera, Maurice Black, Vernon Steele, Noah Young, Dan Maxwell, David Clyde, James Burtis, Brandon Hurst, Olaf Hytten, Marvin Hatley, Claude King, Bill Moore, Art Rowlands, Lionel Belmore, Dick Wessel, Charlie Hall, Bob O'Conor, Leo Willis, Sam Lufkin, Bobby Dunn, Phyllis Barry, Belle Daube, Elizabeth Wilbur, Carlotta Monti, Murdock MacQuarrie, Mary McLaren. 80 minutes.

86. **The Bohemian Girl**—Hal Roach/MGM 1936—James W. Horne and Charles Rogers—Thelma Todd, Jacqueline Wells (Julie Bishop), Antonio Moreno, Mae Busch, James Finlayson, Darla Hood, Harry Bowen, Zeffie Tilbury, William P. Carlton, Harry Bernard, Mitchell Lewis, Antoinette Lees (Andrea Leeds), Margaret Mann, Harold Switzer, James C. Morton, Eddie Borden, Sam Lufkin, Bob O'Conor, Bobby Dunn, Felix Knight, Dick Gilbert, Leo Willis, Jack Hill, Arthur Rowlands, Lane Chandler, Baldwin Cooke, Lee Phelps, Bill Madsen, Frank Darien, Sammy Brooks, Alice Cooke, Eddy Chandler, Charlie Hall. 70 minutes.

87. **On the Wrong Trek**—Hal Roach/MGM 1936—Charles Parrott—Charley Chase, Rosina Lawrence, Bonita Weber, Clarence Wilson, Gertrude Sutton, Jack Egan, Frances Morris, Charles McAvoy, Eddie Parker, Bob O'Conor, Bud Jamison, Leo Willis, Robert Kortman, Harry Wilson, May Wallace, Harry Bowen, Harry Bernard, Dick Gilbert, Robert "Bobby" Burns, Charley Sullivan, Joe Bordeaux, Jack Hill, Lester Dorr, gag appearance by L & H in this Charley Chase short.

88. **Our Relations**—Hal Roach/MGM 1936—Harry Lachman—Sidney Toler, Alan Hale, Daphne Pollard, Betty Healy, Iris Adrian, Lona Andre, James Finlayson, Arthur Housman, Jim Kilganon, Charlie Hall, Harry Bernard, Harry Arras, Charles Bachman, Harry Neilman, John Kelly, Art Rowlands, Harry Wilson, Baldwin Cooke, Nick Copland, James C. Morton, Lee Phelps, George Jimenez, Bob Wilbur, Jim Pierce, Ruth

Warren, Walter Taylor, Constantine Romanoff, Alex
Pollard, Joe Bordeaux, Stanley "Tiny" Sandford, Billy
Engle, Bob O'Conor, Bobby Dunn, Ralf Harolde, Noel
Madison, Del Henderson, Fred Holmes, Jack Hill, Ed
Brandenberg, Jack Egan, Dick Gilbert, Ernie Alexan-
der, Polly Chase, Jay Belasco, Gertrude Astor, Buddy
Messinger, Gertrude Messinger, David Sharpe, Johnny
Arthur, Marvin Hatley, Sam Lufkin, Ray Cooke, Rose-
mary Theby. 74 minutes.

89. **Way Out West**—Hal Roach/MGM 1937—James W.
Horne—James Finlayson, Sharon Lynne, Stanley Fields,
Rosina Lawrence, James Mason, James C. Morton,
Frank Mills, Dave Pepper, Vivien Oakland, Harry
Bernard, Mary Gordon, May Wallace, the Avalon
Boys Quartet (including Chill Wills), Jack Hill, Sam
Lufkin, Tex Driscoll, Flora Finch, Snowflake, Bobby
Dunn, John Ince, Bill Wolf, Denver Dixon, Eddie
Borden, Helen Holmes, Ben Corbett, Jay Wilsey, Cy
Slocum, Fritzi Brunette, Frank Montgomery, Fred
Cady, Lester Dorr. 65 minutes.

90. **Pick a Star**—Hal Roach/MGM 1937—Edward Sedg-
wick—Patsy Kelly, Jack Haley, Rosina Lawrence,
Mischa Auer, Lyda Roberti, Charles Halton, Russell
Hicks, Spencer Charters, Sam Adams, Robert Gleckler,
Johnny Arthur, Joyce Compton, James Finlayson, Wal-
ter Long, James C. Morton, Ralph Malone, Blair Da-
vies, Eddie Kane, Charles Bachman, Charles McMurphy,
Frank O'Connor, Charlie Hall, Ray Cooke, Cully Rich-
ards, Sam Lufkin, John Hyams, Leila McIntyre, Otto
Fries, Howard Brooks, Margie Roanberg, Alice Moore,
Mary Blackwell, Arline Abers, Brooks Benedict, May
Wallace, Jack Norton, Wilma Cox, Barbara Weeks,
Edward Clayton, Bob O'Conor, Sid Saylor, Jack Hill,
Jack Egan, Charley Sullivan, Eddie Hart, Si Jenks,
Wilbur Mack, Murdock MacQuarrie, Mary Gordon,
Al Williams, Jr., Barney Carr, Felix Knight, Patricia
Ka, James Burke. 70 minutes.

91. **Swiss Miss**—Hal Roach/MGM 1938—John G. Blystone—
Walter Woolf King, Della Lind, Adia Kuznetzoff, Ed-
die Kane, Anita Garvin, Franz Hug, Eric Blore,
Ludovico Tomarchio, Sam Lufkin, Tex Driscoll, Charles
Judels, George Sorel, Harry Semels, Etherine Landucci,
Gustav von Seyffertitz, Conrad Seideman, Bob O'Conor,
Michael Mark, Jean de Briac, Agostino Borgato, Doo-
dles Weaver, Hal Gerard, Baldwin Cooke, Ed Brand-

enberg, Jack Hill, Lester Dorr, Charles Gamora. 72 minutes.

92. **Block-Heads**—Hal Roach/MGM 1938—John G. Blystone—Billy Gilbert, Patricia Ellis, Minna Gombell, James C. Morton, James Finlayson, Harry Woods, Tommy Bond, Jean del Val, Henry Hall, Sam Lufkin, Harry Strang, William Royle, Harry Earles, Max Hoffman, Jr., Patsy Moran, Ed Brandenberg, Jack Hill, George Chandler, Harry Stubbs. 58 minutes.

93. **The Flying Deuces**—Boris Morros/RKO—1939—A. Edward Sutherland—Jean Parker, Reginald Gardiner, James Finlayson, Charles Middleton, Clem Wilenchik (Crane Whitley), Jean del Val, Richard Cramer, Michael Visaroff, Monica Bannister, Bonnie Bannon, Mary Jane Carey, Christine Cabanne, Frank Clarke, Eddie Borden, Sam Lufkin, Kit Guard, Billy Engle, Jack Chefe. 69 minutes.

94. **A Chump at Oxford**—Hal Roach/UA 1940—Alf Goulding—Forrester Harvey, Wilfred Lucas, Forbes Murray, Frank Baker, Eddie Borden, Peter Cushing, Charlie Hall, Gerald Fielding, Victor Kendall, Gerald Rogers, Jack Heasley, Rex Lease, Stanley Blystone, Alec Harford. 42 minutes. (A longer version, running 63 minutes, was released in Europe and has since been put into circulation here. It features James Finlayson, Anita Garvin, Vivien Oakland, James Millican, Harry Bernard, Sam Lufkin, Jean de Briac, George Magrill.)

95. **Saps at Sea**—Hal Roach/UA 1940—Gordon Douglas—James Finlayson, Ben Turpin, Richard Cramer, Eddie Conrad, Harry Hayden, Charlie Hall, Patsy Moran, Gene Morgan, Charles Bachman, Bud Geary, Jack Greene, Eddie Borden, Robert McKenzie, Ernie Alexander, Mary Gordon, Jack Hill, Walter Lawrence, Carl Faulkner, Harry Evans, Ed Brady, Patsy O'Byrne, Harry Bernard, Sam Lufkin, Constantine Romanoff, Francesca Santoro, Jackie Horner. 57 minutes.

96. **Great Guns**—20th Century-Fox 1941—Monty Banks—Sheila Ryan, Dick Nelson, Edmund MacDonald, Charles Trowbridge, Ludwig Stossel, Kane Richmond, Mae Marsh, Ethel Griffies, Paul Harvey, Charles Arnt, Pierre Watkin, Russell Hicks, Irving Bacon, Robert Lowery, Fred Kohler, Jr., Lyle Latell, Max Wagner, Billy Benedict, James Flavin, Edward Earle, Dave Willock, Harold Goodwin, Cyril Ring, Bud Geary, Leroy Mason, Alan Ladd, Walter Sande. 74 minutes.

97. **A-Haunting We Will Go**—20th Century-Fox 1942—
Alfred Werker—Dante the Magician (Harry A. Jan-
sen), Sheila Ryan, John Shelton, Elisha Cook, Jr.,
Don Costello, Edward Gargan, Addison Richards,
George Lynn, James Bush, Lou Lubin, Robert Emmett
Keane, Richard Lane, Willie Best, Bud Geary, Eddy
Waller, Walter Sande, Mantan Moreland, Frank Faylen,
Judy Ford (Terry Moore), Tom Dugan, Ralph Dunn,
Edgar Dearing, Wade Boteler, Francis Pierlot, Leon
Tyler. 67 minutes.

98. **Air Raid Wardens**—MGM 1943—Edward Sedgwick—
Edgar Kennedy, Jacqueline White, Horace (Stephen)
McNally, Nella Walker, Donald Meek, Henry O'Neill,
Howard Freeman, Paul Stanton, Robert Emmet O'Con-
nor, William Tannen, Russell Hicks, Phil Van Zandt,
Frederick Worlock, Don Costello, Charles Coleman,
Jules Cowles, Lee Phelps, Joe Yule, Sr., Forrest Tay-
lor, Milton Kibbee, Edward Hearn, Rose Hobart. 67
minutes.

99. **Tree in a Test Tube**—U.S. Government 1943—A World
War II government short, filmed in Technicolor during
a lunch hour at Fox. Narrated by Pete Smith.

100. **Jitterbugs**—20th Century-Fox 1943—Malcolm St. Clair—
Vivian Blaine, Bob Bailey, Douglas Fowley, Noel Mad-
ison, Lee Patrick, Robert Emmett Keane, Charles Halton,
Edwin Mills, James Bush, Anthony Caruso, Jimmy
Conlin, Sid Saylor, Lester Dorr, Francis Ford, Chick
Collins, Hal K. Dawson, Gladys Blake. 74 minutes.

101. **The Dancing Masters**—20th Century-Fox 1943—Malcolm
St. Clair—Trudy Marshall, Bob Bailey, Matt Briggs,
Margaret Dumont, Allan Lane, Robert Mitchum, Nestor
Paiva, George Lloyd, Edward Earle, Charles Rogers,
Sherry Hall, Sam Ash, Bill Haade, Arthur Space,
Daphne Pollard, Ruthe Brady, Hank Mann, Jay Wilsey
(Buffalo Bill, Jr.), Chick Collins, Robert Emmett Keane,
Emory Parnell, Harry Tyler. 63 minutes.

102. **The Big Noise**—20th Century-Fox 1944—Malcolm St.
Clair—Doris Merrick, Arthur Space, Veda Ann Borg,
Bobby Blake, Frank Fenton, Jack Norton, James Bush,
Phil Van Zandt, Esther Howard, Robert Dudley, Edgar
Dearing, Selmer Jackson, Harry Hayden, Francis Ford,
Charles Wilson, Ken Christy, Beal Wong, Louis Arco,
Sarah Edwards, Julie Carter, Billy Bletcher. 74 minutes.

103. **Nothing but Trouble**—MGM 1944—Sam Taylor—Mary
Boland, Philip Merivale, Henry O'Neill, David Leland,

John Warburton, Mathew Boulton, Connie Gilchrist, Chester Clute, Garry Owen, Grayce Hampton, Charles Irwin, Robert Emmet O'Connor, Lee Phelps, Edward Earle, Edward Keane, Forbes Murray, Eddie Dunn, Robert Homans, Olin Howland, Dell Henderson, Joe Yule, Sr., Ray Teal, Steve Darrell, Jean DeBriac, Paul Porcasi. 69 minutes.

104. **The Bullfighters**—20th Century-Fox 1945—Malcolm St. Clair—Margo Woode, Richard Lane, Carol Andrews, Diosa Costello, Ralph Sanford, Irving Gump, Ed Gargan, Lorraine De Wood, Emmett Vogan, Roger Neury, Gus Glassmire, Rafael Storm, Jay Novello, Robert Filmer, Hank Worden, Guy Zanette, Jose Portugal, Max Wagner, Frank McCown (Rory Calhoun), Julian Rivero, Cyril Ring, Joe Dominguez, Steve Darrell. 61 minutes.

105. **Atoll K**—A Sirius Release 1951—John Berry and Leo Joannon—Suzy Delair, Max Elloy, Adriano Rimoldi, Luigi Tosi, Suzet Mais, Felix Oudart, Robert Murzeau, Dalmatoff. Opened in Paris, November 1951. Released in England as ESCAPADE in 1952. Released in U.S. by Franco-London as ROBINSON CRUSOELAND in 1952, and by Exploitation Films as UTOPIA in 1954. 99 minutes.

CLARK and McCULLOUGH

Unless you are old enough to have attended Broadway shows in the 1920's and 30's, you have probably never heard of Clark and McCullogh. For several years they rivaled the Marx Brothers in popularity in New York, and even when they had to support weak material, they captured the hearts of the Broadway critics, who admired their madcap sense of fun and their boundless energy. They worked in Hollywood for seven years, but it is the sad fate of short subjects that they have been buried in obscurity, revived only by the staunchest film buffs. Most of the team's two-reel comedies for RKO, made in the early 1930's, do survive, and prove that Bobby Clark and Paul McCullough were an inspired pair of comedians who deserve more attention than they have received in recent years.

Robert Edwin (Bobby) Clark was born in Springfield, Ohio, in 1888. His father, a Pullman conductor, died when he was six. Bobby had a performing bent from his earliest days; he sang in a local choir, and saved his money to buy a bugle, so he could join the Sons of Veterans Drum and Bugle Corps in Springfield. As he entered fourth grade he was moved to a new elementary school, where he met Paul McCullough, four years his senior. McCullough, also a native of Springfield, loved to tumble, and convinced his new friend to go with him to a local YMCA tumbling class. Clark went along, and liked it very much. He and McCullough continued to meet at every possible opportunity to practice together. After several years of friendship, and countless hours of tumbling, the boys decided they were good enough to make a living taking falls. In 1900 they formed a theatrical partnership and set out to conquer show business.

Show business, it seemed, was not ready to be conquered by two youngsters from Springfield. An advertisement they placed in a local journal brought no results. They finally landed a job with a traveling minstrel troupe. Wrote Robert

Lewis Taylor in an excellent profile of Clark in *The New Yorker*, "The team's contract stipulated that the members blow bugles in the parade, do a song and dance in the first part of the show, present their tumbling in front of the curtain during intermission, and stand ready to do anything, subject to the producer's discretion, from reciting 'Hamlet' to juggling midgets in the 'afterpiece.' " After being stranded by one producer and abused by another, Clark and McCullough tired of the minstrel life and sought jobs in the circus. They were hired by the Hagenbach-Wallace Circus, mainly as tumbling clowns, but gradually the two young men started adding comic routines to their bag of tricks. Clark later admitted that they liked the sound of laughter from the audience, and decided that it wouldn't hurt to mix comedy with their acrobatics. Wrote Taylor, "McCullough would climb up on a table and Clark would attempt to hand him a chair. It would get hung up, however, on the edge of the table, balking their best efforts. 'Complicated, isn't it?' Clark

This jaunty title card introduced each of the RKO Clark and McCullough shorts.

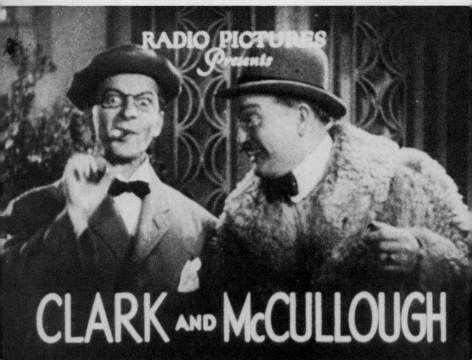

would yell, circling the disaster. 'Really a problem for a scientist, *but* we will attempt it!' The ensuing battle with the chair, the prodigious expenditures of energy (often involving the removal of most of their clothing), the ultimate total collapse of the table, and a fist fight, stopped the show."

In 1906, Clark and McCullough were hired by the Ringling Brothers Circus, in which once again their routines brought down the house every night. They spent six years with circuses, but in 1911, the two performers grew restless and decided to try their luck elsewhere. The following year they broke into vaudeville, in a theater in New Brunswick, New Jersey. Their act was the same table routine that had been a hit in the circus; the material was sure-fire, and Clark and McCullough went over quite well. As they started to tour the United States and Canada, they gradually added new material, and eschewed tumbling for dialogue and sketch comedy. By this time, their costumes and props were also established, the same ones they would use throughout their careers. Brooks Atkinson once described them in this way: "Clark with the flat hat, the cavernous topcoat, the sleight-of-hand cigar and the primeval cane; McCullough with the fur coat, straw hat, and toothbrush mustache."

The team became a modest success in vaudeville, and managed to work steadily with a good salary. But in 1917 Jean Bedini, a famous burlesque impresario, caught their act in Boston and convinced them to join his company as featured comedians. This was at a time when burlesque was not devoted solely to undulating female bodies, but featured some of the greatest comedians of all time. All the comics who came out of burlesque—Bert Lahr and Phil Silvers among them—regarded it as the greatest comedy training ground of all time. It was also extremely popular, and as a result of the burlesque experience, Clark and McCullough became internationally renowned. They even scored a hit in London, where Bedini's show *Peek-a-Boo* attracted the cream of society as well as the standard burlesque devotees.

The team was hired for a musical-comedy revue called *Chuckles of 1922* that became London's biggest hit of the season. Many tempting offers were made by rival London producers, but they were outbid by the American songwriter Irving Berlin, who caught *Chuckles* during a trip to England and hired the team to appear in the second edition of his *Music Box Revue* on Broadway. In the fall of 1922, Clark and McCullough made their Broadway debut in the Berlin show, and were an immediate success. They were featured

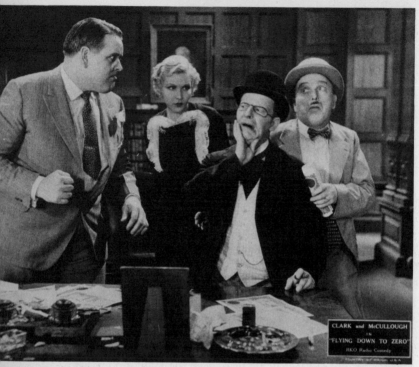

In FLYING DOWN TO ZERO, Clark and McCullough are threatened by Bud Jamison and observed by Constance Bergen.

along with Charlotte Greenwood, William Gaxton, opera star Grace LaRue, and singer John Steel. They stayed with the show for 272 performances, then went on tour with a road-company version. The comics returned for the 1924 edition of *Music Box Revue*, this time with star billing, along with Fanny Brice, Grace Moore, Oscar Shaw, Claire Luce, and the Brox Sisters. This, the fourth revue in the series, was considered the weakest by most critics, although it was generally agreed that Bobby Clark's personality and delivery were such that even stale material sounded good when he mouthed it. An oft-quoted gag from the show had McCullough walking on stage with a toothbrush pinned to his lapel. "It's a college pin," Clark would explain. "He's from Colgate."

On September 20, 1926, Clark and McCullough were promoted to starring status in a Broadway musical comedy. An entrepreneur, Philip Goodman, who had had considerable success when he put another vaudeville comedian, W. C. Fields, on Broadway in *Poppy*, approached Clark and McCullough about a similar move. They were worried, but they accepted. "After all," Clark later recalled, "we were a vaudeville team. How'd we know we could carry a musical? I figured we'd probably be back in burlesque, or maybe the minstrels, within a week." They weren't. *The Ramblers* opened to mixed reviews, but most critics agreed that the lunatic team of Clark and McCullough made the show worth seeing. *The Ramblers* was a hit, and the comedy team was established on Broadway. In December 1926 they were given the singular honor of a dinner at the Friars Club in New York. The soirees held by this actors organization remain social highlights to this day; the dinner for the two comics in 1926 was likewise an impressive affair. After much speechmaking and reminiscences, and some traditional "roasting" by fellow Friars, Bobby Clark made a speech which *Variety* printed in toto. A sample: "This is wonderful, it is amazing to think that Clark and McCullough made so many friends who own

Clark and McCullough are trying to put something over on Gavin Gordon and Anita Garvin in ALL STEAMED UP.

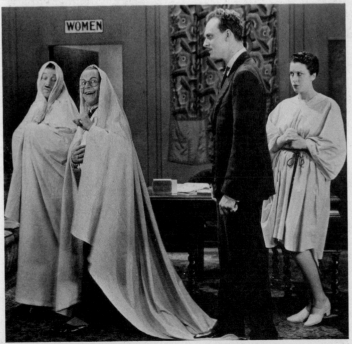

their own dinner clothes . . . A great many people think it is strange that McCullough and I have been together so long. It is not strange at all. We are doing fine, we get along together fine. We don't have fights, we don't have arguments. If a question arises as to how a certain piece of business should be done or how some certain gag should be put over, we don't talk and argue about it like so many people; we sit down quietly and talk it over pro and con. I listen to McCullough's version, and he listens to mine, and then I go out on the stage and do it my way."

Not long after their Broadway success, the talkies hit Hollywood, and the alert studios scanned the Broadway stage for possible film recruits. Clark and McCullough were among the first to make the trip West, to Fox Studios, where they started their film career with several one-reel adaptations of old vaudeville and burlesque sketches. These were made in the summer of 1928. By the end of the year, Fox decided to spend more time and money on the Clark and McCullough shorts (which were among the only talkie films the studio had to offer theaters) and hired two comedy experts to direct: Norman Taurog and Harry Sweet. Taurog started in silent comedies and went on to direct SKIPPY, WE'RE NOT DRESSING, BOYS TOWN, and many other successful films. Harry Sweet specialized in comedy, and in the early 1930's supervised all of RKO's comedy output, originating Edgar Kennedy's long-running series of domestic comedies. Taurog and Sweet alternated on the Clark and McCullough series, which were unusual in that they were not shorts, but featurettes, running thirty to fifty minutes. The team worked on all the scripts, which borrowed heavily from their backlog of routines. One of their collaborators, Sidney Lanfield, later became a prominent director at Fox (SING BABY SING, HOUND OF THE BASKERVILLES, etc.) and recalls Clark and McCullough as "both gentlemen. They were a pleasure to work with—no temperament, and most cooperative." The scripts were, in keeping with the then-popular method of making shorts, loose foundations for what finally appeared on screen. "There always is some freedom with comedy scripts," Lanfield says. "Everyone helps."

The two comics, however, were not pleased with "everyone helping." To be sure, they improvised on stage: Bobby Clark's ad libs were among the classic moments of Broadway comedy. But the Hollywood method of creating comedy films was strange to them, and they felt uncomfortable. After completing their series for Fox in 1929, Clark and

McCullough returned to New York and started rehearsing for a new show. *Strike Up the Band* opened on January 14, 1930, with a book by Morrie Ryskind, based on a libretto by George S. Kaufman. The songs, including the title tune and "I've Got a Crush on You," were by George and Ira Gershwin. With all that talent behind it, and Clark and McCullough on stage, the show should have been better than it was, but it was still good enough to keep Broadway audiences pleased for a long and healthy run. The show was an allegorical satire on the chocolate industry, with prohibitive tariffs endangering the profits of several business magnates. The show had "more wit and satire than one expects to find in a Broadway musical comedy," said one reviewer, and Clark and McCullough put over the material with their traditional gusto.

The following year they returned with another show, *Here Goes the Bride*, written by *New Yorker* cartoonist Peter Arno. Brooks Atkinson, who had not thought the team suitable for Broadway in 1926, was by this time an (avid) admirer. With the Marx Brothers gone, he said, "Clark and McCullough are the logical First Actors for the Stage . . . Their genius rises to its greatest magnificence when they are running in circles around the stage, now and then emitting a staggering bellow of song."

Despite their lukewarm reaction to Hollywood in the late 1920's, they were persuaded to return in late 1931 to do a

Clark and McCullough encounter Dorothy Granger—and her husband, Tom Kennedy—IN THE DEVIL'S DOGHOUSE.

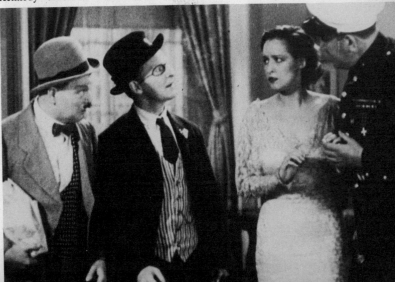

series of shorts for RKO Radio Pictures. RKO was building up its comedy short-subjects department, hiring proven talent as well as promising newcomers, both behind and in front of the camera. The director of the team's earliest RKO effort was Mark Sandrich, who also collaborated on the scripts. Within a few years he was promoted to feature films at the studio, and went on to direct some of the best Fred Astaire-Ginger Rogers musicals, among other hits. Another scenarist on the series, Johnnie Grey, started with Mack Sennett and provided first-rate comedy scripts for several studios throughout the 1930's and into the 40's. Their combined efforts produced a series of two-reelers for Clark and McCullough that ranged from fairly good to hilarious, all of them combining rapid-fire dialogue (often supplied by Clark) with inventive sight gags. Their first film, FALSE ROOMERS, co-starred James Finlayson (Laurel and Hardy's usual nemesis) and other comedy "regulars" Eddie Dunn and Kewpie Morgan. The plot involves them wrecking Morgan's car, and seeking refuge in Finlayson's boarding house. He warns them that there is no cooking allowed in the establishment, but they proceed to pop corn over a gas heater in the room. A young girl mistakes their room for the bathroom and other complications arise as Morgan drives into the house with his car. A slapstick finale has Clark and McCullough driving out of the house with the bed attached to Morgan's automobile.

Director Sandrich loved sight gags and slapstick and worked them into his shorts as much as possible (there's even some pie-throwing in THE ICEMAN'S BALL). But he also appreciated the genuine sense of the bizarre that made Clark and McCullough unique. JITTERS THE BUTLER (1932) is all about a portly servant who graciously—even willingly—makes his derriere available to be kicked! It's certainly the *most* bizarre of all the team's two-reelers. These shorts were also made prior to the introduction of the Production Code, and scripts were rife with risqué material—be it lingeried ladies in THE GAY NIGHTIES or Clark's deathless line to a pretty girl in THE ICEMAN'S BALL: "You know, it's women like you who make men like me make women like you make men like me."

When Sandrich left the series in mid-1933, the films began to rely more on situation and dialogue, most of it written by Bobby Clark. Their first film with director Sam White, KICKIN' THE CROWN AROUND, is a wild spoof of prohibition set in a mythical kingdom where the 18,000th Amendment prohibits

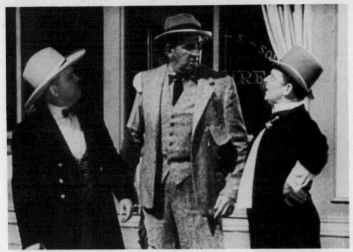

Plug Hardy (Tom Kennedy) isn't in the market for lawyers in ODOR IN THE COURT.

the sale or possession of salami. Some 6 percent garlic salami has been smuggled into the country, however, and Clark and McCullough are hired to track down the culprit (the prime suspect is a strange character named Disputin).

Clark and McCullough filmed their shorts during the summer months, to allow them to perform on Broadway during the regular season. In December of 1932 they opened with Beatrice Lillie in *Walk a Little Faster*, a memorable show that featured such songs as "April in Paris." The money was good at RKO, but the duo did not wish to remain in Hollywood any longer than they had to. RKO continued to release the two-reelers every other month, to good if not overwhelming response. The quality remained fairly high in the series, and in 1934 the team turned out a two-reeler that rates as a comedy classic: ODOR IN THE COURT. The pace and dialogue of this film are so frenetic that one viewing is not sufficient to appreciate the comedy. Fourth and fifth viewings reveal throwaway lines and subtle gags not apparent at first.

The short opens as a young blonde (Helen Collins) tells her husband (Lorin Raker) that their divorce is final, and the trial is set for that afternoon. He doesn't want to pay any alimony, and notices a handbill for Blackstone and Blodgett, two energetic lawyers ("No case too small—No fee too large"). The two would-be attorneys are standing on the sidewalk distributing their leaflets. "Help make our home Europe," cries Blackstone (Clark) as he hands the papers to passersby. Meanwhile, Helen's lover, a boxer named Plug Hardy (Tom Kennedy) has a sidewalk conference with his lawyer, Thackeray D. Ward (Jack Rice), who promises to get $100,000 alimony from Raker and split the bonanza with Kennedy. Walking down the street, Kennedy is nearly knocked over by a speeding car. Sensing a damage suit in the making, Clark and McCullough jump in: to make things look more realistic they tear Kennedy's suit, throw ashes on him, and give him a black eye. Clark then asks him the license number of the car: when Kennedy tells him he doesn't know it, the two lawyers make a fast getaway.

After a confrontation with Thackeray D. Ward, and a visit from husband Raker, the two lawyers determine to win this case. Clark calls in his secretary by ringing a huge bell. "Did you ring?" she asks coyly. "No, but I'm glad you're here. Bring a pad—bring two pads," he commands. "What flavor?" "Six and ⅞," he replies distractedly. She returns with two pillows, tosses one to Clark and they get down to business planning to frame their opposing attorney by having the pretty young secretary kiss him, while Clark and McCullough photograph the event. Ward, it seems, is scheduled to marry the judge's daughter, and this will be their ace in the hole.

Clark and McCullough come to court that afternoon with a large crowd of fans and a thirty-piece marching band. As they parade into the courtroom with their advertising banner ("Watch us Work—Something New in Law") they immediately get on the judge's nerves. As soon as Ward starts to question his witness, Clark interferes:

> Clark: I object!
> Judge: On what grounds?
> Clark: None.
> Judge: Overruled!
> Clark: Content.

After this parlay, Ward continues his examination and Clark continues to confound the judge, yelling "I don't object" after one statement, and later, "It's a lie, but I don't object!" When he is given the chance to cross-examine the witness, the wife in the case, he asks her how long she was married to the defendant. "Two years," she replies. "Two years—hear that, everybody, two years!" he proclaims, striding around the courtroom. Then turning to her, he asks,

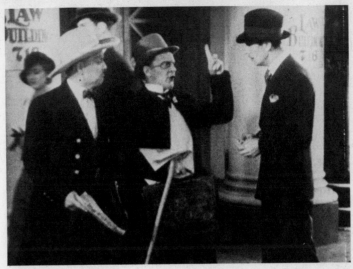

"Mal dicket, mal docket," says Clark, threatening lawyer Jack Rice in ODOR IN THE COURT.

"During that time did he ever beat you?" "Why, no," she answers innocently. "Why?" "Because I never did anything." "Aha!" he shouts. "Married two years and never did anything—a slacker!" The marching band accompanies this triumph with a chord in G.

Helen is granted the divorce, but when it comes time to set the alimony, Clark frustrates Ward by showing him "new evidence," the picture of him kissing the young secretary, and Ward is forced to withdraw his plea for alimony. Outside the courtroom, Ward breaks the new to Plug Hardy, concluding, "We don't get anything." Plug disagrees, and socks Ward in the jaw. Clark and McCullough see this and run over hoping for a damage suit. When they see the victim is Ward, they abandon the idea, but when Hardy recognizes them, Clark yells "I object" and the two lawyers run off into the crowd.

It is difficult to capture the lunacy of ODOR IN THE COURT on paper, with Clark running around the courtroom and the dialogue coming fast and furious. The film belies Clark's recollections, later in life, that their movies weren't any good, and it serves as an excellent testimonial to the comic skill of Clark and McCullough. The team continued to make shorts for RKO, and their last one, in 1935, ALIBI BY BYE, let them go out with a bang, as two "alibi photographers" in Atlantic City who let moonlighting husbands and wives pretend to be anywhere *but* Atlantic City for alibi purposes. The situation gets complicated when a man, his wife, her friend, a hotel manager, the hotel detective, a maid, and Clark and McCullough try to dodge each other by running in and out of four adjoining rooms in the hotel. The timing is split-second, and the result is a hilarious short, one of the best in the series.

After completing their last film for RKO, the two comics took a version of *George White's Scandals* on tour around the country, then returned to New York for a rest. McCullough, suffering from nervous exhaustion, entered a sanitarium in Medford, Massachusetts. He was released in March 1936, and was driving home with a friend when they passed a barber shop. McCullough decided to have a shave, and chatted amiably with the barber. Then, suddenly, he grabbed a razor and slashed his throat and wrists. He was in critical condition when he reached a nearby hospital, and remained in that state for several days, before dying on March 25, 1936. Publicly, Clark and McCullough had been known as one of the closest partnerships in show business. It was said that few teams had been so harmonious. But other stories circulated, and still do, that Clark dominated his straight-man partner and enjoyed flaunting his superiority. Many show-business friends of Clark's tried to convince him that his long-time foil was unnecessary and that Clark would do much better as a single. Clark always pooh-poohed such ideas

A typical Hollywood touch, little short of sacrilege, made Bobby Clark wear real glasses in THE GOLDWYN FOLLIES.

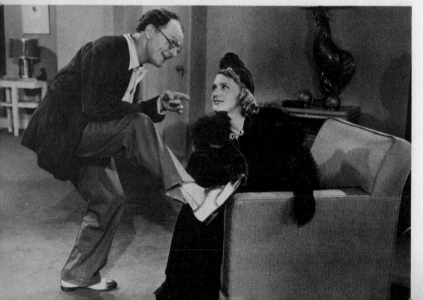

and wouldn't entertain the idea of splitting the team for one minute. After the tragedy of early 1936, he had no choice.

Clark went into seclusion for several months and emerged for the first time to replace Bob Hope in *The Ziegfeld Follies of 1936*, playing opposite Fanny Brice and Gypsy Rose Lee. He was extremely nervous about working "single," but his fears were unwarranted. Clark was a hit, and continued to work on Broadway for many years, in such shows as *Streets of Paris*, *All Men are Alike*, *Star and Garter*, *Sweethearts* and *As the Girls Go*. He became interested in comedy of the Restoration period, and several of his Broadway appearances were in revivals of classics like *Love for Love*, *The Rivals*, and *The Would-Be Gentleman*. Clark, for all his clowning on stage, was seriously interested in this period of theater, and even lectured on it at the American Theater Wing classes.

He returned to Hollywood only once, in 1938, for THE GOLDWYN FOLLIES, a horrendous hodgepodge which Clark later called "the world's longest trailer." He never had worse material, and in true Hollywood fashion, the powers-that-be made him abandon his trademark, painted-on glasses, in favor of an actual pair.

In his last years, Bobby Clark had the satisfaction of being revered as one of the great comedians of all time. He lived comfortably with his wife, a native of Switzerland whom he met when she was in one of Jean Bedini's burlesque shows. A man of boundless energy, Clark lived to be 71, and died in February 1960. His solo career, spanning some twenty years, made many people forget Clark's beginnings, and his long-time partnership with Paul McCullough. While it is true that Clark was always the dominant member of the duo, it is unfair to dismiss his days as half of a comedy team as unimportant. The work of Clark and McCullough was wild, way-out and often inspired. Their kind of humor has all but disappeared, and it is sorely missed.

The Films of Clark and McCullough

(Director's name follows year.)

1. **Clark and McCullough in the Interview**—Fox 1928—(no director credited)—one reel.
2. **Clark and McCullough in the Honor System**—Fox 1928—(no director credited)—one reel.

3. **The Bath Between**—Fox 1929—Ben Stoloff—Carmel Myers, Mack Flouker, Ben Holmes, Elwood Gray, Wally Shartles. Two reels.

4. **The Diplomats**—Fox 1929—Norman Taurog—Marguerite Churchill, Andres De Segurola, Cissy Fitzgerald, John St. Polis, John Baston, Andre Cheron, Joe Marba. Four reels.

5. **Waltzing Around**—Fox 1929—Harry Sweet—Otto Fries, Florence Lake, Ivan Linow, Lillian Halligan, Stanley Blystone, Dan Tobey, Kid Williams, Charles Sullivan. Four reels.

6. **In Holland**—Fox 1929—Norman Taurog—Marjorie Beebe, George Bickel, James Marcus, Ralph Emerson. Five reels.

7. **Belle of Samoa**—Fox 1929—Marcel Silver—Lois Moran, Filoi and her 60 Samoan singers and dancers. Two reels.

8. **Beneath the Law**—Fox 1929—Harry Sweet—Joyzelle, Billy Bletcher, May Boley, George Bickel, Joe Marba. Three reels.

9. **The Medicine Men**—Fox 1929—Norman Taurog—Four reels.

10. **Music Fiends**—Fox 1929—Harry Sweet—Frederick H. Grahame, Harry Adams, Helen Bolton. Three reels.

11. **Knights Out**—Fox 1929—Norman Taurog—Clifford Dempsey, Frederick H. Grahame, Gavin Gordon, Dixie Lee, Jack Jordan, Lucy Beaumont, Charles Eaton, Erin La Bissoniere, Allan Lane. Three reels.

12. **All Steamed Up**—Fox 1929—Norman Taurog— Gavin Gordon, Anita Garvin, Estelle Bradley. Three reels.

13. **Hired and Fired**—Fox 1929—Norman Taurog—Helen Bolton, Jack Baston, Ernest Shields, Bertram Johns. Three reels.

14. **Detectives Wanted**—Fox 1929—Norman Taurog—Sally Phipps, Allan Lane, Jane Keckley, Jack Duffy, Ernest Shields, Charles Sullivan, Dick Dickinson, Ray Turner. Three reels.

15. **A Peep on the Deep**—RKO 1930—Mark Sandrich—the team's first RKO short; no cast information available. Two reels.

16. **Chesterfield Celebrities**—Warner Brothers-Vitaphone 1931—A commercial short. One reel.

17. **Such Popularity**—Warner Brothers-Vitaphone 1931—A commercial short for Chesterfield cigarettes. One reel.

18. **False Roomers**—RKO 1931—Mark Sandrich—James Finlayson, Eddie Dunn, Josephine Whittell, Harry Dunkinson, Nora Cecil, Kewpie Morgan. Two reels.

19. **A Melon-Drama**—RKO 1931—Mark Sandrich—James Finlayson, Nora Cecil, Elise Cavanna, Eddie Dunn, Billy Gilbert, Ethan Laidlaw, Gunnis Davis. Two reels.
20. **Scratch as Catch Can**—RKO 1931—Mark Sandrich—James Finlayson, Phil Dunham, Charlotte Ogden, Walter Brennan, Robert Graves, Jr., Constantine Romanoff, Charles Hall, Vincent Barnett. Two reels.
21. **The Iceman's Ball**—RKO 1932—Mark Sandrich—Vernon Dent, Walter Brennan, James Finlayson, Shirley Chambers, Billy Franey, Fred Kelsey. Two reels.
22. **The Millionaire Cat**—RKO 1932—Mark Sandrich—Nora Cecil, Catharine Courtney, James Finlayson, Carol Tevis, Billy Franey, Anita Garvin, Stuart Holmes. Two reels.
23. **Jitters the Butler**—RKO 1932—Mark Sandrich—James Finlayson, Dorothy Granger, Robert Greig, Stuart Holmes, Maude Truax, Phil Dunham, Gerald Barry. Two reels.
24. **Hokus Focus**—RKO 1933—Mark Sandrich—James Finlayson, James Morton, Julie Haydon, Alf James, Max Davidson. Two reels.
25. **The Druggist's Dilemma**—RKO 1933—Mark Sandrich—James Finlayson, Cecil Cunningham. Two reels.
26. **The Gay Nighties**—RKO 1933—Mark Sandrich—James Finlayson, Dorothy Granger, John Sheehan, Monty Collins, Sandra Shaw, Charles Williams. Two reels.
27. **Kickin' the Crown Around**—RKO 1933—Sam White—Ferdinand Munier, Leni Stengel, Francis McDonald, Charles Irwin, Neal Burns, Bynunsky Hyman, Charles Hall, Franc Yaconelli, Frank O'Connor, Billy Franey, Eddie Baker (Edgar Kennedy seen briefly in stock footage at beginning of film). Two reels.
28. **Fits in a Fiddle**—RKO 1933—Sam White—Herman Bing, Barbara Sheldon, Spec O'Donnell, Curley Wright, Tiny Sandford, Jack Rice, Charles Hall. Two reels.
29. **Snug in the Jug**—RKO 1933—Ben Holmes—Harry Gribbon, Anders Van Haden, Russell Powell, Leila Leslie, James Morton, Harry Bowen. Two reels.
30. **Hey Nanny Nanny**—RKO 1934—Ben Holmes—Thelma White, Nat Carr, Sidney Jarvis, Monty Collins. Two reels.
31. **In the Devil's Doghouse**—RKO 1934—Ben Holmes—Dorothy Granger, Tom Kennedy, Bud Jamison, Jack Rice. Two reels.
32. **Bedlam of Beards**—RKO 1934—Ben Holmes—George Hays, Al Hill, Margaret Armstrong, Vivian Fields. Two reels.

33. **Love and Hisses**—RKO 1934—Sam White—Ferdinand Munier, Maude Truax, Monty Collins, Vivien Reid, Sumner Getchel, Sylvia Picker. Two reels.

34. **Odor in the Court**—RKO 1934—Ben Holmes—Tom Kennedy, Helen Collins, Jack Rice, Lorrin Raker, Gus Reed. Two reels.

35. **Everything's Ducky**—RKO 1934—Ben Holmes—Eddie Gribbon, Joyce Compton, Maude Truax, Phil Dunham, Ed Brady, Dennis O'Keefe. Two reels.

36. **In a Pig's Eye**—RKO 1934—Ben Holmes—Monty Collins, Pearl Eaton, Bud Jamison, Richard Lancaster. Two reels.

37. **Flying Down to Zero**—RKO 1935—Lee Marcus—Eddie Gribbon, Monty Collins, Constance Bergen, Bud Jamison. Two reels.

38. **Alibi Bye Bye**—RKO 1935—Ben Holmes—Dorothy Granger, Tom Kennedy, Bud Jamison, Constance Bergen, Doris MacMahon, Harrison Greene, Jack Rice. Two reels.

Clark and McCullough also appeared in a Movietone Newsreel in 1930 with George Gershwin, in which they rehearsed the "Mademoiselle from New Rochelle" number from their Broadway show *Strike Up the Band*.

Bobby Clark also appeared without McCullough in the following film:

> **The Goldwyn Follies**—United Artists 1938—George Marshall—Adolphe Menjou, Zorina, Andrea Leeds, Kenny Baker, Helen Jepson, Phil Baker, Ella Logan, Jerome Cowan, Nydia Westman, Charles Kullman, the American Ballet of the Metropolitan Opera, Edgar Bergen and Charlie McCarthy, the Ritz Brothers. Color—120 minutes.

WHEELER and WOOLSEY

Wheeler and Woolsey are generally forgotten today, but in the late 1920's they scored an overwhelming success on Broadway and went to Hollywood to star in two dozen films, most of which were disliked by the critics but successful at the box office. They ranged from very enjoyable (HIPS HIPS HOORAY, COCKEYED CAVALIERS) to excruciating (ON AGAIN OFF AGAIN), but they deserve at least one more look.

Bert Wheeler, the slight, wavy-haired member of the team, was born Albert Jerome Wheeler in 1895 in Paterson, New Jersey. His first encounter with show business was as a property boy in his home town's stock company. Eventually he worked himself into the on-stage activities, and was spotted by Gus Edwards, who cast him in his famous schoolboy act with a young George Jessel. With his first wife he became a vaudeville headliner; Bert and Betty Wheeler were a top attraction for eleven years. One of their routines was "Charlie Chaplin and a Girl." In 1924 Florenz Ziegfeld signed Wheeler as a star comedian in his *Follies*. The opening night performance lasted five hours, and Alexander Woolcott noted, "The American girl was glorified . . . by a round-faced little comedian named Bert Wheeler, who has come out of vaudeville and who threatened on Saturday night to take the new Follies and, for all the hot rivalry around him, make it his oyster." In his famous routine Wheeler would sit on the edge of the stage, eating, and talk to the audience. He would start to cry, and at one point he would wipe his eyes with his sandwich and eat his handkerchief. Wheeler stayed with Ziegfeld for six years both in the Follies and in the hit show *Rio Rita*, which teamed him with Robert Woolsey. The year was 1928.

Later in his career, Bert Wheeler appeared as a single, and with various straight men (including Paul Douglas) in vaudeville and on the stage. He made two movies on his own. 1939's COWBOY QUARTERBACK was a disguised remake

81

of ELMER THE GREAT, Joe E. Brown's famous baseball comedy by Ring Lardner. In it, Wheeler plays an aspiring football player who tackles potato sacks in Marie Wilson's grocery store for practice. Coach William Demarest spots him and signs him for the Packers team. Bert becomes involved with gangsters but he redeems himself by winning the big game during the last forty seconds. Joe E. Brown fared better with this material. Bert's other film was LAS VEGAS NIGHTS, a 1941 hodgepodge with little plot but lots of music. Wheeler sang "Dolores" with the Tommy Dorsey band while the regular Dorsey vocalist sat by on the bandstand. His name: Frank Sinatra. Throughout the 1940's and 50's Wheeler appeared in scores of Broadway shows and straw-hat productions. On Broadway he starred with Paul and Grace Hartman in *All for Love*, with Frank Fay in *Laugh Time*, and in Fay's role in *Harvey*. He was a regular on the *Brave Eagle* television series in the 1950's as well. In 1963 Wheeler made a comeback on the nightclub trail in Las Vegas and New York. The last years of his life were spent doing club dates in the New York area. In 1966 a theater bearing his name opened on 44th Street in New York. Wheeler was often quoted as saying that his films with Woolsey "were pretty bad, but they all made money." He died on January 18, 1968, of emphysema.

Wheeler and Woolsey in their heyday in Hollywood.

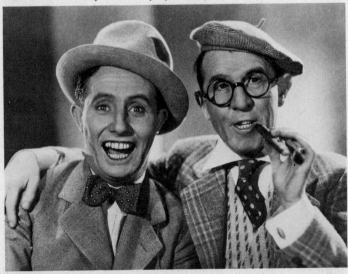

Robert Woolsey, the bespectacled, cigar-chomping member of the team, was born in 1889. At fifteen he became a jockey, but his racing career was curtailed when he was thrown by a horse in 1907. He held a variety of jobs, ending up in a traveling stock company. After gaining valuable experience, he played leads in a Gilbert and Sullivan troupe. From there he went to the Broadway stage, making his debut in 1919. Two years later he scored a hit in *The Right Girl* as star comic. Of this show *The New York Times* wrote, "The life of this party is unquestionably Robert Woolsey, who accomplishes a great deal with a pair of horn-rimmed spectacles and about two jokes." He appeared as Mortimer Pottle with W. C. Fields in *Poppy*, and a few years later joined the *Ziegfeld Follies*. In 1928 Ziegfeld paired him with Bert Wheeler for the show *Rio Rita* and the team of Wheeler and Woolsey was born. In 1936 a press release stated that Woolsey had used 20,000 cigars during his career, which if placed end to end would reach from Chicago to Hollywood. Just why anyone would want to place 20,000 cigars end to end was not made clear, but the article did provide one interesting piece of information. Woolsey had adopted the cigar as a prop because he didn't know what to do with his hands.

In 1929 Radio Pictures (later known as RKO Radio) transformed *Rio Rita* into a lavish musical film, part of it shot in Technicolor. It was to be Radio Pictures' first release, but production was slow and it came out second. For unclear reasons the team was paired with a combination leading lady and straight man, Dorothy Lee, making her second film appearance. Miss Lee, who was born in 1911, came from a nonprofessional family, attended high school in Los Angeles, and after a session at the Los Angeles coaching school went into films. It looked that way. She predated Ruby Keeler by a few years, but the two were evenly matched: her speaking voice was incredibly flat and high-pitched; she could not sing, and her dancing was just fair. However, she possessed a remarkable vitality, the kind associated with the movies' ideal flapper, a few years earlier. She fit into the W & W antics quite well, and indeed, when she left the team, RKO was unable to find a suitable replacement.

RIO RITA was actually Bebe Daniels' and John Boles' film, with Wheeler and Woolsey providing comedy relief. The duo repeated their famous slapping routine from the stage show in one color sequence which exists today as part of the Museum of Modern Art's program of highlights of musical

films of the late 1920's and 1930's. Their second film, THE
CUCKOOS, gave them more chance to display their talents,
although they were still confined to a standard musical-
comedy format. In fact, the film looks exactly like a photo-
graphed stage play, with little imagination in the staging of
musical numbers and comedy sequences. The sketchy plot
involves a wealthy heiress (June Clyde) who is kidnapped by
a nobleman (Ivan Lebedeff) because she refuses to marry
him. W & W are bankrupt fortune tellers who help find her.
Dorothy Lee plays a gypsy girl who becomes involved in the
plot when Bert falls in love with her. He sings one pleasant
song to her, "It's a Wonder You Don't Feel it," and does a
duet with Woolsey, an amusing patter song called "Oh, How
We Love Our Alma Mater." THE CUCKOOS, score intact,
had been a Broadway show with Clark and McCullough
called *The Ramblers*.

Dorothy Lee came to the movies right out of high school, which stands as a
strong argument for higher education. Still, she had great charm.

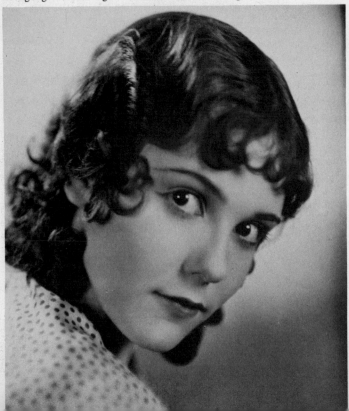

Their third film, DIXIANA, reunited them with Bebe Daniels in a circus story set in old New Orleans, Bebe plays Dixiana, a star performer, and the boys are clearly in support. The conclusion of the film is a Technicolor Mardi Gras sequence featuring Bill "Bojangles" Robinson.

Finally, in 1930, Wheeler and Woolsey were allowed to carry a film by themselves, and they proved capable of succeeding on their own. HALF SHOT AT SUNRISE was not as well-paced as some of their later films, but overall it was quite good. Bert Wheeler liked this one more than some of their later efforts, and was impressed by the fact that RKO built a French village set especially for them. The setting is World War I in France, with W & W as two soldiers wanted by the MP's. One scene, in which the boys disguise as waiters, had some hilarious patter, the kind that was to sustain so many of their films. A customer asks, "Do you have any wild duck?" "No," Woolsey replies, "But if you like we'll bring you a tame one and aggravate him." "I can't eat this duck," the man complains. "Send for the manager." "It's no use," Woolsey assures him. "He won't eat it ei-

A Hollywood-ized Dorothy Lee with Bert Wheeler in a posed still from HIPS HIPS HOORAY.

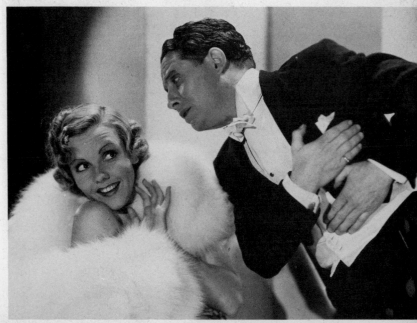

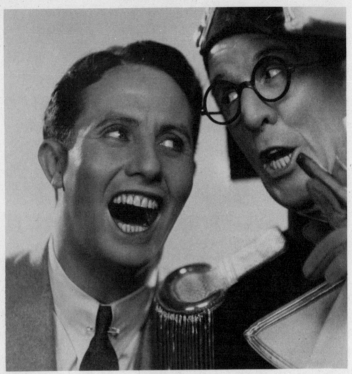

You might say Wheeler and Woolsey had the title roles in CRACKED NUTS.

ther." Dorothy Lee plays the daughter of the boys' colonel, and does one number with them, "Nothing but Love." Near the end of the film are about five minutes of absolutely serious footage, when Bert goes over the top to deliver a message, under fire. Bob worries that he has been gone too long, and goes out after him. It is played straight, and is quite effective. This display of friendship was lacking from their other films, and perhaps accounts for their failure to reach the stature of other comedy teams which depended on human values as a basis for their comedy. Another highlight of the film is a mock ballet with actress Leni Stengel, in the middle of an active sprinkler system. This device was sure-fire, and was repeated in several later films.

HOOK, LINE, AND SINKER is a rapidly paced comedy that stands out as one of their best early efforts. With titles super-imposed over W & W riding a tandem bicycle, it wastes no time in getting to the gags. A cop stops them and says angrily, "You broke the law!" "Well, couldn't you get another one?" Woolsey asks. "I'll give you a ticket," he threatens. "Try to make it up front," Woolsey interrupts. "My partner's eyes aren't so good." Bob then proceeds to sell the cop an insurance policy, proclaiming, "Why, people are dying this year who have never died before!" On the road they meet Dorothy Lee, who is running away from her mother to claim a luxury hotel willed to her by a late relative. The boys decide to go with her to help operate the establishment, but when they arrive they discover an incredibly run-down building inhabited by one very old bellboy (George F. Marion). Searching for a scheme to do something with the hotel, Marion suggests, "It would make a swell fire." Hugh Herbert appears as a mysterious house detective who periodically walks through the lobby and announces, "Ten o'clock and all's well." Through shrewd publicity the hotel becomes a fashionable resort, and the boys become mixed up with gangsters who try to hide stolen goods there. There is a climactic shoot-out during which Bert and Bob exchange some more dialogue: "You know," Bert says, "I'm not as big a fool as I used to be." "Oh?" answers Woolsey, "Did you diet?"

CRACKED NUTS has Bert and Bob vying for the throne of the Kingdom of Eldorania, pitted against corrupt politicians (including Boris Karloff) and military men (including Stanley Fields). Ben Turpin appears in one scene as an aerial bomber, assuring Karloff as the camera takes a close-up of his marvelously crossed eyes that he'll hit his target. Dorothy Lee is Edna May Oliver's niece, brought to Eldorania to escape the wooing of Bert Wheeler, never dreaming that he, too, is headed for Eldorania. One scene includes an ancestor of the Abbott and Costello "Who's on First" routine, as W & W examine a map of the country with the towns of What and Which. After some byplay involving the towns' names, Bert explains, "The town of Which is where General Diddy died." "Diddy?" repeats Woolsey. "Yes, he did," says Bert. "Now we come to the river, but it's impossible to ford the river here." "Why?" "For divers reasons." For musical fans there is also one so-so number, "Dance and Let the World Dance With You."

Following CRACKED NUTS in 1931, the team decided to split and try one solo film each. Woolsey starred in EVERYTHING'S ROSIE, with Anita Louise as Rosie, an orphan adopted by Bob, a circus medicine man. *The New York Times* said that ROSIE was "inflicted" upon a small audience at its premiere, and that it lacked wit, intelligence, and taste. Wheeler did not fare much better with TOO MANY COOKS, based on Frank Craven's play about newlyweds (Bert and Dorothy Lee) trying to build a house, with too much interference from other family members. Bert and Dorothy were scheduled to star in another film, IF I WAS RICH, but plans were cancelled when the team decided to rejoin for another film together. This was CAUGHT PLASTERED, originally titled FULL OF NOTIONS, and it was quite enjoyable. The boys are vaudevillians stranded in a small town who meet a kindly old woman about to lose her failing drugstore. Bert and Bob take over and subdue their scheming landlord (Jason Robards, Sr.), making the drugstore a success. A stream of one-liners and puns makes up much of the script. Talking about their last performance Bert recalls, "The manager said he didn't allow any profanity in his theater." "We didn't use any profanity," Bob replies. "No, but the audience did." Later, in the store, a dowager tries to flirt with Woolsey, and asks him for a racy book. "How about *The Four Horsemen?*" he suggests. Then she tells him that she went to the radio station to have her voice tried. "I bet it was found guilty," he snaps. Woolsey inaugurates his own radio station in the drugstore, but the gag call letters are not explained until the end when Bob signs off from YMI Broadcasting.

Wheeler and Woolsey's 1931 film, PEACH O'RENO, was liked by the critics, for a change, but it is hard to see why this was favored over their other efforts. W & W play Wattles and Swift, cut-rate divorce lawyers in Reno who have their customers take numbers while they wait for consultations. Bert spends much of the film in drag acting as correspondent for a male client's divorce case, and many of the jokes are wildly double entendre. A woman, seeing Bert, comments that she (he) looks like a loose woman. "Don't worry," says Woolsey, "she'll be tight before the evening is over."

Wheeler and Woolsey's next film should have been a smash: it was based on the Broadway hit GIRL CRAZY, with a George and Ira Gershwin score including "I've Got Rhythm," "Embraceable You," and "But Not for Me." Instead, the film was plagued with production problems and emerged a solid mediocrity—with notably inferior renditions of those Gershwin gems. (The one highspot was Bert and Dorothy Lee's rendition of a song written especially for the film, "You've Got What Gets Me.") Perhaps mercifully, the film was kept from circulation for many years because of the 1943 MGM remake with Mickey Rooney and Judy Garland.

The team was back in its element in HOLD 'EM JAIL later that year, despite the absence of Dorothy Lee, who was busy with her married life for the next two W & W films as well. Her replacement in HOLD 'EM JAIL was young Betty Grable, minus most of the personality she later displayed. She played the daughter of Edgar Kennedy, the warden of Bidermore Prison; Edna May Oliver played Edgar's sister. Though prisoners, Woolsey does some fast talking and secures unusual privileges for Bert and himself; they become handymen for Kennedy's family. While cleaning one room, Edna May Oliver is vocalizing (horrendously) at the piano. Woolsey approaches and asks where she learned to sing. "I spent four years in Paris," she replies, adding, "Of course, I'm not a virtuoso." "Not after four years in Paris," comments Woolsey. The climax of the film is a football game, with an abundant supply of sight gags.

Columbia borrowed the team—and gave them a veteran comedy director in Eddie Cline—for an agreeable farce called SO THIS IS AFRICA, about a pair of vaudevillians who are hired for a photographic expedition into the jungle with Mrs. Johnson-Martini. Their second film of 1933 is an unheralded gem called DIPLOMANIACS. Bert and Bob play barbers on an Indian reservation (!) who are sent as emissaries

A production still from SO THIS IS AFRICA with director Eddie Cline giving instructions from the ladder-top.

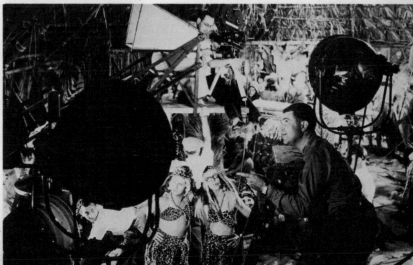

to a Geneva peace conference. Written by a decidedly pre-
ALL ABOUT EVE Joseph L. Mankiewicz and Henry Myers
(who were responsible for the 1932 nonsense classic MILLION
DOLLAR LEGS), it also bears some resemblance to the Marx
Brothers' DUCK SOUP . . . and even features two of its memorable costars, Edgar Kennedy, as the head of the world's
most violent peace conference, and Louis Calhern, as a
villain who breaks into song ("Annie Laurie") without
provocation—or purpose! The film is a heady combination
of satire, slapstick, parody, and puns . . . with an entire song
number in pig-Latin!

1934 was the bumper-crop year for Wheeler and Woolsey.
They appeared in three films which are not only their best,
but remain three excellent examples of comedy of the 1930's.
Much of the credit goes to the two directors responsible for
these films. Mark Sandrich (best known for the Fred Astaire-
Ginger Rogers musicals) and George Stevens; Sandrich directed the first two. HIPS HIPS HOORAY brought back Dorothy
Lee, and for good measure added Thelma Todd as love
interest for Woolsey, and Ruth Etting for a song, "Keep
Romance Alive." RKO spent quite a bit of money on this
production, and allowed Sandrich to stage an elaborate production number with a few dozen chorus girls who wore very
little indeed. HIPS HIPS HOORAY, as well as the other two
1934 films, does not depend on one-line jokes; instead, it

The boys are obviously rooting for Thelma Todd as she argues with Noah
Beery in a scene from COCKEYED CAVALIERS.

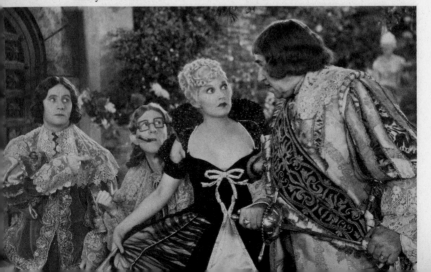

has stronger construction, more music, and some elaborate sight gags. The best scene in the film is another beautiful mock ballet with Bert, Bob, Dorothy and Thelma Todd. The climax of the film is a cross-country race with W & W at the helm of a wild racing car. Last, but not least, this film features the best song to come from a Wheeler and Woolsey film, "Keep on Doing What You're Doing." Don Koll, who knew Bert Wheeler for the last years of his life, recalls that Bert had an amazing faculty for remembering lyrics. When he first met Wheeler, he started singing "Just Keep on Doing What You're Doing." Bert's reaction was "How in the

Betty Grable joins Wheeler and Woolsey in THE NIT WITS.

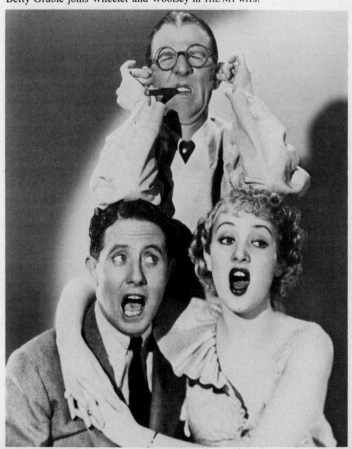

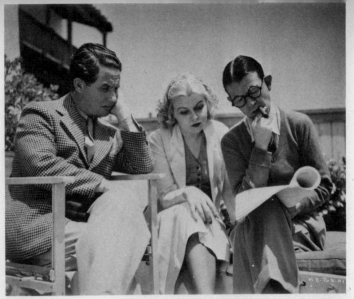

Bert and Bob review the script of MUMMY'S BOYS with costar Barbara Pepper. Bert's expression matched those of most viewers upon seeing the finished product.

hell do you know *that* song?" but he was able to sing the rest of it without forgetting a word.

HIPS HIPS HOORAY was followed by another Sandrich production which in many ways was even better than his first: COCKEYED CAVALIERS, an elaborate period piece. Thelma Todd joined the boys again, as the wife of Baron Noah Beery. The film opens with an operetta motif; Franklin Pangborn, as the town crier, sings the local gossip. Bert and Bob are wandering vagabonds, the former suffering from kleptomania. "Well," advises Woolsey, "take something for it!" "I've already taken everything," Bert answers. They disguise as the king's physicians in order to crash into society, and meet Dorothy Lee, who is disguised as a boy to escape from her impending marriage to Duke Robert Greig. There is one excellent novelty song, "I Went Hunting," performed by W & W in Billy Gilbert's tavern, with Noah Beery joining in on one chorus.

Critic Richard Watts, Jr., hardly a fan of Wheeler and Woolsey, had this to say for the film: "The important news of the new Wheeler and Woolsey comedy is, to this prejudiced observer, that it is fairly funny. It has always seemed to me that the chance for these decidedly minor-league comedians to achieve hilarity lay in the possibility that some day they would become so bad that they would seem almost festive, somewhat in the manner of a fabulously bad pun.

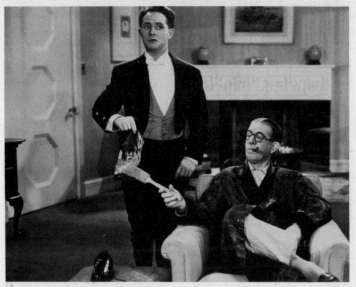

This is one of the funniest scenes from ON AGAIN. OFF AGAIN, which gives you an idea of how funny *that* picture is.

That, I think, is what happened in COCKEYED CAVALIERS. Some of the gay bits of banter are so incredibly awful and the two stars, particularly Mr. Woolsey, strive so grimly to capture the antic quality of almost every comic from Groucho Marx to probably even Milton Berle, that the effect is not without its fascination. In addition, the film possesses a properly insane mood and is aided by the presence of such lively young women as Miss Dorothy Lee and Miss Thelma Todd in the cast. Heaven help me, I thought the new work at the Rialto Theater had its points, some of them intentional."

The last film in this outstanding trio was KENTUCKY KERNELS, one of the early efforts of director George Stevens, who started with Laurel and Hardy and later directed such fine pictures as A PLACE IN THE SUN and SHANE. Stevens had a great comedy sense, and liberal training in the art of *visual* humor, which made this W & W film a success. Much of the credit must also go the film's prime scene stealer, little Spanky McFarland. Even Noah Beery, an actor not remembered for his subtlety, didn't have a chance next to Spanky. The plot has the boys adopting Spanky and traveling down South with him to claim an inheritance. On arrival, they find themselves in the middle of an age-old family feud between Spanky's family (headed by Lucille LaVerne) and Mary Carlisle's kin, led by Noah Beery. There is a hilarious chase climax with W & W being led by a drunken horse, and a battle scene with the boys shooting berries instead of bullets. The film also has a good song. "One Little Kiss," with one chorus sung by everyone in the cast from Woolsey to Noah Beery.

THE NITWITS was George Stevens' second film with W & W, and also Betty Grable's second film with the team; she still did not impress the critics, but the film turned out to be one of W & W's best. In this one Bert and Bob ran a cigar stand in the music publisher's building where Betty works. The publisher is murdered. Betty thinks Bert did it; he thinks *she* did it, so he confesses to save her. Then Bob confesses to try to save Bert. In the end, of course, the real killer is caught. One gimmick of the film is the boy's invention, an electric chair that compels its victim to speak the truth. The film's hilarious chase climax borrows liberally from several "Boy Friends" comedies directed by Stevens when he was with Hal Roach.

The team's winning streak was broken by director Fred Guiol, who made their next three films, three of their lesser efforts. THE RAINMAKERS has them trying to produce rain during a California dry spell, with Berton Churchill and George Meeker as conmen selling phony elixirs to the local farmers. Its only distinction was that it brought Dorothy Lee back as their leading lady, SILLY BILLIES is incredibly slow, and even Miss Lee can't save the proceedings. There is a good climax with Bert and Bob saving their wagon train by shooting cotton balls soaked in ether at the Indians, but it comes too late to salvage the sinking film. Understandably, it was Dorothy Lee's last with the team.

ON AGAIN, OFF AGAIN, released in 1937, could have easily been cut up and used for protection leader, but instead it was released as a feature film. The script, by gagman Nat Perrin and comic Benny Rubin, might have served as a two-reeler, but as a feature it left much to be desired. Even Bert's famous crying routine was condensed to nothing. Marjorie Lord (twenty years before her tenure as Danny Thomas' TV wife) made a stab at leading lady, but she was too deadpan to arouse any excitement. Even though he was ill with kidney disease, Robert Woolsey decided to work on HIGH FLYERS the following year. The film had more going for it than ON AGAIN, OFF AGAIN, but it was still a disappointment. The few highlights of this mystery about the boys unintentionally covering up for a gang of jewel thieves, are Bob's

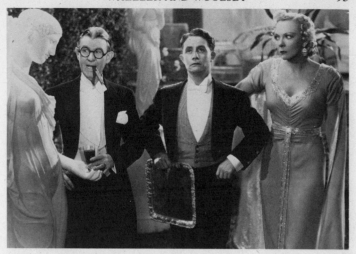

Bert becomes Bob's butler after losing a bet in ON AGAIN, OFF AGAIN. The statuesque blonde at right is Esther Muir, best remembered as the girl wallpapered by the Marx Brothers in A DAY AT THE RACES.

Jack Carson threatens Wheeler and Woolsey in a scene from their final film together, HIGH FLYERS.

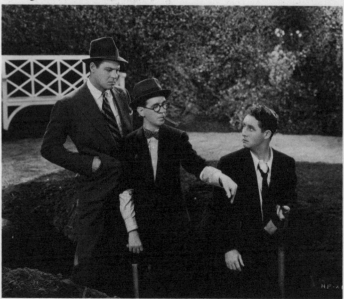

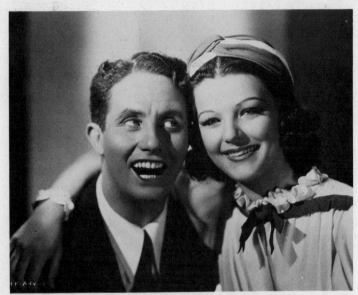

Bert Wheeler's leading lady in HIGH FLYERS is Marjorie Lord, later to gain fame as Danny Thomas' wife in his long running TV series.

dance scene with Lupe Velez, and Bert's imitation of Charlie Chaplin.

Woolsey finished HIGH FLYERS, and was confined to his bed for over a year after its completion. He died of complications from his chronic disease on October 31, 1938; he was forty-nine.

Wheeler and Woolsey were products of vaudeville and the stage, where they spent years perfecting a few special routines until they glistened before appreciative audiences. The transition to Hollywood was not an easy one. Years after their stay there, Bert Wheeler complained that the abrupt change from working before a live, laughing audience to performing for a sullen camera crew proved very disconcerting. In films, their time-worn stage routines were used up immediately, and Wheeler and Woolsey had to put themselves in the hands of Hollywood writers and directors. When provided with first-rate material and guidance, as in such efforts as COCKEYED CAVALIERS, they were more than capable of producing some very entertaining films, which stand as testimony to their talent to this day.

The Films of Wheeler & Woolsey
(Director's name follows year.)

1. **Rio Rita**—RKO 1929—Luther Reed—Bebe Daniels, John Boles, Dorothy Lee, Georges Renevant, Don Alvarado, Sam Nelson, Fred Burns, Sam Blum, Eva Rosita, Nick De Ruiz, Tiny Sandford, Helen Kaiser. 127 minutes; part-color.

2. **The Cuckoos**—RKO 1930—Paul Sloane—June Clyde, Hugh Trevor, Dorothy Lee, Ivan Lebedeff, Marguerita Padula, Mitchell Lewis, Jobyna Howland. 70 minutes; color sequences.

3. **Dixiana**—RKO 1930—Luther Reed—Bebe Daniels, Everett Marshall, Joseph Cawthorn, Jobyna Howland, Dorothy Lee, Ralf Harolde, Edward Chandler, George Herman, Raymond Maurel, Bruce Covington, Bill "Bojanles" Robinson, Eugene Jackson. 98 minutes; color sequence.

4. **Half Shot at Sunrise**—RKO 1930—Paul Sloane— Dorothy Lee, Hugh Trevor, Edna May Oliver, Eddie de Lang, Captain E. H. Calvert, Alan Roscoe, John Rutherford, George MacFarlane, Roberta Robinson, Leni Stengel, the Tiller Sunshine Girls. 79 minutes.

5. **Hook, Line, and Sinker**—RKO 1930—Edward Cline— Dorothy Lee, Natalie Moorhead, Jobyna Howland, Ralf Harolde, William B. Davidson, George Marion, Sr., Hugh Herbert, Stanley Fields. 72 minutes.

6. **Cracked Nuts**—RKO 1931—Edward Cline—Dorothy Lee, Edna May Oliver, Leni Stengel, Stanley Fields, Harvey Clark, Boris Karloff, Ben Turpin, Frank Thornton, Frank Lackteen, Wilfred Lucas, Edward Peil, Sr. (Hugh Herbert receives billing, but does not appear in this film). 78 minutes.

7. **The Stolen Jools**—Paramount/National Screen Service 1931—William McGann—An all-star short to benefit the National Variety Artists, featuring Eddie Kane and in cameo appearances Norma Shearer, Wallace Beery, Buster Keaton, Edward G. Robinson, George E. Stone, Stan Laurel, Oliver Hardy, Our Gang, Polly Moran, Hedda Hopper, Joan Crawford, William Haines, Dorothy Lee, Edmund Lowe, Victor McLaglen, El Brendel, Joyce Compton, Charlie Murray, George Sidney, Winnie

Lightner, Fifi D'Orsay, Warner Baxter, Irene Dunne, Richard Dix, Claudia Dell, Lowell Sherman, Eugene Pallette, Stuart Erwin, Skeets Gallagher, Gary Cooper, Wynne Gibson, Charles "Buddy" Rogers, Maurice Chavalier, Loretta Young, Douglas Fairbanks, Jr., Richard Barthelmess, Louise Fazenda, Charles Butterworth, Bebe Daniels, Ben Lyon, Barbara Stanwyck, Frank Fay, Jack Oakie, Fay Wray, Joe E. Brown, George "Gabby" Hayes, Mitzi Green. Two reels.

8. **Hollywood on Parade**—Episode A-3—1932—no director credited—W & W make a gag appearance in this short along with Tom Mix, Bebe Daniels, Ben Lyon, Roscoe Ates, Anna May Wong, Douglas Fairbanks Jr., Billie Dove, Jimmy Durante, Bromley's Puppets, and m.c. Eddie Kane. One reel.

9. **Caught Plastered**—RKO 1931—William A. Seiter— Dorothy Lee, Lucy Beaumont, Jason Robards, Sr., DeWitt Jennings, Charles Middleton, Bill Scott, Nora Cecil, Josephine Whittell, Arthur Houseman. 68 minutes.

10. **Oh! Oh! Cleopatra**—RKO 1931—A Masquers Club Comedy—Joseph Santley—Dorothy Burgess, Robert Fraser, Tyler Brooke, Tom McGuire, Claude Gillingwater, Mitchell Lewis, Montagu Love, Alec B. Francis, Crawford Kent, Kenneth Thomson, Richard Carlyle, Georgie Harris, Tom Wilson, Eddie Sturgis, William Farnum, Walter Hiers, Hale Hamilton, Edmund Breese, Paul Nicholson, William Arnold, James Finlayson, Max Davidson, Maurice Black, William C. Camp. Two reels.

11. **Peach O'Reno**—RKO 1931—William A. Seiter— Dorothy Lee, Zelma O'Neal, Joseph Cawthorn, Cora Witherspoon, Sam Hardy, Arthur Hoyt, Mitchell Harris, Bill Elliott, Monty Collins. 63 minutes.

12. **Girl Crazy**—RKO 1932—William A. Seiter—Eddie Quillan, Mitzi Green, Kitty Kelly, Arline Judge, Dorothy Lee, Stanley Fields, Brooks Benedict, Lita Chevret, Chris Pin Martin, Monty Collins. 75 minutes.

13. **Hold 'Em Jail**—RKO 1932—Norman Taurog—Betty Grable, Edgar Kennedy, Edna May Oliver, Roscoe Ates, Paul Hurst, Warren Hymer, Robert Armstrong, John Sheehan, G. Pat Collins, Jed Prouty, Spencer Charters, Stanley Blystone, Monty Banks, Leo Willis, Ben Taggart, Lee Phelps, Charles Sullivan, Jim Thorpe, Johny Kelly, Ernie S. Adams, Monty Collins. 74 minutes.

14. **So This is Africa**—Columbia 1933—Edward Cline—

Raquel Torres, Esther Muir, Berton Churchill, Clarence Moorehouse, Henry Armetta. 68 minutes.

15. **Signing 'em Up**—RKO 1934—Leigh Jason—promotional short for the NRA (National Relief Organization) filmed on the RKO lot, starring W & W and featuring such contract players as Bruce Cabot, Pert Kelton, Roscoe Ates, and Dorothy Lee. 4 minutes.

16. **Diplomaniacs**—RKO 1933—William A. Seiter—Marjorie White, Phyllis Barry, Louis Calhern, Hugh Herbert, Edgar Kennedy, Charles Coleman, Richard Carle, Charlie Hall, Dewey Robinson, Neely Edwards, Billy Bletcher, William Irving, Vernon Dent, Constantine Romanoff, Carrie Daumery, Grace Hayle, Artie Ortega, Blackie Whiteford, Harry Schultz, Dick Alexander, John Kelly. 76 minutes.

17. **Hips Hips Hooray**—RKO 1934—Mark Sandrich— Dorothy Lee, Thelma Todd, Ruth Etting, George Meeker, James Burtis, Matt Briggs, Spencer Charters, Dorothy Granger, Stanley Blystone, Marion Byron. 68 minutes.

18. **Cockeyed Cavaliers**—RKO 1934—Mark Sandrich— Thelma Todd, Dorothy Lee, Noah Beery, Franklin Pangborn, Robert Greig, Henry Sedley, Alf P. James, Jack Norton, Snub Pollard, Billy Gilbert, Charlie Hall. 72 minutes.

19. **Kentucky Kernels**—RKO 1934—George Stevens—Mary Carlisle, Spanky McFarland, Noah Beery, Lucille LaVerne, Sleep 'n' Eat (Willie Best), William Pawley, Louis Mason, Frank McGlynn, Jr., Dick Alexander, Paul Page, Margaret Dumont, Dorothy Granger, Harrison Greene, Charlie Hall. 75 minutes.

20. **The Nitwits**—RKO 1935—George Stevens—Betty Grable, Hale Hamilton, Evelyn Brent, Fred Keating, Erik Rhodes, Charles Wilson, Lew Kelly, Arthur Aylesworth, Willie Best, Arthur Treacher, Edgar Dearing. (Although credited, Dorothy Granger was cut from the final release print of this film.) 81 minutes.

21. **The Rainmakers**—RKO 1935—Fred Guiol—Dorothy Lee, Berton Churchill, George Meeker, Frederic Roland, Edgar Dearing. 75 minutes.

22. **Silly Billies**—RKO 1936—Fred Guiol—Dorothy Lee, Harry Woods, Ethan Laidlaw, Chief Thunderbird, Delmar Watson, Richard Alexander, Lafe McKee, Tommy Bond. 64 minutes.

23. **Mummy's Boys**—RKO 1936—Fred Guiol—Barbara Pepper, Moroni Olsen, Frank M. Thomas, Willie Best, Fran-

cis McDonald, Frank Lackteen, Charles Coleman, Mitchell Lewis, Frederick Burton, Tiny Sandford, Dewey Robinson. 68 minutes.

24. **On Again, Off Again**—RKO 1937—Edward Cline— Marjorie Lord, Patricia Wilder, Esther Muir, Paul Harvey, Russell Hicks, George Meeker, Maxine Jennings, Kitty McHugh, Hal K. Dawson, Alec Hartford, Pat Flaherty, Jane Walsh, Alan Bruce. 68 minutes.

25. **High Flyers**—RKO 1937—Edward Cline—Lupe Velez, Marjorie Lord, Margaret Dumont, Jack Carson, Paul Harvey, Charles Judels, Lucien Prival, Herbert Evans, Herbert Clifton, George Irving, Bud Geary, Bruce Sidney. 70 minutes.

Bert Wheeler appeared without Woolsey in the following films:

1. **Small Timers**—Warner Brothers-Vitaphone 1929—one of the "Vitaphone Acts" series, a sketch about a theatrical hotel, with Bernice Speer and Al Clair. One reel.

2. **The Voice of Hollywood**—Tiffany—Bert hosted reel #13 in the 1929 series, with Ken Maynard, and reel #9 in the 1930 series. One reel each.

3. **Too Many Cooks**—RKO 1931—William S. Seiter— Dorothy Lee, Sharon Lynne, Roscoe Ates, Robert McWade, Hallam Cooley, Florence Roberts, Clifford Dempsey, George Chandler. 77 minutes.

4. **Hollywood Handicap**—Universal 1932—Charles Lamont—A Thalians comedy with many cameo appearances; James Burke, Vernon Dent, Monty Collins, Jack Duffy, Anita Garvin, Marion Byron, Dickie Moore, Ivan Lebedeff. Two reels.

5. **A Night at the Biltmore Bowl**—RKO 1935—A chronicle on Hollywood nightlife with Bert and such other RKO contractees as Betty Grable, Joy Hodges, Edgar Kennedy, Lucille Ball, Grady Sutton, Anne Shirley, Preston Foster, Dennis O'Keefe; with the Jimmy Grier Orchestra. Two reels.

6. **Sunday Night at the Trocadero**—MGM 1937—George Sidney—Reginald Denny, George Hamilton's Music Box Music, Louis and Celeste, Medina and Mimosa, (Peter) Lind Hayes, Gaylord Carter, Connee Boswell, and guest stars Arthur Lake, Dick Foran, John Howard, Margaret Vail, Chester Morris, Sally Blane, Norman Foster, Robert Benchley, Mr. and Mrs. Groucho Marx, Frank Mor-

gan, Eric Blore, Toby Wing, Stuart Erwin, June Collyer, Russell Gleason, Glenda Farrell, Frank McHugh, Benny Rubin. Two reels.

7. **Cowboy Quarterback**—Warner Brothers 1939—Noel Smith—Marie Wilson, Gloria Dickson, DeWolf Hopper, William Demarest, Eddie Foy, Jr., William Gould, Charles Wilson, Frederick Tozere, John Harrison, John Ridgely, Eddie Acuff, Clem Bevans, Sol Gross, Don Turner. 56 minutes.

8. **Las Vegas Nights**—Paramount 1941—Ralph Murphy— Phil Regan, Constance Moore, Virginia Dale, Lillian Cornell, Hank Ladd, Betty Brewer, Frank Sinatra, Tommy Dorsey and Orchestra. 89 minutes.

9. **Innocently Guilty**—Columbia 1950—two-reeler starring Bert with Christine McIntyre, Vernon Dent. Remake of Andy Clyde's *It Always Happens*.

10. **The Awful Sleuth**—Columbia 1951—Richard Quine— Christine McIntyre, Minerva Urecal, Tom Kennedy. Remake of Charley Chase's *The Big Squirt*. Two reels.

Robert Woolsey appeared without Wheeler in the following films:

1. **The Voice of Hollywood**—Tiffany 1930—Woolsey hosted entry #10 in this series. One reel.

2. **Everything's Rosie**—RKO 1931—Clyde Bruckman— Anita Louise, John Darrow, Florence Roberts, Frank Beal, Alfred P. James, Lita Chevret, Clifford Dempsey. 67 minutes.

3. **Hollywood on Parade**—B-7—Paramount 1933—Off-screen moments of the stars, with Johnny Mack Brown, Willy Pogany, Harry Green, Bebe Daniels, Mary Pickford, John Boles, Buster Collier, and the 1932 Wampas Baby Stars (Ruth Hall, Patricia Ellis, Lillian Bond, Boots Mallory, Evalyn Knapp, Dorothy Layton, Dorothy Wilson, Mary Carlisle, Marion Shockley, Toshia Mori, Gloria Stuart, Eleanor Holm, Ginger Rogers, Lona Andre). One reel.

THE MARX BROTHERS

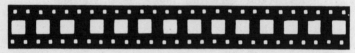

There will never be anyone to compare with the Marx Brothers. Other comedians used satire, and most comics today poke fun at certain sacred cows. But only the Marx Brothers made fun of absolutely everything; that is why they are still popular today, as funny and pungent as ever. The crime is that the Marxes weren't allowed to function at full steam in more than a handful of pictures. Their first film forced them to share the running time with several musical and romantic subplots; then it seemed as if they were going to be given carte blanche to work on their own. When they came to MGM in 1935 the subplots returned, until the brothers were inundated by them, and the scripts became insipid. "Come-back" films were made, but they failed to capture the old flair and spirit. By this time the brothers had achieved success in other areas and weren't concerned with maintaining their status as movie stars. Thus, in less than two decades, Hollywood suppressed one of the most brilliant comedy teams of all times.

Marx Brothers movies are the world's greatest cure for modern-day hangups; we all get vicarious pleasure from watching the brothers get away with things we'd love to do ourselves. Harpo chasing after various blondes, Chico swindling supposed con man Groucho, Groucho insulting everyone in sight, all provide us with untold satisfaction. Even their musical interludes—often the most serious moments in their films—are fun, because Harpo, and especially Chico, seem to be enjoying their instruments so much.

Groucho's steady flow of dialogue included the greatest collection of puns and nonsense patter ever recorded on film. Chico's conversations with Groucho reveal the logic that can be found in illogical thinking—one absurdity leads to another. (In NIGHT AT THE OPERA Groucho tells Chico to sign his name to a contract; "I can't write," Chico confesses. "That's all right," says Groucho, "there's no ink in the pen

anyway.") Harpo's mind, with one of the outstanding imagi-
nations of all time, conceives the kind of eye-popping gags
one expects to see in cartoons, but never on film. (A moment in HORSEFEATHERS comes to mind when Harpo is watching two sharpsters play poker in a dingy speakeasy. The
deck is in the center of the table, and one fellow tells the
other to cut the cards. From under his jacket Harpo produces an ax and quickly chops the entire table in half.)
Zeppo, the amiable but hopelessly lost fourth brother, will
not be analyzed. Let us say at the outset that Zeppo, who
reputedly possessed a natural wit that rivaled Groucho's,
was merely a victim of circumstance in being the "straight"
member of the team. He had no chance working against the
combined lunacy of his brothers, and wisely decided to leave
the act after DUCK SOUP. We hereby acknowledge his presence in the team's early films, and leave it at that.

The Marx Brothers never could have been created or
invented. They simply had to *be*. Over years of touring in
vaudeville and the theater, the brothers grew and developed
their respective personalities. They were a close-knit family,
and for the rapport which they developed, the world can pay
belated thanks to that valiant woman, Minnie Marx, who
gave birth to Julius, Adolph, Leonard, Milton and Herbert,
and stood by them as they developed into Groucho, Harpo,
Chico, Gummo and Zeppo. She was determined to see her
boys successful in show business, and helped them every
step of the way until they were. Chico (Leonard) was the
eldest son, born in 1891: Harpo (Adolph, later known as
Arthur) followed in 1893: Groucho (Julius) in 1895; and
Zeppo (Herbert) in 1901. Gummo (Milton) was with the act
during its vaudeville days, but left when the Marx Brothers
invaded Broadway; he was the family's youngest son.

In vaudeville the brothers, along with assorted outsiders
and various members of the family, tried out a wide variety
of acts. As with most of the successful entertainers who
came out of vaudeville, their final polished routines and
established methods came out of constant trial and error.
Music was always a part of the proceedings, with comedy
added later. The brothers received encouragement and advice from their uncle, Al Shean, who himself was part of the
early 20th-century's most popular American duo, Gallagher
and Shean ("Absolutely, Mr. Gallagher?" "Positively, Mr.
Shean"). The road to success in those days was a slow one,
however, even for good acts. The brothers started performing around 1908, but they received little recognition until the

mid-1920's. The turning point was in 1924 with a show called
I'll Say She Is! which exposed them and their brand of
nonsense to Broadway for the first time. The results were
excellent, and the Marxes finally reached the top; their
reputation was enhanced by a second, more resounding hit,
The Cocoanuts, and then a third, *Animal Crackers*. By the
late 1920's the Marx Brothers were the darling of Broadway,
thanks to such staunch supporters as Alexander Woollcott
and his Algonquin Hotel crowd, which also adopted Harpo
as a member in good standing.

In 1929, while playing in the long-running *Animal Crackers*
on Broadway, the brothers were hired to film their stage hit
Cocoanuts for Paramount Pictures. This was not the team's
first encounter with movies, however. In 1925, Harpo appeared briefly in a Richard Dix film called TOO MANY KISSES.
During the COCOANUTS shooting at Paramount's studios in
Astoria, New York, Harpo told an interviewer about his
film debut (which was also filmed in Astoria) and claimed
that his part was so abbreviated in the final version of the
film that at the premiere, he bent down to pick up his hat
and missed his own movie debut! At the risk of debunking a
cute story, it must now be reported that TOO MANY KISSES
has been found and preserved (by the American Film Insti-
tute) and reveals Harpo in a surprisingly *visible*—if not completely comprehensible—role, in this entertaining yarn that
finds all-American hero Dix in a sleepy Spanish village.
Harpo is an incidental character who pops in and out of
several scenes, sporting his wig and familiar puckish grin
and, in one scene, "strumming" on the rungs of a ladder. He
received screen billing as "The Village Pan." The following
year, the brothers helped finance and star in a short called
HUMORISK, which was never released; finding details on this
obscure venture is virtually impossible. All Groucho had to
say about it was, "It was never finished and it wasn't very
good. Luckily there are no copies available."

In 1929, the Four Marx Brothers finally burst onto the
screen. The Paramount Astoria studio had been used since
the early days of silent movies, but with the advent of talkies
it became a haven for Broadway stars who wanted to appear
in films without leaving the stage. Most of them commuted
to Astoria every morning, put in a full day's work before the
cameras, then returned to New York that evening to perform on the stage. Thus, the Paramount studio served a very
useful purpose through the early 1930's; its chief fault was

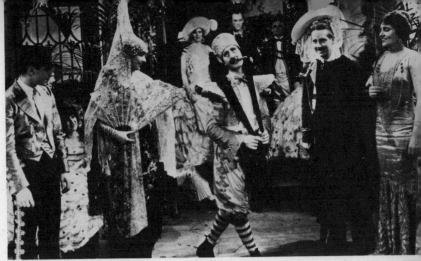

Groucho is the center of attention in this scene from THE COCOANUTS. Zeppo, Kay Francis, Cyril Ring, and Margaret Dumont look on.

that it required all the films shot there to use indoor settings almost exclusively.

The Marx Brothers are very funny in COCOANUTS; some of the routines are among their funniest. But the film bears the indelible mark of the Astoria studio: staginess. Two directors were employed on the film, Robert Florey and Joseph Santley. The latter's career was undistinguished, but it is difficult to understand the film's static quality under the guidance of Florey, who was a very competent and visually oriented director. It has been speculated that he really didn't understand or appreciate the Marxes; Florey himself has explained that it was impossible to work with them because they could not stand still for five minutes. Whatever the reasons, COCOANUTS' success as a film is due entirely to Groucho, Harpo, Chico and Zeppo, and not to the musical co-stars or apparently helpless directors. The plot is too complicated to explain in a few words, but basically Groucho (as Mr. Hammer) is a hotel proprietor in Florida who took advantage of the land boom months back, but now faces bankruptcy. His only hope is the wealthy Mrs. Potter, his sole paying guest, played by the indomitable Margaret Dumont. As in most of their films, Groucho tries to win her over with his peculiar brand of lovemaking ("I'll meet you tonight under the moon. Oh, I can see you now. You and the moon . . . You wear a necktie so I'll know you.")

Groucho's other prospect for money making in COCOANUTS is an auction of some property he owns. He corners one of his nonpaying guests, Chico, to help him rig the auction, and engages in one of the best verbal exchanges ever dreamed up for the two. It starts innocently enough as Groucho is giving Chico directions to reach the auction site and tells him he must go by a viaduct. "Why a duck?" asks Chico, and the ball starts rolling. Groucho finally settles things with Chico, who is to start the bidding and keep it going. When the auction is held later that day, Chico not only keeps it going, but outbids everyone else and ruins Groucho's perfectly planned scheme. As auctioneer, Groucho becomes desperate. "What am I offered for lot twenty-five?" No answer is heard. "What am I offered for lot twenty-five and a year's subscription to *Youth Companion?*" Then, "Will somebody take a year's subscription? I'm trying to work my way through college." When this fails, he offers, "Will somebody take a six months' subscription? I'll go to high school." With no bids, he volunteers, "Does anybody want to buy a lead pencil?" With this final rebuff, Groucho announces, "I'll wrestle anybody in the crowd for five dollars!" Another scene in the film comes close to a wrestling match, with slinky villainess Kay Francis inviting Harpo to her room, hoping to use him as a fall guy in her robbery scheme, but finding instead a constant flow of Marx Brothers in and out of her room and the one adjoining it. This double-room mayhem predated a similar scene with detective Robert Emmet O'Connor in A NIGHT AT THE OPERA.

COCOANUTS is full of funny scenes, but its most distressing one is the last, where after all the film's conflicts and plots are neatly tied up, the Marxes are shown waving inanely at the camera, after which the two young lovers get the final close-up of the film. Wrote Allen Eyles, "One feels they ought to have advanced and split the screen wide open, or thrown cocoanuts at Bob and Polly as they throw apples at Margaret Dumont in DUCK SOUP." This is something the studios, both Paramount and MGM, could never understand about the Marx Brothers. By making them conform to the framework of a sickly romantic plot, they negated the whole Marx appeal—the idea that *nothing* was sacred, certainly not a silly boy-meets-girl story line. The fault does not lie entirely with the film companies, of course. This was the convention of the day in stage musicals. But the fact remains that scenes like the final one of COCOANUTS (and the closing shot in DAY AT THE RACES) seriously mar the total effect of the film.

COCOANUTS was made while the brothers were performing *Animal Crackers* on Broadway. In 1930, they journeyed

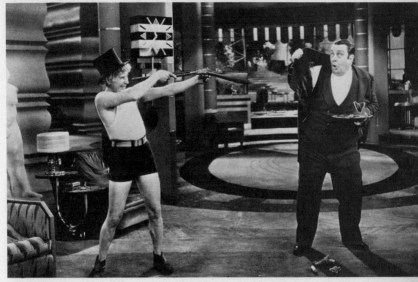

Harpo takes aim, in a manner of speaking, at butler Robert Greig in ANIMAL CRACKERS.

Chico doesn't want to be interrupted when he's performing, as indicated in this scene from ANIMAL CRACKERS.

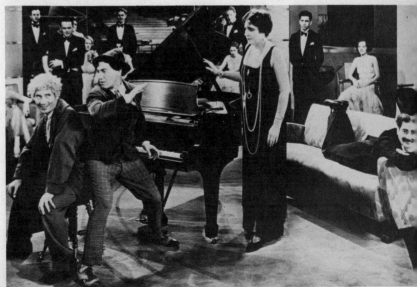

back to Astoria to put this second show on film. The resulting film has its faults, but in general, ANIMAL CRACKERS is
one of the team's best comedies. One of its many distinctions is that it gives Zeppo a better break than any other
Marx film; he is the one who introduces the immortal song
"Hooray for Captain Spaulding," and later he shares a hilarious scene with Groucho as the latter dictates a letter to the
law office of Hungerdunger, Hungerdunger, Hungerdunger
and McCormack. "Captain Spaulding" is Groucho's most
famous number; it subsequently became his theme song on
radio and TV. Following the song, later in the film, is a fine
patter routine about the Captain's journey ("After fifteen
days on water, and six on the boat . . ."). In fact, that is
ANIMAL CRACKERS' strongpoint: an abundance of first-rate
dialogue. One of the best scenes has Chico playing a monot-
onous series of chords on the piano. "Say, if you get near a
song, play it," says Groucho. Caught up in the routine of the
song, Chico says, "I can't think of the finish." "Funny, I
can't think of anything *but*," replies Groucho.

A dated but ingenious gimmick has Groucho satirizing the
then-popular O'Neill play *Strange Interlude* with periodic

The captain has arrived—which is the guests' cue to sing "Hooray for Captain
Spaulding" and Groucho's cue to reply, "Hello, I must be going" in ANIMAL
CRACKERS.

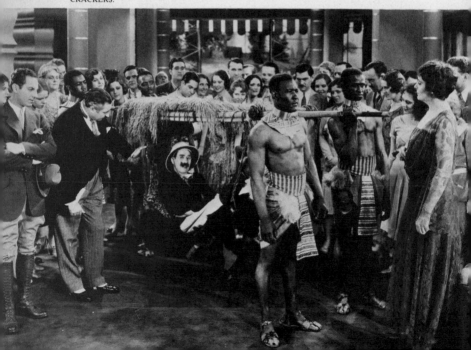

nonsense asides. They start when Groucho tells another character. "If I were Eugene O'Neill I'd tell you what I really think of you. You're lucky the Theatre Guild isn't putting this on." Then, after a moment he adds, "And so is the Guild." Harpo shines in a deliciously crooked bridge game which he plays with Chico, Margaret Dumont and Margaret Irving. He is told to sit wherever he wants, so he hops onto Miss Irving's lap. When it is his turn to deal, he licks one thumb, and deals with the other hand. He chooses the good cards for himself and Chico, holding them up for Chico's approval, then tossing the other cards to the unsuspecting ladies. The ladies begin to suspect some dirty work when Harpo keeps producing the ace of spades. "He's got a thousand of them," Chico says with a laugh.

After ANIMAL CRACKERS, the brothers decided to abandon Broadway for Hollywood, where they appeared in their first film written especially for the screen, MONKEY BUSINESS. While it could hardly be called a classic, it moves swiftly and allows the brothers to engage in some memorable routines. The film's best, and most famous, scene has the four stowaways—Groucho, Harpo, Chico and Zeppo—trying to go through ship's customs using Maurice Chevalier's passport. Each brother wears a straw hat and sings "You Brought a New Kind of Love to Me" to prove his identity: one by one they are tossed aside. Then Harpo strolls along, flashes his Chevalier passport, and begins to sing in the Frenchman's voice (he's got a record player tied to his back). The scheme is exposed when the record slows down and he has to rewind the turntable. MONKEY BUSINESS also includes Groucho's first encounter with lovely Thelma Todd, as the girl friend of a gangster on board their ship. Groucho hides in her closet, dances the tango with her, and eventually tries to make love to her, all in vain. And, as usual, Groucho and Chico have their running conversations, the longest one involving a discourse on Columbus. Groucho tries to show Chico where Columbus sailed, and draws a circle on the globe. "Oh, Columbus Circle," Chico says triumphantly. MONKEY BUSINESS loses steam after the brothers leave their ship and go to a Long Island estate where the plot thickens, so to speak. The climactic fight in a barn near the estate isn't quite as hilarious as it should be, with Zeppo doing most of the work and the other brothers providing the laughs.

Their next film, HORSE FEATHERS, rates as one of the team's best, with ample doses of all four brothers, fine dialogue, and imaginative sight gags. It opens as Groucho

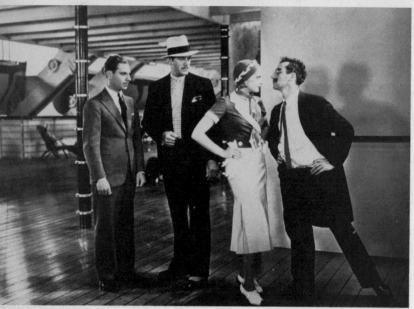

Groucho makes an advance toward Thelma Todd as her boyfriend, Harry Woods, watches uneasily. Zeppo is noncommittal. A scene from MONKEY BUSINESS.

Chico and Harpo try to impress their boss, Rockcliffe Fellows, in the party scene from MONKEY BUSINESS. Groucho doesn't believe them; Zeppo is noncommittal. Leo Willis is seen again over Fellows' shoulder.

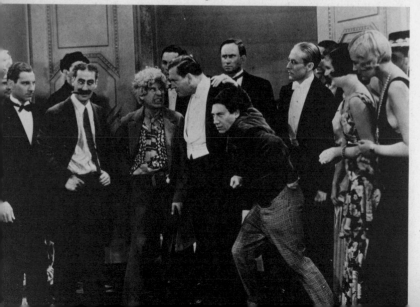

(Professor Quincey Adams Wagstaff) assumes the presidency
of Huxley College, singing a tune that sums up his feelings
about everything, "I'm Against It," accompanied by a panel
of distinguished colleagues. From that point the film goes in
several directions: Zeppo is in love with the "college widow,"
Thelma Todd; Harpo and Chico spend most of their time at
a speakeasy; and Groucho decides that he must build up his
football team to score a victory over their rival, Darwin
College. He arranges to talk to two young athletes at the
same bar frequented by Harpo and Chico, and mistakes them
for the men he is supposed to meet. The speakeasy sequence
is one of the film's best, with Harpo strolling from one end
to the other as he pulls all sorts of odd tricks (the aforementioned cutting of cards, using a pay telephone as a slot
machine, etc.). He and Chico go through several exasperating
minutes involving the club password, "swordfish." Later,
Harpo and Chico venture into a biology class at Huxley
where Groucho decides to lecture on the human body. When
he sees that Harpo's only interest is in the female body he
counsels the student, "My boy, as you grow older, you'll

An apple for the teacher. Professor Robert Greig looks unimpressed, a scene
from HORSE FEATHERS.

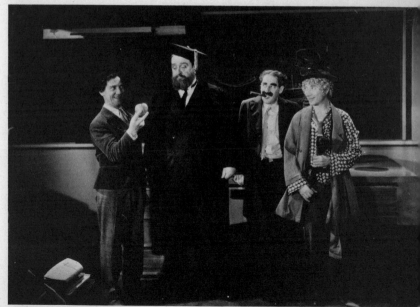

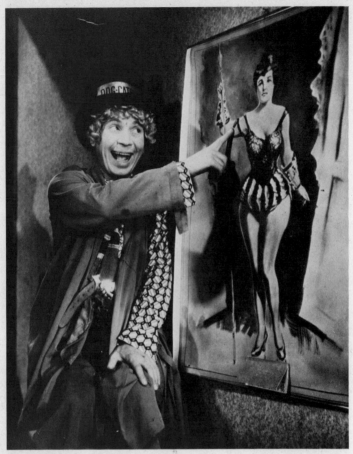

A stirring moment from HORSE FEATHERS.

find you can't burn the candle at both ends." At this, Harpo reaches into his cavernous pocket and produces a candle, burning of course at both ends. Groucho watches for a minute and comments, "Well, I knew there was *something* you couldn't burn at both ends!"

Later there is a lightning-paced scene in Thelma Todd's apartment. Scenes like this seem to have been choreographed, rather than directed, with Chico, Harpo and Groucho running in and out at odd moments, each anxious to cuddle up with the beautiful blonde (for a while, Harpo only runs through to deliver a cumbersome piece of ice). In this same scene, Harpo and Chico sit down at their respective instruments to go into a serious musical interlude. Groucho walks all the way up to the camera and tells the audience, "Listen, I have to stay here, but why don't you folks go out to the lobby for a smoke until this thing blows over?" This is one of the best-remembered gags from any Marx Brothers picture—indeed, Bob Hope and Bing Crosby remembered it twenty years later when, in ROAD TO BALI, Hope turned to the audience and commented, "He's going to sing, folks; now's the time to go and get your popcorn." Another classic gag comes in HORSE FEATHERS when Groucho takes Thelma out for a ride on a secluded lake. She tries to make love to him, but winds up toppling out of the rowboat into the water. "Throw me a life saver," she screams; Groucho obliges by taking out a pack of the candy and tossing her one. The film's climax is a wild football scene with all four brothers joining forces for Huxley, and engaging in the most ingenious forms of cheating ever imagined. Football is one of the many comedy staples, used at one time or another by most comedians (Wheeler and Woolsey and the Ritz Brothers both used gridiron games as highlights of films), but few others succeeded in making such a shambles of the game as did the Marx Brothers.

Many consider DUCK SOUP (1933) the Marx Brothers' most nearly perfect film; it is a comedy classic by any standards. One reason for the film's success is that it is better constructed than most Marx efforts, which jump from comedy scene to musical number to romantic interlude with no rhyme or reason. DUCK SOUP has continuity, although it is just as frantic as any of the team's other films. Groucho stars as Rufus T. Firefly, who becomes the president of Freedonia when the country's principal financial backer, Mrs. Teasdale (Margaret Dumont), insists on the move. The rest of the film involves Mrs. Teasdale's herculean efforts to keep Firefly from getting their country into war with neighboring Sylvania. This proves impossible, for Groucho has an overwhelming distaste for the Sylvanian representative, Ambassador Trentino (Louis Calhern). Groucho's instincts are right on target, of course: Trentino is actually a conniving opportunist trying to win over Mrs. Teasdale and gain control of Freedonia. Harpo and Chico enter the proceedings as private detectives hired by Trentino to get the goods on Firefly. Zeppo, as usual, has little to do, his main scene being the opening one where he introduces President Firefly to a throng of loyal Freedonians.

The film is pure Marx Brothers, with no time wasted on

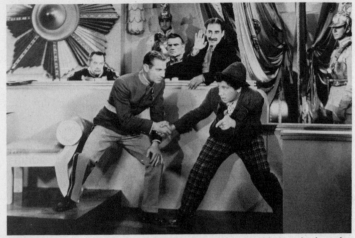

Chicolini on trial in DUCK SOUP—though Chico looks as if he's poised to play the piano.

superfluous trivialities like young lovers. The musical numbers are part of the plot (Groucho warns Freedonians about his reign as president with a song called "Just Wait Till I Get Through With It"), and the action moves at a brisk pace. Credit for this goes to DUCK SOUP'S director, Leo McCarey, who received his comedy training at the Hal Roach studios in the 1920's, where he collaborated with comedian Charley Chase on some classic two-reelers, and later worked with Laurel and Hardy. McCarey's heart was still in sight-gag comedy when he did DUCK SOUP, and he provided the brothers with their all-time best visual sequences, while the four scenarists (Bert Kalmar, Harry Ruby, Arthur Sheekman, Nat Perrin) counterbalanced them with first-rate dialogue. It is safe to assume that McCarey was also responsible for casting Edgar Kennedy in DUCK SOUP, as the lemonade vendor who engages in a running battle of wits with Harpo. The height of the feud comes when Harpo rolls up his pants and, while Kennedy isn't looking, wades into his vat of lemonade, immediately dispersing a crowd of customers. The conclusion comes later in the film when Harpo comes to see an attractive young girl in her apartment. Kennedy is seen walking upstairs and it becomes apparent that the girl is his wife. She shoos Harpo out of the living room and into the bathroom. Kennedy arrives home in a grouchy mood, and goes immediately to take a bath. Settled in the tub, he hears the sudden honk of a horn. He does a take, settles down again, and hears the sound once more. Suddenly, Harpo emerges from the other end of the tub, blowing a cavalry charge, and runs out the door.

DUCK SOUP's memorable moments are too numerous to detail here, but the mirror sequence and the announcement of war are probably the film's true highlights. The mirror idea was hardly new in 1933 (two people thinking they are looking into a mirror when they are actually looking at each other) and had been used several times, notably in Charlie Chaplin's THE FLOORWALKER (1917). But, as usual, the Marxes outdid the original gag many times over, first by adding many inventive touches to the initial scene (Harpo and Chico are both disguised as Groucho, and try to "expose" each other by doing various unexpected movements) and then having the real Groucho show up and make the group a threesome! The war sequence takes place during the trial of Chico, when Groucho goes one step too far with Ambassador Trentino and war is declared. The entire assembly—the four brothers, the guards, the court officials and scores of

Harpo and Edgar Kennedy engage in a battle of wits in DUCK SOUP.

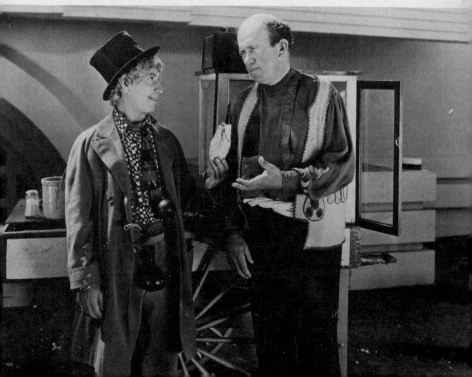

spectators—all join in a musical hosanna to the country's entry into war. The number is lavishly staged, and the lyrics are appropriately ridiculous.

One reason DUCK SOUP is admired over and above the other Marx Brothers films is that it is one of the few successful political travesties ever filmed. But in 1933 it was not appreciated. Audiences and critics liked the brothers better when they were merely being ridiculous, poking fun at stuffed shirts and letting loose a healthy barrage of puns and sight gags. They did not crave political satire, and the mood of the country in 1933 was too somber to take it in stride. Thus, DUCK SOUP was neither a critical nor a financial success at the time of its release, and it lost the Marx Brothers their berth at Paramount Pictures.

The brothers were rescued, a year later, by Irving Thalberg, the "boy wonder" of MGM whose productions were typified by one word: class. Thalberg was a showman, but he had great integrity; this was backed up by the MGM production team that guaranteed the most stylish finished products in Hollywood. Thalberg was responsible for giving the Marx Brothers the film that turned out to be their biggest success, and in this writer's opinion, their best film, A NIGHT AT THE OPERA. Thalberg wanted to retain the brothers' basic comic style, but at the same time he was determined to give them pace and production to back it up. A NIGHT AT THE OPERA was the happy medium for both the brothers and Thalberg,

Unemployment faces the Marx Brothers and Allan Jones in this scene from A NIGHT AT THE OPERA.

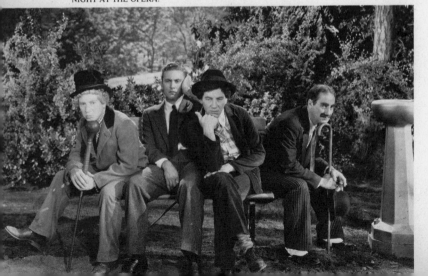

for it included comedy sequences that were among the Marxes' best, and at the same time featured a romantic, musical subplot tied to co-stars Allan Jones and Kitty Carlisle. The latter aspect of the film was not intrusive because it was woven so well into the brothers' antics. It worked as an asset instead of a liability, because the players were sincere, and the music they were given to perform was first-rate.

The film wastes no time in getting down to business; even DUCK SOUP takes several minutes before the Marxes are introduced. A NIGHT AT THE OPERA gets moving immediately, with Margaret Dumont complaining that she has been waiting several hours for Groucho to meet her for dinner, then discovering that he has been sitting behind her (with a young blonde) all evening. The lines come fast and furious as Groucho asks a waiter if he has any milk-fed chicken. When the answer is yes, Groucho snaps, "Well, squeeze one and bring me a glass." He finally sits down with his perennial vis-a-vis, here portraying a "Mrs. Claypool" who is anxious to sponsor an opera company. Groucho introduces her to Hermann Gottlieb, the head of the New York Opera Company, who tries to woo Mrs. Claypool to invest in his company, and launch his protégé, Rodolfo Lasparri. Gottlieb is played by Sigfried (later known as Sig) Rumann, who specialized in playing Viennese doctors for thirty years in Hollywood. His protégé Lasparri (Walter Woolf King) is a vain young man who beats his valet (Harpo) and tries unsuccess-

Allan Jones and Chico backstage at A NIGHT AT THE OPERA.

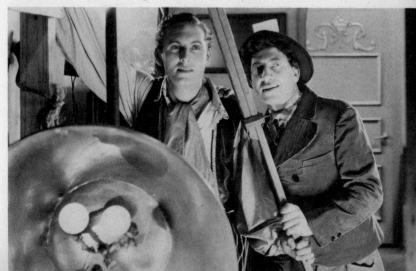

fully to woo another member of the troupe, Kitty Carlisle. She prefers down-to-earth chorus-boy Allan Jones.

A NIGHT AT THE OPERA is the most coherent of all the Marx Brothers films; everything ties together as Groucho tries to outwit Gottlieb by signing his protégé to an exclusive contract, but instead signing Allan Jones after a classic encounter with Jones' "manager," Chico. The two try to work out an agreeable contract that bogs down when Chico objects to the opening phrase, "The party of the first part shall be referred to in this contract as the party of the first part." Before their argument is over, the contracts are just tiny slips of paper and the agreement is settled by a handshake. The entire troupe sails for New York, but Groucho is distressed to find that he has been given a cabin the approximate size of a broom closet. Things get worse when he opens his trunk and finds Harpo, Chico and Allan Jones inside, all stowaways who plan to share the cabin with Groucho on the way over. This leads into the brothers' most famous sequence of all time, the stateroom scene, in which two maids, two repairmen, a girl looking for her aunt, a manicurist, a washerwoman and four waiters all crowd into the impossibly small enclosure. Margaret Dumont arrives for an appointment with Groucho, opens the door, and the inhabitants billow out.

Midway through the incomparable stateroom scene in A NIGHT AT THE OPERA.

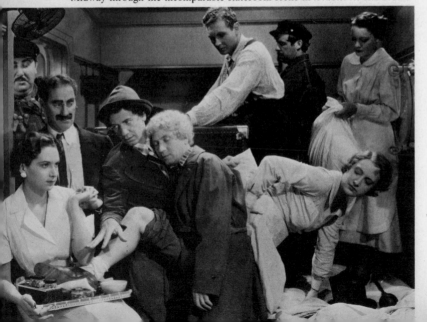

The musical scenes flow along with the picture, as in the sequence that takes place in the ship's steerage section. The stowaways (Harpo, Chico, Allan Jones) have decided to take their chances by sneaking out of the cabin and into this part of the boat, where they help themselves to food served by the happy immigrants on board. After dinner, Jones starts to sing "Cosi, Cosa" and the people around him join in for a lively, entertaining production number. After this, Chico sits down at the piano and plays "All I Do Is Dream of You" with his typical pistol-shooting-finger technique, much to the delight of the children around him. The kids also have fun watching Harpo try his luck at the piano, before moving over to the harp, where he turns serious for a rendition of "Alone." Because of their indiscretion, however, the stowaways are caught, and the plot takes off from there.

Thalberg's idea paid off, for A NIGHT AT THE OPERA was the Marx Brothers' most resounding success to date, both critically and at the box office. From what had been termed a "slump" only a year before, they shot back to become top money-making stars in Hollywood. Then came A DAY AT THE RACES. It looked like a sure bet, reteaming the Marx Brothers with their OPERA director Sam Wood, and three of the film's principal players: Allan Jones, Sig Rumann and, of course, Margaret Dumont. The same testing procedure was used to perfect the film's script, sending the cast on tour to various parts of the country, playing the scenario live on stage and eliminating material that did not go over with the various audiences. All signs pointed to success for A DAY AT THE RACES. Then, three weeks into production, Irving Thalberg died. It was a terrific blow to everyone at MGM, including Groucho, who has said many times that his interest in making films vanished when the producer passed away. But the film had been virtually set when Thalberg died, and his absence should have had no effect on the final outcome of the picture. What was missed was Thalberg's keen eye for polishing and repolishing a finished product. He was known to make changes in a film after shooting had completed, and frequently went to great expense to redo comparatively minor scenes if he felt they would improve the film. Perhaps if he had been alive he would have spotted some of the flaws in A DAY AT THE RACES; perhaps not.

Oddly enough, there is nothing wrong with the film's comedy scenes. In fact, most of them are uproarious. What is wrong with A DAY AT THE RACES is that it has none of the

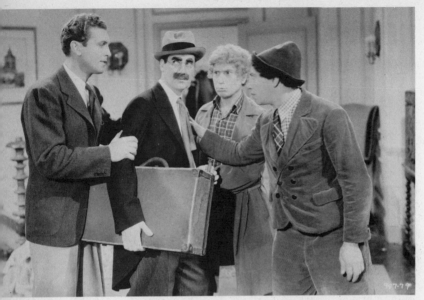

Dr. Hackenbush (Groucho) wants to make a hasty retreat, but Allan Jones, Harpo and Chico have a different idea in A DAY AT THE RACES.

This started out as a cozy tête-à-tête between Groucho and seductive Esther Muir, until Chico and Harpo arrived. A DAY AT THE RACES.

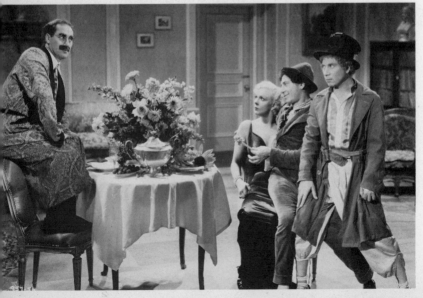

pace of its predecessor. When the film breaks for a musical sequence, everything stops dead in its tracks, and the effect is that of an intermission, instead of a musical number that is part of a whole. In addition, the songs simply aren't as good as those in OPERA. Allan Jones' singing of "Blue Venetian Waters" is very nice, but the song has no charm at all, and Vivien Fay's ballet, which follows it, is incongruous to the point of absurdity. The Marx Brothers would no more put up with a ballet than they would with a pompous singer or a stuffy speech maker. In addition, both this and the later number, "Tomorrow Is Another Day," are far too long, and completely destroy the film's continuity. The latter sequence, which segues into a production number, involves a group of blissfully happy, crap-shooting Negroes, singing and dancing through shantytown as Harpo plays pied piper with his flute.

The crime is that these unnecessary musical numbers break up a series of hilarious comedy routines that show the Marxes at their peak. Margaret Dumont (as Mrs. Upjohn) insists that Maureen O'Sullivan hire the illustrious Dr. Hugo Hackenbush (Groucho) to head her sanatorium. As Mrs. Upjohn's money is the only hope for keeping the sanatorium in business, Hackenbush is hired. This thwarts the plans of mortgage holder Douglass Dumbrille, who had planned to take over the property and turn it into a gambling casino; he determines to obtain the property by whatever means are necessary. Meanwhile Allan Jones, Maureen's boyfriend, has spent his last cent on a racehorse, Hi Hat, and with the help of hustler Chico and jockey Harpo, hopes to make a lot of money with it. The racetrack is the backdrop for the film's classic sequence where Groucho encounters racing tout Chico, peddling "tootsie-frootsie ice cream." He stops Groucho from making a bet in order to sell him a hot tip. "Two dollars and you'll remember me all the rest of your life," says Chico. "That's the most nauseating proposition I've ever heard," replies Groucho, but he goes along with the idea anyway. Within ten minutes, he has been forced to buy a dozen additional books and guides to decipher the name of the horse he is to bet on, and when Chico continues to sing out, "Get your tootsie-frootsie ice cream," Groucho mutters, "I think I'm getting a tootsie-frootsie-ing right here!" The racetrack is also the setting for the film's fast-paced climax, where Chico and Harpo must delay the start of the race until Hi Hat is found. They try everything: Harpo turns on a fan and blows hundreds of spectators' hats onto the track; Groucho leads a train of cars from the parking lot

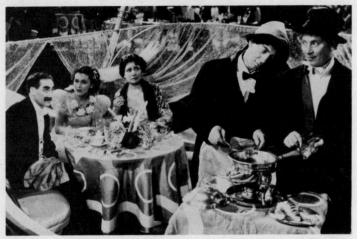

This scene never appeared in the final print of A DAY AT THE RACES; Groucho,
Maureen O'Sullivan and Margaret Dumont are worried about the new waiters.

onto the field; and Harpo dislodges the outer railing of the
track, sending the horses off into an adjacent meadow.

This fine scene is preceded by others just as funny: Groucho
pretending to be the Florida medical board on the telephone
when one of Dumbrille's henchmen calls up to check on Dr.
Hackenbush's credentials; Dr. H. conducting a checkup on
Margaret Dumont with the dubious help of Harpo and Chico,
under the watchful eye of Viennese specialist Sig Rumann;
and Groucho trying to engage in a midnight tryst with man-
trap Esther Muir, while Harpo and Chico, aware that she is a
decoy for the villains, try to break up the romantic meeting
by wallpapering everything in sight, including Miss Muir. All
these sequences, and others, are screamingly funny, but the
mood is spoiled by the intrusive production numbers. Then,
after the marvelous racetrack climax, the final insult is added
by having Harpo, Groucho, Chico and the rest of the cast
walking triumphantly toward the camera, along the track,
singing excerpts from the film's songs and smiling inanely.
This is an ending unworthy of even THE COCOANUTS, and
goes against everything the brothers stand for. It buckles
them firmly into the standard musical-comedy format, which
everyone hoped they had abandoned after ANIMAL CRACKERS.

Critics were generally cold to RACES, despite its top-notch
comedy sequences, but the film was a bigger commercial
success than A NIGHT AT THE OPERA. This meant little to the
Marxes, who felt lost without Irving Thalberg. The follow-

ing year, 1938, the brothers made a bold move: they accepted RKO's offer to do a picture on loan from MGM, and the film they signed to do was ROOM SERVICE, a long-running Broadway comedy. Up until this time, every film the brothers had done was hand-tailored for them (even if the results were less than perfect). ROOM SERVICE had a regular cast of characters and a very definite, complicated plot to follow. Most people have deemed the experiment of putting the Marxes into such a situation a failure. It is not quite that bad; ROOM SERVICE suffers from claustrophobia, it is true (the one set, a hotel room, serves for 99 percent of the film), but it is still entertaining, with particularly fine work from Donald MacBride as the frantic hotel supervisor who is driven to the brink of insanity by the Marxes' wheeling and dealing to prevent their eviction. There are some funny lines (Groucho tries to get rid of young Frank Albertson by telling him his mother is probably sitting by the fireside at home, crying her eyes out. "But we haven't got a fireside," Albertson protests. "Then how do you listen to the President's speeches?" Groucho snaps) and a few especially funny sequences (Harpo's medical examination where a squeeze doll is used to simulate his voice saying "Ah"), but the film does get tangled up in an unusually large number of plot devices. Indeed, the funniest line of the film is unintentional. Near the end, Ann

Ann Miller is beginning to understand; but now Frank Albertson and Groucho look confused in ROOM SERVICE.

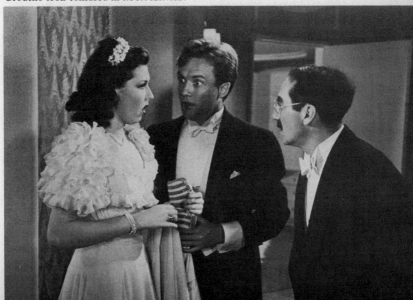

Miller, as Albertson's girl friend, appears in the brothers' apartment. Like co-star Lucille Ball, Miss Miller has virtually nothing to do in the film, and has been absent for most of the proceedings. Now, after more than an hour of intricate goings on, she arrives and is given a five-second rundown of the scheme they are trying to hatch. "Oh, now I understand," she beams, and runs off to help the situation, probably no more aware of what is going on than when she came in.

The Marx Brothers returned to MGM and starred in three more vehicles: AT THE CIRCUS, GO WEST and THE BIG STORE. They all have their moments, but generally speaking, these films are pale shadows of the past, and cannot match even the weakest of the brothers' Paramount vehicles. Their main problem is that they have none of the old lunatic spirit that made the Marx Brothers films unique. They conform more and more to standard story lines, and milder humor. The dialogue is limp where it ought to be bristling, the action scenes are phony where they ought to be fun, and the subplots and romantic scenes are more intrusive and annoying than ever before. Indeed, at times it seems that they are the focal points of the films, and the brothers' comedy is just incidental.

The Marx Brothers might have taken aim at the writers in GO WEST.

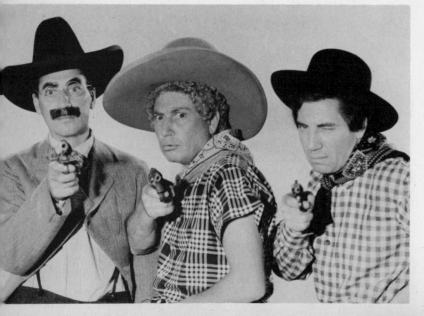

The main distinction of AT THE CIRCUS is Groucho's rendition of "Lydia, The Tattooed Lady," a delightful specialty song composed by Harold Arlen and E. Y. Harburg. Groucho continued to sing it for years to come, and it never failed to delight audiences. He sings the tune near the beginning of CIRCUS, and everything that follows is anticlimactic by comparison. Especially annoying is Kenny Baker, who shares the romantic spotlight with Florence Rice; they are as unappealing a duo as MGM ever concocted, and provide a genuine detriment to the film's enjoyment. In addition, their songs, written by Arlen and Harburg hot on the heels of WIZARD OF OZ, are nothing special. Most of the comic sequences in the film are rather contrived, lacking the fresh spark that made their previous adventures so enjoyable. If the film has a highlight, it is probably Groucho's antics at a society party given by Margaret Dumont. Hearing that the 400 have been invited, Groucho counts heads to make sure everyone is present. "It looks like they all showed up," he concludes. "There'll be no second helpings." Then, as he stalls the party from breaking up by forcing the guests to remain while he finishes an extra cup of coffee, Harpo and Chico knock out the villains and save the circus from sabotage. They also detach a floating platform that is holding the society orchestra, which floats out to sea as the musicians play *Lohengrin*.

GO WEST is better than AT THE CIRCUS, but practically anything would be. It too has many weak moments, and a dreary romantic plot, but it holds up fairly well because of several inspired sequences. One can *almost* forgive the dead space in between these highlights, because the comedy sequences are so well done. The first is the film's opening scene in an eastern train station where Groucho, Harpo and Chico are all trying to buy tickets out West. Groucho finds himself ten dollars short, while Harpo and Chico aren't quite as well off. Groucho decides to make the extra money by selling various things to the two open-faced suckers standing near him. Groucho proceeds to interest them in a coonskin cap and a moth-eaten jacket, among other items, each selling for one dollar. Chico pays him with a ten-dollar bill, and as Groucho counts out nine dollars change, Harpo pulls a string and the ten-spot flies back into his hand. After several repeats of this same procedure, Groucho begins to suspect that something is wrong. Finally, he believes he has gotten the money he needs, and bids his two customers good-bye. "Wait a minute," says Chico. "We forgot to pay you the

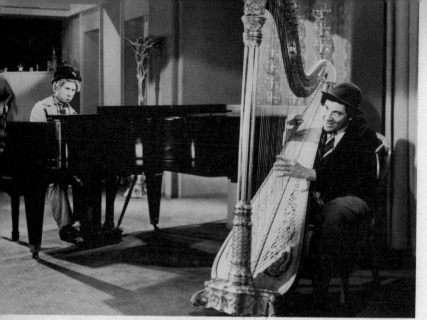

When in doubt, enter harp and piano, but here the roles were reversed; a posed shot from THE BIG STORE.

sales tax." The tax, it seems, is one dollar. "No thanks," replies Groucho, "I couldn't afford it." The second highspot comes as the brothers embark on a stagecoach trip, along with other passengers including Walter Woolf King (Lasparri from A NIGHT AT THE OPERA) as a conniving businessman trying to buy a supposedly worthless piece of land from Groucho. The scene is reminiscent of the stateroom scene from OPERA as the brothers, King, two lady passengers, and several babies participate in a wildly funny commotion brought on by Harpo's determination to confound the pompous King. He repeatedly knocks King's hat off and into a duffel bag which he quickly closes. As King goes to grab for it. Harpo further confuses matters by switching hats around. The hat-removing procedure gets faster and faster, and other passengers are driven into the melee before Harpo is through. From here the film goes downhill, with straight leads John Carroll and Diana Lewis failing to make their scenes worthwhile, especially on the "outdoor" sets that are obviously interiors. A prolonged sequence at an Indian reservation produces no laughs, and Harpo's harp sequence is made pointless by having him "play" on an Indian weaving loom. The scenes inside a western saloon affer the most opportunities, and result in the film's most disappointing sequences. GO WEST doesn't pick up steam until the famous climactic sequence where the brothers take over a train carrying the villains East to collect their fortune on the deed they have stolen from its rightful owner, Carroll. At first, the brothers do everything they can to stop the train so Carroll, riding alongside in a wagon, can get on. Then, once the villains (King and Robert Barrat) get off and start to ride East in their own carriage, the brothers' efforts are concentrated on keeping the train going at full speed. This becomes difficult when all the fuel is consumed, so in desperation, they wreck the train and feed all the wood they can chop into the furnace. Everything ends happily, of course, except for Marx Brothers fans, who rightly feel that they have been cheated out of a potentially fine film by incompetent scripting.

THE BIG STORE is no better. Like the previous two MGM films, it has some moments of humor, mostly at the beginning of the film, but like the other two, it is forced and mostly unfunny. The final scene, designed as a comic highlight, is not, due to the fact that it looks artificial. It features the brothers on roller skates, but all of the gags are performed in long-shot where we know that doubles are being used. This procedure negates all the potential humor of the sequence, and it falls flat. Indeed, except for the opening scene of Groucho's fly-by-night detective office, where Harpo helps him to seem busy to impress customer Margaret Dumont, the film has no laughs. It is the worst of their MGM films, and perhaps the worst film they ever made.

With THE BIG STORE the Marx Brothers decided to end their movie career. For five years they found other activities to keep them busy: Groucho and Chico made frequent appearances on various radio programs, and in the early 1940's, Chico formed a band which toured the country. Chico "starred" on piano, and told jokes in between musical selections. The band featured, as drummer and sometimes-vocalist, a young man named Mel Torme. Harpo did USO tours and made a guest appearance in *Stage Door Canteen*. He also appeared in a promotional short called ALL STAR BOND RALLY produced in 1945 by 20th Century-Fox. As host Bob Hope is talking on stage, a scream is heard and a young pretty blonde runs down the aisle of the theater. She is followed by Harpo, eyes gleaming and horn honking. She races on stage, and he follows by trampling over the piano. As he follows her, however, he notices a harp in the center of the stage, and decides to forsake the young girl in favor of a musical piece.

After the war the brothers decided to give movies another try. Produced by David L. Loew for United Artists release,

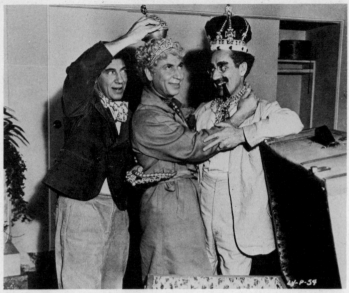

The Marx Brothers (reunited on screen after a five-year absence in A NIGHT IN CASABLANCA) fool around for the still photographer.

A NIGHT IN CASABLANCA lacks the slick production values of MGM, and the usual cast of familiar character actors (except for Sig Rumann, wisely cast as the heavy). It also lacks the imposing presence of Margaret Dumont, whose appearance in even the worst of the MGM features guaranteed at least a few moments of hilarity with Groucho out to woo her. CASABLANCA also has a pair of inconsequential romantic leads (Charles Drake and Lois Collier). But with all this going against it, it manages to retain much of the old verve with a formidable supply of one-liners from Groucho, and some memorable pantomime from Harpo. It could hardly rate as one of their best films, but to repeat James Agee's oft-quoted line, "The worst they might ever make would be better worth seeing than most of the things I can think of." As with most Marx films, CASABLANCA starts off well, with a cop accosting Harpo for loitering. Harpo is slouching against the side of a building, and the cop asks sarcastically if he thinks he's holding the building up. Harpo nods, and when the cop pulls him away, the structure topples over! This gag was contributed by Frank Tashlin, who is credited with "additional material" in the film's titles. Tashlin started in Hollywood as an animator, went on to direct some great Warner Brothers cartoons, and eventually secured a position as a first-rate comedy director. For A NIGHT IN CASABLANCA he not only contributed the building gag, but one of the film's funniest sequences, where Harpo, Chico and Groucho drive Sig Rumann crazy by intercepting his every move as he tries to pack his clothes in a suitcase. With lightning speed and perfect timing, they manage to keep shirts, coats and other articles from landing in his valise, as they "float" them across the room into a closet.

Except for Agee, most of the critics were unimpressed with A NIGHT IN CASABLANCA; Groucho was frustrated because he and his brothers had invested in the film and hoped to see some profits, which never appeared. Even critics who had championed the Marx cause when they first burst onto Broadway, and later into films, deserted them by the 1940's. The trouble was that while the Marxes superficially remained the same, their humor, particularly Groucho's, lost most of its bite as time went on. He was still delivering funny dialogue ("I'm Beatrice Rheiner, I stop at the hotel," says

A candid photo taken moments after Groucho completed a memorable scene with a then-unknown Marilyn Monroe in LOVE HAPPY.

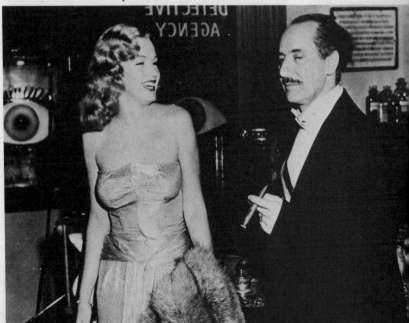

seductive Lisette Verea; "I'm Ronald Cornblow, I stop at nothing," replies Groucho), but puns were only part of the Groucho character. The Marx Brothers were never pretentious, and anyone accusing them of offering social commentary might have been roundly lambasted by Groucho, but in effect, that is what they were doing. Their humor was based on satire in its purest form, poking fun at all kinds of sacred institutions. In 1946 and CASABLANCA, however, the puns were simply puns for their own sake and nothing more. This doesn't mean that they weren't funny, but it does help to explain why most reviewers found the Marx Brothers "tired" in their later vehicles, especially this one.

After three years, they tried one more time, with another independent production (produced by Mary Pickford's company), LOVE HAPPY. It certainly isn't top-drawer Marx comedy, but on the other hand, it is more pleasant than, for instance, THE BIG STORE. The spotlight in LOVE HAPPY is on Harpo, with Chico in support, and Groucho making little more than a token appearance as detective Sam Grunion, who introduces and narrates the story. There's plenty of footage that doesn't involve the Marxes, as slinky spy Ilona Massey tries to retrieve a sardine can that contains some valuable jewels (Harpo has unwittingly stolen it, along with other food supplies) and as Vera-Ellen and others try to finance their Broadway musical show. This seems to be a necessary evil, but for all the sugary pathos that evolves from the relationship of Harpo and Vera-Ellen, it is easier to stomach than similar sequences from some of the MGM films. Critics in 1949 had the right idea when they generally agreed that even a diluted version of the Marx Brothers was worth seeing, and far better than other comedies being made at the same time. The statement is still true today, even more so than in 1949, and LOVE HAPPY remains a pleasant diversion.

One of LOVE HAPPY's best scenes comes when Harpo discovers that Vera-Ellen has been kidnapped, and runs to alert Chico. He decides to relate his message in pantomime, jumping around and whistling to egg Chico on with his guesses as to the meanings. Harpo pretends to be a dog. Chico ventures a few names, but Harpo gestures that it is a big dog. "A St. Bernard?" No, Harpo says, a *big* dog. Finally Chico guesses "Great Dane" and Harpo shakes his hand feverishly. Then he punches Chico, who demands to know what's going on. Finally, from this demonstration he realizes that Harpo's word is "jaw." Whistling happily, Harpo

then tells Chico to put the two words together. Great Dane—
Jaw. Great Danejaw. Great danger. "Ah!" shouts Chico
when he discovers the right phrase, and goes off with Harpo
to catch the villains. Such moments are not plentiful in LOVE
HAPPY, but it's still fun to watch Groucho deliver leering
glances at a beautiful customer (played by Marilyn Monroe),
Chico playing the piano, and Harpo cavorting on the electric
signs over Times Square in the film's climax.

The Marxes had said they were through many times, but
this time it looked like the real thing. After LOVE HAPPY, the
act broke up. Groucho inaugurated a highly successful radio
show, which later moved to TV, called *You Bet Your Life* (and
later shown as *The Best of Groucho*), an informal quiz show
which allowed Groucho to trade quips with his contestants.
The formula remained successful for over ten years. A later
program, *Tell It to Groucho*, didn't work out as well, and
barely lasted one season. Harpo tried to retire, but he could
seldom resist a good offer. He spent five weeks shooting
ANDROCLES AND THE LION in 1952 for producer Gabriel
Pascal, who thought him the perfect person to play Shaw's
hero. But RKO's boss at the time, Howard Hughes, dis-
agreed, and replaced Harpo with Alan Young. Harpo did
occasional TV guest appearances throughout the 1950's, including one memorable episode of *I Love Lucy* in which he
and Lucille Ball made an unforgettable team. Of the three
brothers, Chico was the least active in the 1950's, preferring
to play cards and talk with his friends than to work.

In 1957 producer-director Irwin Allen hired all three brothers to take roles in his all-star extravaganza, THE STORY OF
MANKIND. This unique production attempted to cram the
history of the world into 100 minutes, with some of the
oddest casting Hollywood ever concocted (Hedy Lamarr as
Joan of Arc, Harpo as Sir Isaac Newton, etc.) The brothers
appeared in separate sequences which gave them little opportunity to generate much excitement. Harpo and Chico
got together a nightclub act that played Las Vegas in the
1950's, and Chico even accepted a straight role in a CBS-TV
Playhouse 90. Then, in 1959, the *G.E. Theater* TV series
presented a half-hour episode, *The Incredible Jewel Robbery*, starring Harpo and Chico. Directed by film veteran
Mitchell Leisen, the show was played in pantomime, with a
musical score and an obtrusive laugh track. In it, Harpo
and Chico are would-be crooks who lead a small-time, but
profitable, life of crime. They decide to put all their energy
into one big heist, and plan their scheme carefully. The two

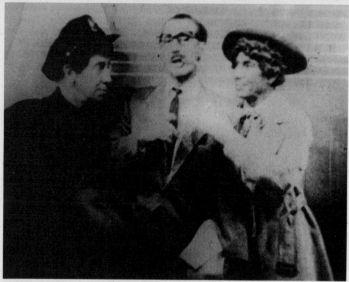

Chico, Groucho and Harpo—together again, if only for a TV segment from
THE INCREDIBLE JEWEL ROBBERY.

thieves disguise their car as a police vehicle, with Harpo
using a round salami as a stencil for the police emblem on
the door, and doughnut holes to help him dot the *i*'s. The
next day, Harpo approaches a jewelry store and dons a
perfect disguise—that of Groucho! He enters and snatches
several gems from the store proprietor (Benny Rubin), who
sounds a police alarm. Chico, in police uniform, drives up
and takes Harpo away. As they are leaving, another police
car arrives, but seeing that the situation is well in hand,
drives on. Everything works perfectly, but as Harpo and
Chico drive away, they are stopped by a woman outside a
home for the deaf and dumb. She explains, in pantomime,
that another woman is lying on the ground nearby, about to
have a baby. They take the woman to the hospital, and are
about to drive off again, when another police car pulls up
alongside Chico's. The officer inside waves hello, then notices his colleague's car door. Chico's police emblem is painted
white-on-black, while the real officer's is black-on-white.
After an exchange of glances, the cops catch on and take the
two culprits to jail. Store-owner Benny Rubin watches the
lineup and immediately recognizes Chico, but because Harpo
is no longer wearing a disguise, he doesn't spot him. Just

then, Groucho strides in, and Rubin points the finger at him. Harpo and Chico rush up to Groucho (Harpo hands him his leg in characteristic fashion) to give him moral support. "We don't talk until we see our lawyer!" The brothers smile in triumph, and the Groucho duck from *You Bet Your Life* is lowered with a "The End" sign attached. *The Incredible Jewel Robbery* is more a curio than a great piece of comedy, but its sheer novelty made it a success in 1959. Its only lasting significance is that it presents the final appearance of the three Marx Brothers on-screen in that wonderful closing shot. (Groucho and Chico worked together the year before in a commercial short called SHOW-DOWN AT ULCER GULCH; Chico and Harpo subsequently made a TV pilot that was never aired, called DEPUTY SERAPH.)

Chico died on October 14, 1961, forever putting to an end the hope that someday someone would reunite all three brothers for a new, free-wheeling film in the old tradition (Billy Wilder announced such plans, but unfortunately they never came to fruition). Harpo lived in semiretirement for the next few years, occasionally doing a TV show or a benefit concert. He died September 28, 1964, and more regrets were voiced that he and his brothers had not been given a chance to do much clowning in the previous decade.

Groucho lived to see the worldwide Marx Brothers revival, and enjoyed various tributes including an honorary Academy Award. Despite failing health, he continued to perform into his eighties, and died on August 19, 1977. He may have lost some of his vigor, but he never surrendered his sense of irreverence. At one Marx Brothers festival he was asked what it felt like to be an elder statesman of comedy, and he replied, "Like an old jerk."

The Films of the Marx Brothers

(Director's name follows year.)

1. **The Cocoanuts**—Paramount 1929—Robert Florey and Joseph Santley—Groucho, Harpo, Chico, Zeppo, Margaret Dumont, Mary Eaton, Oscar Shaw, Kay Francis, Cyril Ring, Basil Ruysdael, Sylvan Lee, Gamby-Hale Ballet Girls, Allan K. Foster Girls, Barton MacLane. 96 minutes.

2. **Animal Crackers**—Paramount 1930—Victor Heerman—Groucho, Harpo, Chico, Zeppo, Margaret Dumont, Lillian Roth, Louis Sorin, Hal Thompson, Margaret Irving, Kathryn Reece, Robert Greig, Edward Metcalf, The Music Masters, Ann Roth, Gerry Goff. 98 minutes.

3. **Monkey Business**—Paramount 1931—Norman Z. McLeod—Groucho, Harpo, Chico, Zeppo, Thelma Todd, Rockcliffe Fellowes, Tom Kennedy, Ruth Hall, Harry Woods, Ben Taggart, Otto Fries, Evelyn Pierce, Maxine Castle, Cecil Cunningham, Douglass Dumbrille, Rolfe Sedan, Leo White, James Bradbury, Jr., Leo Willis, Ethan Laidlow, Constantine Romanoff. 77 minutes.

4. **Horse Feathers**—Paramount 1932—Norman Z. McLeod—Groucho, Harpo, Chico, Zeppo, Thelma Todd, David Landau, Robert Greig, James Pierce, Nat Pendleton, Reginald Barlow, Florine McKinney, F. J. LeSaint, Captain E. H. Calvert, Vince Barnett, Sid Saylor, Ben Taggart, Edgar Dearing, Frank Rice, Theresa Harris, Phil Tead. 68 minutes.

5. **Hollywood on Parade**—A-9—Paramount 1932—off-screen footage of Groucho, Harpo and Chico with their families; also Skeets Gallagher, Eddie Lambert and his orchestra, Ivan Lebedeff, Lois Wilson, Claire Windsor, Vivian Duncan, Fifi D'Orsay. One reel.

6. **Duck Soup**—Paramount 1933—Leo McCarey—Groucho, Harpo, Chico, Zeppo, Margaret Dumont, Louis Calhern, Raquel Torres, Edgar Kennedy, Edmund Breese, William Worthington, Edwin Maxwell, Leonid Kinsky, Verna Hillie, George MacQuarrie, Fred Sullivan, Davison Clark, Charles B. Middleton, Eric Mayne, Dennis O'Keefe, Dale Van Sickel, Wade Boteler, Captain E. H. Calvert. 70 minutes.

7. **A Night at the Opera**—MGM 1935—Sam Wood—Groucho, Harpo, Chico, Margaret Dumont, Sigfried Rumann, Kitty Carlisle, Allan Jones, Walter Woolf King, Edward Keane, Robert Emmet O'Connor, Lorraine Bridges, Billy Gilbert, Purnell Pratt, Jonathan Hale, Leo White, Jay Eaton, Rolfe Sedan, Frank Yaconelli, John Lipson, Gino Corrado, George Irving, Selmer Jackson, Wilbur Mack, Philips Smalley, Stanley Blystone, Rodolfo Hoyos, Sr., Rita and Rubin, Inez Palange, Harry Tyler, Alan Bridge, Fred Malatesta, Sam Marx (extra), William Gould. 92 minutes.

8. **A Day at the Races**—MGM 1937—Sam Wood— Groucho, Harpo, Chico, Margaret Dumont, Sigfried Rumann, Al-

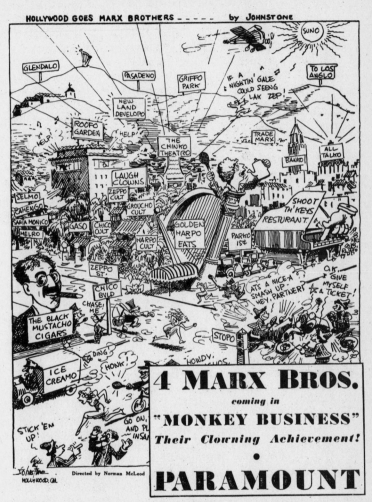

A trade advertisement drawn by Will Johnstone, whose association with the Marxes dated back to Broadway; he wrote their first play, *I'll Say She Is*.

Ian Jones, Maureen O'Sullivan, Douglass Dumbrille, Leonard Ceeley, Esther Muir, Robert Middlemass, Vivien Fay, Ivie Anderson and The Crinoline Choir, Frankie Darro, Charles Trowbridge, Pat Flaherty, Frank Dawson, Max Lucke. Si Jenks, Wilbur Mack, William Irving, Johnny Hyams, Harry Wilson, Hooper Atchley, Edward Earle, Mary McLaren, Edward LeSaint, Jack Norton, Byron Foulger, Carole Landis (extra); reportedly Dorothy Dandridge is seen in one of the production numbers. 109 minutes.

9. **Room Service**—RKO 1939—William A. Seiter—Groucho, Harpo, Chico, Lucille Ball, Ann Miller, Frank Albertson, Donald MacBride, Cliff Dunstan, Philip Loch, Alexander Astro, Charles Halton, Philip Wood, Donald Kerr, Stanely Blystone. 78 minutes.

10. **At the Circus**—MGM 1939—Edward Buzzell—Groucho, Harpo, Chico, Margaret Dumont, Florence Rice, Kenny Baker, Eve Arden, Nat Pendleton, Fritz Feld, James Burke, Jerry Marenghi, Barnett Parker, Jack McAfee, Little Bozo, Amanda Randolph, Granville Bates, Irving Bacon, John Dilson, Barlowe Borland, Emory Parnell, Frank Orth, Willie Best, Forbes Murray, Harry Hayden, Sid Miller, Mickey Daniels, Eugene Jackson, Byron Foulger, Mariska Aldrich, Matt McHugh, Frank Darien, Charles Gemora, The Escelante Family Troupe, Slicker the Seal, the Pena Family, the Juggling Normans. 87 minutes.

11. **Go West**—MGM 1940—Edward Buzzell—Groucho, Harpo, Chico, John Carroll, Diana Lewis, Robert Barrat, Walter Woolf King, June MacCloy, George Lessey, Mitchell Lewis, Tully Marshall, Clem Bevans, Joe Yule, Iris Adrian, Joan Woodbury, Edgar Dearing, Billy Wayne, Ed Gargan, Harry Tyler, Frederick Burton, Baby Quintanilla, Barbara Bedford, Arthur Housman. 80 minutes.

12. **The Big Store**—MGM 1941—Charles Riesner—Groucho, Harpo, Chico, Margaret Dumont, Douglass Dumbrille, Tony Martin, Virginia Grey, William Tannen, Marion Martin, Virginia O'Brien, Henry Armetta, Anna Demetrio, Paul Stanton, Russell Hicks, Bradley Page, Charles Holland, Charles Lane, Christian Rub, Edward McWade, Lee Kohlmar, Joe Yule, Etta McDaniel, Bob Perry, Al Hill, George Lloyd, Lee Phelps, Edgar Dearing, Eddy Chandler, Hal Le Seuer, Jan Duggan, Harry C. Bradley, Victor Potel, Mitchell Lewis, Dewey Robin-

son, William Newell, Milton Kibbee, Clara Blandick, Kay Deslys. 83 minutes.

13. **Screen Snapshots #8**—Columbia 1943—Ralph Staub—Gene Autry, Tyrone Power, Lou Holtz, Ritz Brothers, Annabella, Kay Kyser, Alan Mowbray. 10 minutes.

14. **A Night in Casablanca**—David Loew-United Artists 1946—Groucho, Harpo, Chico, Sig Rumann, Lisette Verea, Charles Drake, Lois Collier, Dan Seymour, Lewis Russell, Frederick Gierman, Harro Mellor, David Hoffman, Hall Harvey, Ruth Roman. 85 minutes.

15. **Love Happy**—United Artists 1949—David Miller—Harpo, Chico, Groucho, Vera-Ellen, Ilona Massey, Marion Hutton, Raymond Burr, Melville Cooper, Paul Valentine, Leon Belasco, Eric Blore, Bruce Gordon, Marilyn Monroe, Ed Gargan. 85 minutes.

16. **The Story of Mankind**—Warner Brothers 1957—Irwin Allen—Ronald Colman, Hedy Lamarr, Virginia Mayo, Agnes Moorehead, Vincent Price, Peter Lorre, Charles Coburn, Cedric Hardwicke, Cesar Romero, John Carradine, Dennis Hopper, Marie Wilson, Helmut Dantine, Edward Everett Horton, Reginald Gardiner, Marie Windsor, George E. Stone, Cathy O'Donnell, Franklin Pangborn, Melville Cooper, Henry Daniell, Francis X. Bushman, Jim Ameche, David Bond, Nick Cravat, Dany Crayne, Richard Cutting, Anthony Dexter. Toni Gerry, Austin Green, Alexander Lockwood, Bart Mattson, Don Megowan, Marvin Miller, Nancy Miller, Leonard Mudie, Burt Nelson, Tudor Owen, Ziva Rodann, Harry Ruby, William Schallert, Reginald Sheffield, Abrahama Sofaer, Bobby Watson. Groucho as Peter Minuet, Harpo as Sir Isaac Newton, Chico as a monk, Groucho's wife Eden Hartford as Laughing Water, Groucho's daughter Melinda Marx as an Early Christian Child. Color—100 minutes.

17. **Showdown at Ulcer Gulch**—Shamus Culhane Productions 1958—Ernie Kovacs, Edie Adams, Groucho, Chico, Bob Hope, Bing Crosby, Salome Jens, Orson Bean. A commercial short for *Saturday Evening Post*.

18. **The Incredible Jewel Robbery**—Revue Productions 1959—Mitchell Leisen—Harpo, Chico, Groucho, Benny Rubin, Joy Rogers. A half-hour segment of the *G. E. Theater* television series, with Harpo and Chcio starred, and Groucho making an unannounced appearance in the final scene.

The Marx Brothers also appeared in THE HOUSE THAT
SHADOWS BUILT, a promotional short for upcoming Paramount product in 1931, plugging MONKEY BUSINESS by
performing a skit adapted from their Broadway show *I'll
Say She is*.

Groucho appeared without his brothers in the following
films:

1. **Sunday Night at the Trocadero**—MGM 1937—George
   Sidney—Reginald Denny, George Hamilton's Music Box
   Music, Louis and Celeste, Madina and Mimosa, (Peter)
   Lind Hayes, Gaylord Carter, Connee Boswell, and guest
   stars Arthur Lake, Dick Foran, John Howard, Margaret
   Vail, Chester Morris, Sally Blane, Norman Foster, Robert Benchley, Mr. and Mrs. Groucho Marx, Frank Mor-
   gan, Bert Wheeler, Eric Blore, Toby Wing, Stuart Erwin,
   June Collyer, Russell Gleason, Glenda Farrell, Frank
   McHugh, and Benny Rubin. Groucho appears without
   his greasepaint mustache in this nightclub short. Two
   reels.
2. **Screen Snapshots #2**—Columbia 1943—Ralph Staub—
   Groucho does a radio broadcast with Carole Landis; this
   footage repeated in Snapshot entry HOLLYWOOD'S GREAT
   COMEDIANS ten years later. One reel.
3. **Copacabana**—United Artists 1947—Alfred W. Green—
   Carmen Miranda, Andy Russell, Steve Cochran, Gloria
   Jean, Louis Sobel, Abel Green, Earl Wilson. 92 minutes.
4. **Mr. Music**—Paramount 1950—Richard Haydn—Bing
   Crosby, Nancy Olson, Charles Coburn, Ida Moore, Ruth
   Hussey, Robert Stack, Tom Ewell, Charles Kemper,
   Donald Woods, Marge and Gower Champion, Claude
   Curdle, (Richard Haaydn), Dorothy Kirsten, Peggy Lee,
   The Merry Macs. 113 minutes.
5. **Double Dynamite**—RKO 1951—Irving Cummings, Jr.
   —Frank Sinatra, Jane Russell, Don McGuire, Howard
   Freeman, Nestor Paiva, Frank Orth, Harry Hayden,
   William Edmunds, Russ Thorson. 80 minutes.
6. **A Girl in Every Port**—RKO 1952—Chester Erskine—
   William Bendix, Marie Wilson, Don DeFore, Dee Hart-
   ford, Gene Lockhart, George E. Stone, Rodney Wooten,
   Percy Helton, Hanley Stafford, Teddy Hart. 86 minutes.
7. **Will Success Spoil Rock Hunter?**—20th Century-Fox
   1957—Frank Tashlin—Jayne Mansfield, Tony Randall,
   Betsy Drake, Joan Blondell, John Williams, Henry Jones,

Lili Gentle, Mickey Hargitay, Georgia Carr, Dick Whittinghill, Ann McCrea, Alberto Morin, Louis Mercier. Color—94 minutes.

8. **Skidoo**—Paramount 1968—Otto Preminger—Jackie Gleason, Carol Channing, Frankie Avalon, Fred Clark, Michael Constantine, Frank Gorshin, John Philip Law, Peter Lawford, Burgess Meredith, George Raft, Cesar Romero, Mickey Rooney, Austin Pendleton, Alexandra Hay, Luna, Arnold Stang, Doro Merande, Phil Arnold, Slim Pickens, Robert Donner, Richard Kiel, Tom Law, Jaik Rosenstein, Stacy King, Renny Roker, Roman Gabriel, Stone Country, The Orange Country Ramblers. Color—98 minutes.

Harpo appeared without his brothers in the following films:

1. **Too Many Kisses**—Paramount 1925—Paul Sloane— Richard Dix, Frances Howard, Frank Currier, William Powell, Paul Panzer, Joe Burke, Alyce Mills.

2. **La Fiesta de Santa Barbara**—MGM 1936—a Technicolor short featuring such entertainers as the Gumm Sisters (including Judy Garland), Maria Gambarelli, Eduardo Durant's Spanish Orchestra, the Spanish Troubadors, the Dude Ranch Wranglers, Staffi Duna, Paul Porcasi, m.c. Leo Carrillo, and such famous spectators as Robert Taylor, Buster Keaton, Gary Cooper, Warner Baxter, Adrienne Ames, Mary Carlisle, Chester Conklin, Binnie Barnes, Edmund Lowe, Toby Wing, Gilbert Roland, Ida Lupino, Ralph Forbes, Shirley Ross, Irvin S. Cobb, Andy Devine, Rosalind Keith, Joe Morrison, Cecilia Parker, narrated by Pete Smith. Two reels.

3. **Stage Door Canteen**—United Artists 1943—Frank Borzage—Cheryl Walker, William Terry, Marjorie Riordan, Lon McCallister; guest stars Judith Anderson, Henry Armetta, Benny Baker, Kenny Baker, Tallulah Bankhead, Ralph Bellamy, Edgar Bergen and Charlie McCarthy, Ray Bolger, Helen Broderick, Ina Claire, Katharine Cornell, Lloyd Corrigan, Jane Cowl, Jane Darwell, William Demarest, Virginia Field, Dorothy Fields, Gracie Fields, Lynn Fontaine, Arlene Francis, Vinton Freedley, Billy Gilbert, Lucile Gleason, Vera Gordon, Virginia Grey, Helen Hayes, Katharine Hepburn, Hugh Herbert, Jean Hersholt, Sam Jaffe, Allen Jenkins, George Jessel, Roscoe Karns, Virginia Kaye, Tom Kennedy, Otto Kruger, June Lane, Betty Lawford,

Gertrude Lawrence, Gypsy Rose Lee, Alfred Lunt, Bert Lytell, Aline MacMahon, Elsa Maxwell, Helen Menken, Yehudi Menuhin, Ethel Merman, Ralph Morgan, Alan Mowbray, Paul Muni, Elliott Nugent, Merle Oberon, Franklin Pangborn, Helen Parrish, Brock Pemberton, George Raft, Lanny Ross, Selena Royle, Martha Scott, Ethel Waters, Ed Wynn. 132 minutes.

4. **All-Star Bond Rally**—20th Century-Fox 1945—Michael Audley—Bob Hope, Bing Crosby, Fibber McGee and Molly, Frank Sinatra, Harry James Band, Betty Grable, Jeanne Crain, Linda Darnell, Fay Marlowe, Carmen Miranda, Glenn Langan, Frank Latimore. Two reels.

Chico appeared without his brothers in the following:

1. **Hollywood on Parade**—B-7—Paramount 1933—Chico, Buster Crabbe and W. C. Fields were seen chasing after the Earl Carroll girls in this one-reel short.

2. **Hollywood—The Second Step**—MGM 1936—Felix E. Feist—Chico appears briefly as himself in this fictitious story of a young actress's struggles in Hollywood. Maureen O'Sullivan also makes an appearance. One reel.

THELMA TODD-ZASU PITTS
THELMA TODD-PATSY KELLY

Since the beginning of movies there have been only a handful of top-notch comediennes. Many of them have suffered because of poor material, and others have turned to singing or acting to further their careers. In the 1930's, however, three comediennes were given a rare opportunity to star in their own short subjects which, while varying in quality, gave the ladies an opportunity to display their remarkable talents and affinity for pure comedy. The ladies were Thelma Todd, one of the screen's great beauties, ZaSu Pitts, whose helpless gestures and expressive hands were in demand for almost fifty years, and Patsy Kelly, whose presence in any film of the 30's was a guarantee that there would be some lively doings.

Hal Roach's stars at the outset of the 1930's were Laurel and Hardy, Our Gang and Charley Chase. Roach was anxious to inaugurate new comedy series to keep his studio busy; one idea that came to him was a "natural." Why not develop a female counterpart to Laurel and Hardy? For teammates he chose Thelma Todd, who was already working as leading lady for his other comics, and ZaSu Pitts, who was keeping busy in supporting roles in feature films. His production team went to work, and over the next three years they produced 17 shorts with ZaSu and Thelma as inseparable pals who always managed to get into some sort of trouble.

Thelma Todd was born in 1905 in Lawrence, Massachusetts. She attended the State Normal School, working part-time as a model. Upon graduation she became a schoolteacher, but her career in education was interrupted when she won a beauty contest and was named "Miss Massachusetts." A talent scout from Paramount Pictures spotted her and brought her to New York to attend that studio's acting school. She was given minor roles in Paramount silents like GOD GAVE ME TWENTY CENTS (1926) and FASCINATING YOUTH (1926), the latter film designed to showcase the studio's new talent.

141

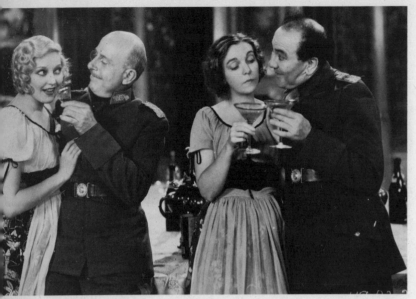

Behind German lines. Thelma and ZaSu try to win over German officers
Stuart Holmes and Charles Judels in WAR MAMAS.

From there she was cast in a series of forgettable films, with
occasional good roles in movies like NEVADA (1927) opposite Gary Cooper, and SEVEN FOOTPRINTS TO SATAN (1928).
In 1929 she was seen by Hal Roach, who was impressed with
her beauty and vivacity. He signed her to a contract and put
her to work immediately in Harry Langdon's two-reel comedies (THE KING, THE FIGHTING, PARSON, etc.), and other comedies with Laurel and Hardy (UNACCUSTOMED AS WE ARE,
ANOTHER FINE MESS, etc.), and Charley Chase (THE REAL
MCCOY, DOLLAR DIZZY, etc.). Sound proved no problem for
Thelma, who had a pleasant, cultured voice, and she took to
comedy with relish. While she did her short-subject series
for Roach, she accepted roles in other studios' feature films.
Her attempts to achieve stardom as a dramatic actress were
doomed to failure, for she was cast mostly in low-budget
melodramas and love stories. Her biggest success, again, was
in comedies, and she worked opposite practically every funny
man in Hollywood: Joe E. Brown (BROAD-MINDED and SON
OF A SAILOR), Buster Keaton and Jimmy Durante (SPEAK
EASILY), the Marx Brothers (MONKEY BUSINESS and HORSE-
FEATHERS), and Wheeler and Woolsey (HIPS HIPS HOORAY

and COCKEYED CAVALIERS). Like it or not, Thelma was best loved as a comedienne; she brought to every film a charm and vitality that have seldom been equaled.

ZaSu Pitts was born in Parsons, Kansas, in 1900. Her family soon moved to California, where ZaSu grew up and eventually found her life's work. Her name was fashioned from the last two letters in the name of one aunt, Eliza, and the first two letters in the name of another aunt, Susan. ZaSu made her movie debut in Mary Pickford's THE LITTLE PRINCESS in 1917 and subsequently appeared in fifty silent films. The story goes that ZaSu's comic possibilities were never realized until the 1930's, but one need only see a 1918 film, A SOCIETY SENSATION, to disprove this legend. It stars Carmel Myers and a young Rudolph Valentino, and it is only ZaSu's fourth movie, yet she is playing the same kind of comedy relief she was to do for the next four decades, and already using those inimitable hands with the same hilarious results. In 1925, director Erich von Stroheim saw the actress' dramatic potential and cast her as the shrewish wife in his masterpiece, GREED. It was Miss Pitts' finest hour, in a vivid portrayal that helped to make the film a classic. Von Stroheim employed her again in THE WEDDING

The girls tangle with burly Bud Jamison in a theatrical boarding house; from STRICTLY UNRELIABLE.

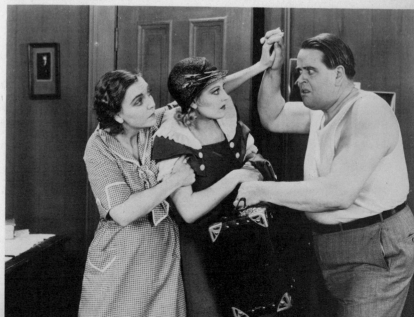

MARCH (1928), but his high regard of her dramatic ability was not shared by many others in Hollywood, who refused to think of ZaSu as anything but a comedienne. She was doing well in feature films when Hal Roach approached her to co-star in a short-subject series with Thelma Todd in 1931. ZaSu accepted, but did not curtail her feature-film activity, working in thirty features while appearing in the Roach shorts over the next few years.

The first Pitts-Todd short was an oddity called LET'S DO THINGS, directed by Roach himself. The second short in the series was CATCH AS CATCH CAN. Guinn "Big Boy" Williams co-starred as a prizefighter who falls in love with ZaSu, and Reed Howes played his manager, who is also Thelma's boyfriend. To direct this short, Roach hired Marshall "Mickey" Neilan, who had been one of Hollywood's top directors in the silent era, and who, through unfortunate circumstances, had skyrocketed downward by the end of the 1920's. CATCH AS CATCH CAN proves that he had not lost his touch, for it is one of the most charming Pitts-Todd shorts, and one of the few that shows filmmaking know-how. Many Hal Roach comedies were handicapped by budget restrictions that necessitated process screens or limp alibis to avoid expensive location shots or large crowd scenes. In this short, the

Thelma tries to remain dignified on this embarrassing situation; from SHOW BUSINESS.

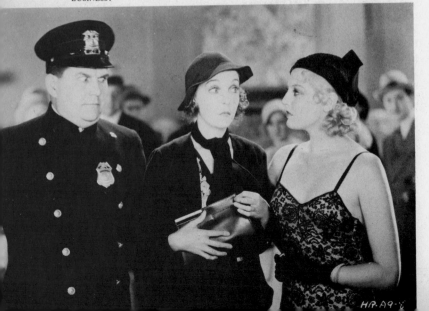

fight scenes take place at a real arena, with a full audience, and the results are gratifying. Neilan also uses a traveling camera, a rarity in Roach comedies. The film itself is quite simple, with ZaSu and Thelma playing switchboard operators in a hotel. Fighter Williams is tired of city life and wants to give up boxing, but his manager (Howes) is trying to dissuade him. Williams perks up when he meets ZaSu and discovers they are both from the same part of the Midwest. As he gets to like her, he renews his interest in fighting the championship bout that night. He buys ZaSu a hat and tells her to wear it to the fight so he will spot her in the crowd. An angry spectator sitting behind her tries to get ZaSu to remove the hat, but she refuses. He finally grabs it and tosses it away, causing a confusing chain reaction as ZaSu clambers over several rows to retrieve the bonnet. She finally does, catches Guinn's attention, and he wins the fight. The comedy is simple, and the sincere performances put it over. The emphasis is on ZaSu, rather than Thelma, as she sighs for the carefree life of Joplin, Missouri, and later engages in a wild battle to retrieve her hat.

The next short in the series went in a different direction, with equally pleasing results. THE PAJAMA PARTY has Thelma and ZaSu driving down to Long Beach to meet their boyfriends (including popular singer Donald Novis) when a reckless driver causes them to run off the road into a lake. The driver, a wealthy society matron, insists that they return to her home, a luxurious mansion. She gives each girl a French maid and has them stay for a party that evening. Everything goes wrong from the start—Thelma falls into a sunken bathtub with her clothes on, and ZaSu misunderstands a party prank later that evening. She has been told to observe the guests and do as they do; when she joins the party, the society guests are wishing one of their friends a happy birthday by kicking him. The hostess has the last turn, and cheerfully cries, "One to grow on!" as she goes through her paces. For the rest of the evening, ZaSu, wanting to seem natural, kicks various guests in the derrière, pushing several of them into the pool, smilingly adding, "One to grow on" as she follows through.

Eight different directors worked on the Pitts-Todd shorts, with extremely variable results. After these first successes, the comedies became unpredictable. Some of them were quite good, while others were very, very weak. There was no consistency, and apparently no successful formula to follow. Marshall Neilan, who had made the team's second

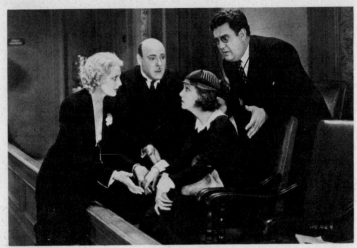

ZaSu has swallowed a bomb; Thelma, James C. Morton and Billy Gilbert
don't know what to do. From SNEAK EASILY.

short, tried again with WAR MAMAS, but the results were
only fair. As WAC's during World War I, the girls' best gag
was ZaSu's salute—a combination of regulation Army greeting and ZaSu's own special hand-flutter. SEALSKINS had two
directors, but neither could make the short anything more
than passable. And so it went, for the next two years—a
charming short would be followed by a dog.

In 1932 George Marshall started directing the Pitts-Todd
shorts, and tried a different approach. The Roach publicity
for the series read thusly: "ZaSu Pitts, the girl whose comedy steals the feature from the stars, and Thelma Todd, the
ravishing blonde fun-maker who makes men wish they were
in the movies too. ZaSu, a bit of dumb, forlorn helplessness
is the perfect foil for the brilliant, dynamic Thelma. Pals, but
what a pair! Their adventures together constitute a grand,
new comedy series and, as well, another glowing chapter
among the achievements of the Hal Roach Studios. Truly,
the Laurel and Hardy of comediennes." Director Marshall
took the publicity literally and decided to give ZaSu and
Thelma a Laurel and Hardy look by having them do physical, knockabout comedy. His films with the girls—STRICTLY
UNRELIABLE, THE OLD BULL, ALUM AND EVE, and THE SOIL-
ERS—consist mainly of ZaSu getting stuck in something or
other, and Thelma trying to bail her out. This type of humor
really doesn't suit Pitts and Todd, and simply isn't funny.

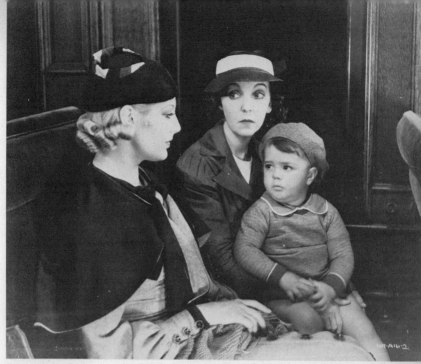

Little Spanky McFarland is left in the care of Thelma and ZaSu in ONE TRACK MINDS.

Billy Gilbert doesn't know what he's in for when he collects the girls' tickets in ONE TRACK MIND.

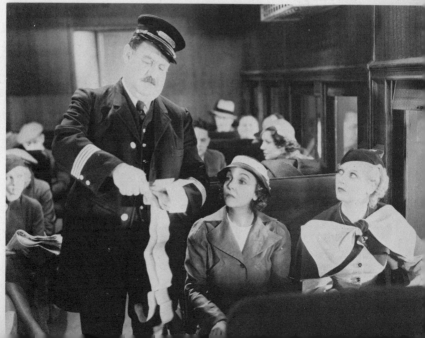

With Laurel and Hardy in the same situations, it might be hilarious, but when ZaSu gets stuck in a hospital cart in ALUM AND EVE, and Thelma, a cop, and two male orderlies become intertwined, the impact is nil.

When Gus Meins took over the series in 1933, he found a better formula for the girls—situation comedy with slapstick undertones. Thus, in SNEAK EASILY, juror ZaSu swallows the evidence at the trial of a mad scientist—a time bomb that's liable to go off any minute! A wild scramble follows to get ZaSu to the scientist's laboratory so he can deliver an antidote. Thelma, attorney Billy Gilbert, and judge James Morton tie pillows to her feet, and try to ease her down the courthouse steps into an ambulance. When ZaSu trips and looks as if she's going to fall over, an assembled crowd gasps and runs off in all directions. In the end, it turns out the scientist was bluffing all along, and the bomb was never made. ASLEEP IN THE FEET is one of the girls' most delightful shorts, with ZaSu and Thelma taking temporary jobs as dancers in Billy Gilbert's dime-a-dance emporium to earn enough money to keep a neighbor from being evicted. Thelma is very popular, but nobody dances with ZaSu except the

A tug-of-war for bedsheets at a bargain sale, with ZaSu, Thelma and James Burtis; from THE BARGAIN OF THE CENTURY.

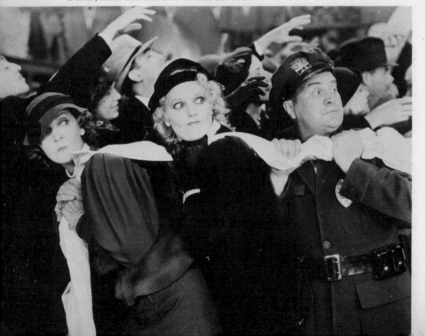

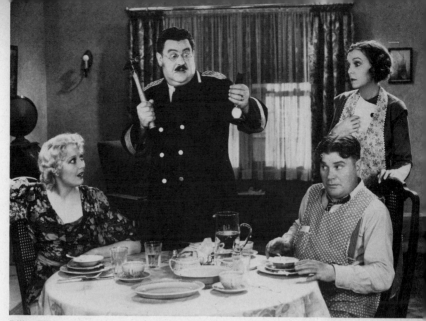

Billy Gilbert goes berserk after James Burtis has broken his watch in THE BARGAIN OF THE CENTURY.

oddballs who can't find any other partners. One of the veterans in the establishment (Anita Garvin) decides to jazz ZaSu up and teach her how to be a sexpot. The results are hilarious as ZaSu plays siren just when proprietor Gilbert is trying to convince some visiting inspectors that he runs a sedate, respectable place.

In mid-1933, the girls did their best short, with the help of Roach's all-purpose comedian, Billy Gilbert, and the direction of one of his top comedians, Charley Chase. Chase's know-how, and some liberal borrowing from his backlog of material, produced a hilarious short called THE BARGAIN OF THE CENTURY. In it, the girls are rushing to a big sale when a cop flags them down; he follows them to the store and is persuaded to help them push through the violent crowd and obtain three bedsheets. When the ruckus dies down, the girls have their sheets, but the bedraggled cop is spotted by his lieutenant and fired. The ex-officer (James Burtis) moves in with the girls and creates havoc in their apartment with his nutty inventions. ZaSu goes downstairs to get some groceries and runs into Billy Gilbert, whom she thinks is the police captain who can restore Burtis' job. Gilbert, a bogus policeman with a hilarious German accent, comes up to the girls' apartment, where they try to win him over. Everything goes haywire when Burtis tries to do a trick with Gilbert's watch, which somehow ends up falling into an ice-cream

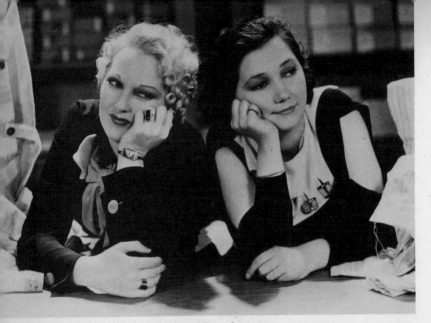

A lovely shot of Thelma and Patsy from BABES IN THE GOODS.

batter ZaSu is preparing. When the dessert is served, the girls keep spotting pieces of the watch in their dishes, and try to cover up Gilbert's bowl so he won't discover the damage. He finally does, and goes crazy, attacking every timepiece in the apartment with a hammer until the real cops arrive and take him away.

Throughout their sixteen shorts, there was never any doubt that ZaSu Pitts and Thelma Todd were both fine comediennes. They had first-rate support from such comic experts as Billy Gilbert, Anita Garvin, Sterling Holloway, little Spanky McFarland and most of the Hal Roach stock company. But the material was often quite weak, and even top-notch people couldn't overcome it. The girls were always a delight, but their shorts took some patience to stomach. In mid-1933, ZaSu Pitts left the Hal Roach studio for bigger and better things (returning twenty years later as comedy foil on TV's *Gale Storm Show*). Thelma Todd was also going to leave, but Roach liked her, and the shorts were, in spite of everything, quite popular. He made it worth her while to remain with a lucrative contract, and for a new teammate, he hired Patsy Kelly.

Patsy Kelly was born in 1910, the youngest child of two Irish immigrants who had come to New York at the turn of the century. Patsy showed great dexterity at an early age, and was a prize pupil at a New York dancing school, along with another girl named Ruby Keeler. Patsy was so good that while still in her teens she was made a dance instructress, coaching younger children and working with her brother, who had show-business aspirations. The story goes that she was working with him backstage one day when comedian Frank Fay saw her and hired her on the spot, ignoring her brother. Working with Fay was unpredictable, but good training for the novice, and within a few years Patsy was a featured player in such Broadway hits as *Three Cheers*, with Will Rogers, *Earl Carroll's Sketch Book* and *Earl Carroll's Vanities*. By the time of *Wonder Bar* with Al Jolson and *Flying Colors* with Clifton Webb, the young Miss Kelly was receiving star billing. She appeared on a Vitaphone short in 1931, as did many Broadway performers, but it was Hal Roach who brought Patsy to Hollywood in 1933 and gave her a start in movies. Once she teamed with Thelma Todd, she was in great demand and added her Irish sparkle to many feature films, usually playing the leading lady's wisecracking friend.

Loud-mouthed, dynamic Patsy was a perfect partner for poised, charming Thelma, and their first shorts indicated that they would be dynamite together. Their films as a whole

The girls escort screwy inventor Don Barclay aboard a plane in this scene from AIR FRIGHT.

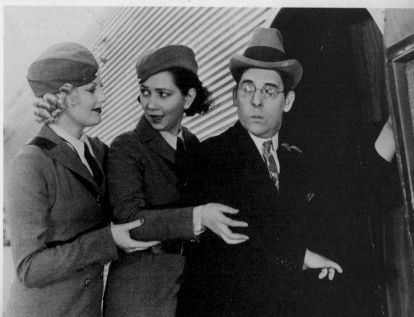

were better than the Pitts-Todd shorts, but once again it was
a case of the stars making material seem better than it was.
Nevertheless, the Todd-Kelly shorts were slickly made, entertaining little comedies, with the duo as working girls
trying to get ahead, but somehow always winding up behind
the eight ball. Their first film together, BEAUTY AND THE
BUS, has the girls winning a car at a movie raffle, and
through a chain of events, causing a mammoth traffic jam.
At one point Patsy tries to stop a burly truck dirver ("Tiny"
Sandford) from doing any damage, and addresses him as
"King Kong." BACK TO NATURE, their second film, has the
girls spending their vacation out in God's Country, where
Thelma yearns for peace and quiet as Patsy manages to do
everything wrong (she chops down a tree that collapses their
tent, takes aim on a rabbit but shoots a hole in their coffee-
pot instead, etc.). AIR FRIGHT is one of their better efforts,
with the girls as stewardesses on an experimental flight where
inventor Don Barclay is going to demonstrate his special
ejection seats. Before the flight is over, everyone has fallen
from the plane, with parachutes attached to their flying
seats.

BABES IN THE GOODS is an amusing outing with the girls
working as salesgirls in the women's wear section of a department store. One obnoxious customer gives them an awful time as she makes them pull out every nightgown they

Billy Gilbert, visiting royalty, is enchanted with Thelma in SOUP AND FISH.

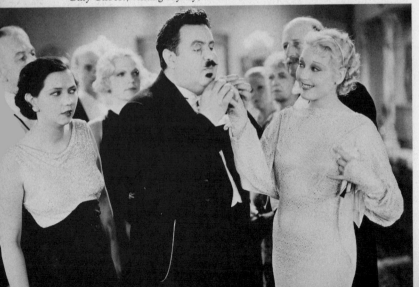

have in stock. "Will the colors run?" she asks about one nightie; "Not till they see you in it," Patsy replies under her breath. Thelma turns to the Amazonian lady and suggests something in battleship gray. Finally their workday is over, and they prepare to leave, when the store manager (Jack Barty) tells them to take over for the two girls who demonstrate a dishwasher in the store window. He leaves them there and instructs them to keep demonstrating the machine as long as they have an audience on the sidewalk. One of movies' most delightful drunks, Arthur Housman, stumbles by at this point and becomes intrigued with the girls; he stays all night to watch them as they wearily go through the motions of washing dishes and showing the convenience of the new machine. At midnight the blinds automatically descend in the windows and the girls are saved—except that they are locked in and can't leave the window showcase! They decide to make the best of the situation by sleeping in the bed in the next portion of the showcase, hoping to wake up early before the store opens the next day. Unfortunately, the blinds open automatically early the next morning, and from inside the window we see none other than drunken

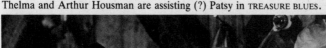

Thelma and Arthur Housman are assisting (?) Patsy in TREASURE BLUES.

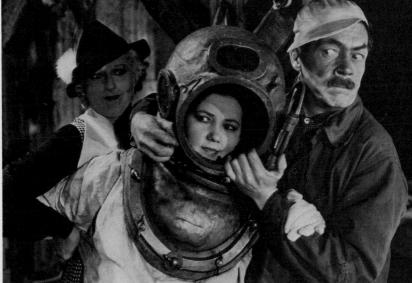

Housman, who's been sitting on a fire hydrant all night waiting to catch a glimpse of the scantily clad girls in the window display. The girls are caught in an embarrassing position, and grab the bed's blankets to cover themselves. The manager arrives for the day and fires the girls, telling them to drop their blankets and leave. The girls obey orders, and the gathered crowd of males outside cheers as the girls unveil themselves and walk out for good.

Other entertaining shorts in the series include I'LL BE SUING YOU, with shyster lawyer Eddie Foy, Jr. trying to collect damages for the girls when they have a near-accident. Patsy has to pretend to have a broken leg, but the scheme backfires when the insurance inspectors come to get a good look at the injured limb. In ONE HORSE FARMERS, a huckster corners the girls on a crowded New York subway car and interests them in a little farm out in the country. "Heaven on Earth." he proclaims, and Patsy falls for it hook, line and sinker. They arrive at their little paradise only to find it one huge sandtrap, with sand pouring out of every corner, flooding every room of the house. A storm brews during their first night in the house, and helpless neighbors come to the girls' place for shelter. By the next morning the house is filled with several dozen neighbors, all milling about as the girls lose a good night's sleep. All Thelma can say is, "So this is Heaven!" In TREASURE BLUES, Patsy's uncle, Salty Harbour (shown in a photo to be James Finlayson) leaves her a full line of sea-diving equipment and a valuable treasure map. The girls, with their friend Arthur Housman, decide to give the map a whirl, and go out to sea. The best gag comes when Housman goes underwater and finds a case of "Old Gold" liquor; the girls think he's found the precious ore, but Housman is even happier with his discovery of the booze.

In THE MISSES STOOGE the girls end up as stooges for magician Herman Bing, with predictably disastrous consequences. Bing does at least one trick too well, and in levitating Thelma, sends her flying out of the house and off into the night. Patsy follows her and finally brings her back, tugging her into the house with a rope tied to her feet as she floats on air. SLIGHTLY STATIC gives Patsy a chance to show the fine footwork that got her started on Broadway, as she and Thelma try to crash radio station LOCO. This film features several musical acts in addition to Thelma and Patsy. One group is The Sons of the Pioneers, with its lead singer a young man later known as Roy Rogers. TWIN TRIPLETS has Thelma an enterprising newspaper reporter who goes to a

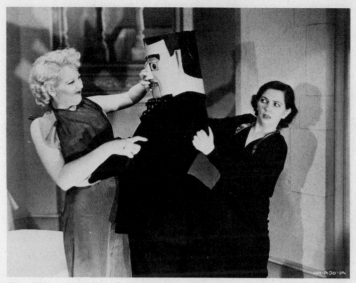

The girls battle a robot whose orders are to destroy every woman in his path, in THE TIN MAN.

maternity hospital and misunderstands a nurse's message. She is positive that a German woman in one room has had six babies. Patsy goes in to get the facts from the woman, and engages in a hilarious round of double-talk as the woman is asked if she had six babies and replies "Nein." "Well, which is it, nine or six?" Patsy asks in amazement. Thelma sets up a photo session, and is ready to be promoted for scooping every paper in town on this event, when Patsy discovers that the woman has only had twins. She scurries about the hospital to find four more babies to pose in the newspaper picture, and after many mishaps, lines everything up. Thelma's raise is in the bag until closer inspection reveals that one of the babies is black. No explaining can get the girls out of this one, and the jig is up.

One of the girls' last shorts is one of their best: TOP FLAT (the title, like most of short subjects, is a spoof of a then-current movie, TOP HAT). Thelma is a dreamy-eyed poet, reciting nonsensical verse that doesn't sell, and driving Patsy crazy. The two decide to split up, and Thelma predicts that she'll soon be living on Park Avenue. Within a few weeks, she is—as a French maid to a wealthy society couple. Patsy sees her being driven in a limousine one day (she's just on

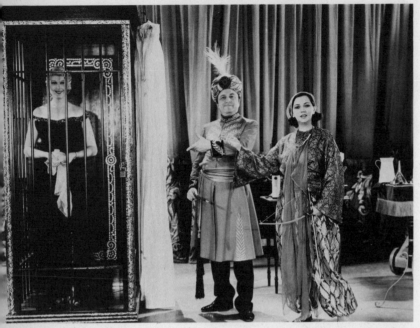

Presto! Magician Herman Bing and assistant Patsy are about to perform some sort of feat involving Thelma, in THE MISSES STOOGE.

an errand for her employer) and thinks Thelma has hit it big. That night she comes to visit her at the penthouse with two rowdy friends—Fuzzy Knight and Gary Owen. The owners are away for the evening, but when the boys start cavorting at the piano, there are complaints from downstairs, and Thelma gets worried. She tries to explain to Patsy that she doesn't own the penthouse, but Patsy won't listen. She's too busy eyeing the luxurious apartment, especially the elegant bathroom. Meanwhile, Fuzzy and Gary are having fun dropping water bombs on well-dressed pedestrians on the sidewalk below (they hit a young couple in the middle of a kiss, but the lovers don't bat an eyelash). When they douse a cop, the trouble begins. The apartment owners come home, and Thelma tries to hide her friends. Patsy's clothes are accidentally thrown down a laundry chute, and as she seeks some other covering, she jumps into one of the beds. The man of the house (Ferdinand Munier) thinks it is Thelma looking for some fun, and tells her to leave. Patsy escapes unnoticed, but then Munier's real wife (Grace Goodall) comes in and goes to sleep. Munier returns, sees the figure in bed, and thinks it is Thelma again. He tells her that they'll go out the next night and "make whoopee." When the wife hears this she explodes and chases her husband through the apartment, anxious to clobber him. With that diversion, the girls grab the two fun-loving boyfriends and race out of the penthouse. TOP FLAT is a delight from start to finish, with Thelma looking more beautiful than ever, and Patsy particularly amusing as she eyes her girl friend's lavish apartment.

Not long after the release of that two-reel comedy, Thelma Todd was dead. Friends worried when she didn't appear at a party one Saturday night in 1935. The next day a maid found her slumped over in the seat of her car, parked in the garage, where she had died of carbon monoxide poisoning. A long and involved investigation followed, but it was never determined if the death was murder, suicide or an accident. The tragedy was not *how* it happened, but that it *had* happened, cutting down the life of a thirty-year-old actress at the peak of her beauty and at a highpoint in her career.

Hal Roach was obligated to give theater exhibitors three

When Patsy goes to meet Lyda Roberti, she tangles with immigration inspector Robert Emmet O'Connor in AT SEA ASHORE.

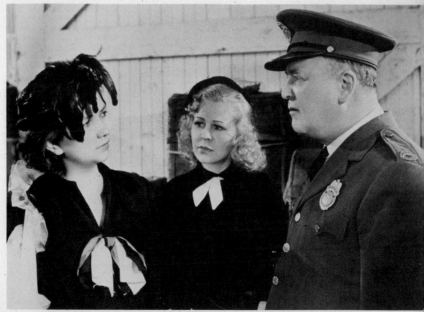

more Todd-Kelly shorts on his release schedule for 1936. Actress Pert Kelton, a deft and versatile comedienne, was recruited as Patsy Kelly's partner for the first short, PAN HANDLERS. Unfortunately, the script was not tailored for her, and she acted as little more than straight man for the amusing antics of her partner. Miss Kelton had been on the Roach lot for Patsy's feature film, KELLY THE SECOND, and seemed a logical choice for a partner, but PAN HANDLERS was her first and last film with Patsy. Roach's next idea was to use the bombastic musical-comedy star Lyda Roberti, who had achieved success in musicals for Paramount Pictures during the 1930's. A two-reeler, AT SEA ASHORE, was tailor-made for her, and gave her a chance to sing "Sweet and Hot" and dance to "Broadway Rhythm" as sung by the Avalon Four (including young Chill Wills). The short also gave Patsy a chance to go through her paces as she comes to meet immigrant Lyda at the dock and hides out from an irate cabdriver in the immigration section of the dock. Inspector Robert Emmet O'Connor won't let Patsy through without a passport, and refuses to believe that she's an American who only came down to meet a friend. Patsy tries to hide in Lyda's trunk, which then gets tossed about by various porters. AT SEA ASHORE is very pleasant, and a good introduction to Lyda Roberti. The duo's second short together, HILL TILLIES, is a weak follow-up, with the girls "roughing it" in the woods for ten days as a publicity stunt, and ending up crazy when they are forced to spend their time with a hallucination-haunted hermit. The short has no music, and practically no laughs.

Patsy and Lyda went on to co-star in the pleasant feature film NOBODY'S BABY, one of a series of comedies that Hal Roach produced with his various stars when he decided that the era of short subjects was over. Interest in Patsy and Lyda was not strong enough to keep them together, however, and they went their separate ways. A year after their last film's release, Lyda Roberti was dead of a heart attack, at age twenty-nine.

Patsy Kelly stayed with Hal Roach, appearing in feature films for the producer through the early 1940's. In a strange coincidence, she was teamed with ZaSu Pitts, after a fashion, in a 1941 feature, BROADWAY LIMITED. She and ZaSu had worked together in a cross-country personal-appearance tour several years earlier, and worked well together in the Roach film. Almost twenty years later, Patsy Kelly announced that she and ZaSu were planning to team together in a new TV series. "What television needs is two old biddies hanging over a back fence," she explained. "ZaSu and I would make a great team now. We're old friends and anxious to put the show on the road. ZaSu and I would play it for sight gags, too, and that doesn't especially mean the old pie-in-the-face routines." Unfortunately, the series never came to fruition (ZaSu Pitts died in 1963); it would have been fun to have these old comedy pros working together, but more than that, it would have been a much-needed boost for the sagging career of Miss Kelly.

After doing DANGER—WOMEN AT WORK in 1943, Patsy left movies for some time, returning only for an occasional bit or a short subject. She was active in radio, summer stock and even on Broadway during the 1940's and early 1950's, but by the end of that decade, she was living in semiretirement. A featured role as a maid in PLEASE DON'T EAT THE DAISIES (1960) started things rolling again, and Patsy found occasional work in features and TV shows like *Valentine's Day*. She even did a TV pilot film that was shown as a one-shot special when it failed to develop into a series. Nothing dimmed the lady's cheerfulness, and sharp sense of humor, and her minor role in ROSEMARY'S BABY (1968) as one of the witches was noticed by many moviegoers who recalled Patsy's heyday in the 1930's and 40's.

Patsy Kelly and ZaSu Pitts, who both co-starred with Thelma Todd in two-reelers, were paired in a 1941 feature film, BROADWAY LIMITED, with Victor McLaglen. Hal Roach produced the film.

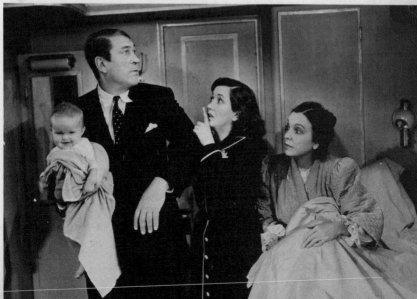

Patsy made some other film and TV appearances, but her career hit high gear again on Broadway, where she joined her old friend Ruby Keeler for a revival of *No, No, Nanette* in 1971. The show was a tremendous hit, and Patsy won a Tony Award for her delightful comic performance. She followed up with a similar supporting role in *Irene* with Debbie Reynolds. Interviewed about her days on the Hal Roach lot, she said, "We all had such a good time I didn't feel right taking the money. It was just a ball all the time. Mr. Roach was a wonderful man; kind, considerate. The best boss I've ever had, and I've had quite a few." She bemoaned the demise of the two-reeler, but explained, "The double feature was the end of short subjects, so Mr. Roach had to start making features. I enjoyed the short comedies much more." And of her long-ago partner Thelma Todd, Patsy said, "She was a wonderful person; beautiful, talented, delightful. There aren't enough adjectives to describe her, God bless her."

Lucille Ball took the art of slapstick into the television era, and Carol Burnett carried on the tradition, mastering the fine art of physical comedy. They may have had better material than Thelma Todd, ZaSu Pitts, and Patsy Kelly— but no one ever had more talent, verve, or sheer comic know-how than these three gifted women.

The Thelma Todd-ZaSu Pitts Shorts

All the following films are two-reelers, except #1, and all were produced by Hal Roach for MGM release. Director's name follows year.

1. **Let's Do Things**—1931—Hal Roach—Donald Novis, Bill Elliott, Mary Kornman, Mickey Daniels, David Sharpe, Gertrude Messinger, Dorothy Granger, Maurice Black, Jerry Mandy, Harry Bernard, Charlie Hall, Eddie Dillon. Three reels.
2. **Catch As Catch Can**—1931—Marshall Neilan—Guinn "Big Boy" Williams, Reed Howes, Billy Gilbert.
3. **The Pajama Party**—1931—Hal Roach—Elizabeth Forrester, Eddie Dunn, Donald Novis, Billy Gilbert, Lucien Prival, Charlie Hall.
4. **War Mamas**—1931—Marshall Neilan—Charles Judels,

Allan Lane, Guinn "Big Boy" Williams, Stuart Holmes,
Carrie Daumery, Harry Schultz, Charlie Hall.

5. **Seal Skins**—1932—Gil Pratt, Morey Lightfoot—Charlie
Hall, Leo Willis, Billy Gilbert.

6. **On the Loose**—1932—Hal Roach—John Loder, Claud
Allister, Billy Gilbert, (billed as William Gilbert in this
short); guest stars Laurel and Hardy.

7. **Red Noses**—1932—James W. Horne—Blanche Payson,
Wilfred Lucas, Billy Gilbert.

8. **Strictly Unreliable**—1932—George Marshall—Billy Gilbert, Charlie Hall, Charlotte Nemo, Bud Jamison,
Symona Boniface.

9. **The Old Bull**—1932—George Marshall—Otto Fries, Robert Burns.

10. **Show Business**—1932—Jules White—Anita Garvin,
Monty Collins, Charlie Hall.

11. **Alum and Eve**—1932—George Marshall—James C. Morton, Almeda Fowler.

12. **The Soilers**—1932—George Marshall—Bud Jamison,
James C. Morton, Charlie Hall, George Marshall (in a
bit role).

13. **Sneak Easily**—1933—Gus Meins—Robert Burns, James
C. Morton, Billy Gilbert, Rolfe Sedan, Harry Bernard,
Charlie Hall.

14. **Asleep in the Feet**—1933—Gus Meins—Billy Gilbert,
Eddie Dunn, Anita Garvin.

15. **Maids a la Mode**—1933—Gus Meins—Billy Gilbert, Harry
Bernard, Kay Deslys, Charlie Hall.

16. **Bargain of the Century**—1933—Charley Chase—Billy
Gilbert, James Burtis, Harry Bernard.

17. **One Track Minds**—1933—Gus Meins—Billy Gilbert,
Lucien Prival, Jack Clifford, Sterling Holloway, Charlie
Hall, Spanky McFarland.

The Thelma Todd-Patsy Kelly Shorts

All the following films are two-reelers. Director's name follows year.

1. **Beauty and the Bus**—1933—Gus Meins—Dan Barclay,
Charlie Hall, Tiny Sandford, Tommy Bond, Eddie Baker,
Ernie Alexander, Robert McKenzie.

2. **Backs to Nature**—1933—Gus Meins—Don Barclay, Charlie Hall.
3. **Air Fright**—1933—Gus Meins—Don Barclay, Billy Bletcher, Charlie Hall.
4. **Babes in the Goods**—1934—Gus Meins—Jack Barty, Arthur Housman, Charlie Hall, Fay Holderness.
5. **Soup and Fish**—1934—Gus Meins—Gladys Gale, Billy Gilbert, Don Barclay, Charlie Hall.
6. **Maid in Hollywood**—1934—Gus Meins—Eddie Foy, Jr., Don Barclay, Alphonse Martell, Charlie Hall, James C. Morton, Charles Rogers, Billy Bletcher, Ted Stroback, Carlton E. Griffin, Constance Bergen, Jack Barty, Billy Nelson.
7. **I'll Be Suing You**—1934—Gus Meins—Eddie Foy, Jr., Douglas Wakefield, Billy Nelson, Benny Baker, Charles Rogers, Charles McAvoy, William Wagner, Fred Kelsey.
8. **Three Chumps Ahead**—1934—Gus Meins—Benny Baker, Frank Moran, Eddie Phillips, Harry Bernard.
9. **One Horse Farmers**—1934—Gus Meins—James Morton, Charlie Hall.
10. **Opened by Mistake**—1934—James Parrott—William Burress, Nora Cecil, Fanny Cossar, Charlie Hall, Ronald Rondell, Allen Caven, James Eagles, Rose Plummer, Virginia Crawford, Mary Egan, Robert McKenzie.
11. **Done in Oil**—1934—Gus Meins—Arthur Housman, Eddy Conrad, Leo White, William Wagner, Rolfe Sedan.
12. **Bum Voyage**—1934—Nick Grinde—Adrian Rosley, Constant Franke, Albert Petit, Germaine De Neel, Francis Sayles, Noah Young, Charles Gemora.
13. **Treasure Blues**—1935—James Parrott—Sam Adams, Arthur Housman, Tiny Sandford, Charlie Hall; photo of James Finlayson used.
14. **Sing, Sister, Sing**—1935—James Parrott—Arthur Housman, Harry Bowen, Charlie Hall, Barbara Webster.
15. **The Tin Man**—1935—James Parrott—Matthew Betz, Clarence Wilson.
16. **The Misses Stooge**—1935—James Parrott—Herman Bing, Esther Howard, Rafael Storm, Adrian Rosley, Harry Bayfield, Harry Bowen, Henry Roquemore, James C. Morton, Ward Shattuck.
17. **Slightly Static**—1935—William Terhune—Harold Waldrige, Dell Henderson, Ben Taggart, Louis Natheaux, Sydney de Grey, Eddie Craven, Kay Hughes, Aileen Carlyle, Dorothy Francis, Harry Bowen, Nora Cecil, Carlton E. Griffin, Bobby Burns, Elinor Van Der Veer,

Lorene Carr, Carl Le Viness, Brooks Benedict, Randall Sisters, The Vitaphone Four, Sons of the Pioneers (including Roy Rogers).

18. **Twin Triplets**—1935—William Terhune—John Dilson, Greta Meyer, Bess Flowers, Billy Bletcher, Charlie Hall.

19. **Hot Money**—1935—James W. Horne—James Burke, Fred Kelsey, Hooper Atchley, Louis Natheaux, Brooks Benedict, Charlie Hall, Sherry Hall, Anya Tiranda, Lee Prather, Lee Phelps, Monty Vandegrift.

20. **Top Flat**—1935—William Terhune and Jack Jevne— Grace Goodall, Fuzzy Knight, Ferdinand Munier, Gary Owen, Harry Bernard.

21. **All American Toothache**—1935—Gus Meins—Mickey Daniels, Johnny Arthur, Duke York, Dave Sharpe, Charlie Hall, Ben Hall, Bud Jamison, Billy Bletcher, Ernie Alexander, Ray Cooke, Si Jenks, Sue Gomes, Manny Vezie, Buddy Messinger.

After Thelma Todd's death, Patsy Kelly made three more shorts, the first one paired with Pert Kelton, the other two with Lyda Roberti:

1. **Pan Handlers**—1936—William Terhune—Grace Goodall, Rosina Lawrence, David Sharpe, Harry Bowen, Willie Fung, Larry Steers.

2. **Hill Tillies**—1936—Gus Meins—Toby Wing, Harry Bowen, Jim Thorpe, Sam Adams, James C. Morton.

3. **At Sea Ashore**—1936—William Terhune—Al Shean, Robert Emmet O'Connor, Joe Twerp, The Avalon Four (including Chill Wills), Harry Bowen, Fred Kelsey.

Patsy and Lyda Roberti also co-starred in the following feature film:

Nobody's Baby—Roach—MGM 1937—Gus Meins— Lynn Overman, Robert Armstrong, Rosina Lawrence, Don Alvarado, Tom Dugan, Si Wills, Dora Clement, Laura Treadwell, Tola Nesmith, Herbert Rawlinson, Florence Roberts, Chick Chandler, Jimmie Grier's Orchestra with the Rhythm Rascals, The Avalon Boys, Orrin Burke, Joan Woodbury. 65 minutes.

BURNS and ALLEN

Few comedy teams enjoyed the sustained popularity of Burns and Allen. George and Gracie started entertaining vaudeville audiences in 1922, and continued their successful careers through 1958, when Gracie retired from show business. Few entertainers were as well-loved, both by the public and show-business colleagues, as Burns and Allen. They worked hard, but always made it seem easy. Their format seldom varied, yet they always seemed fresh.

George Burns entered the world as Nathan Birnbaum in 1896, the youngest of twelve children living in a small apartment on the Lower East Side of New York. His father died when he was seven, but his mother, a warm, loving woman, lived to see her son a headliner at the Palace Theater some years later. George got his first taste of show business on the sidewalks outside his home, where organ-grinders were always on duty, and impromptu dancers performed for passersby. At the age of seven, he and three friends formed the Pee Wee Quartette, a makeshift but dedicated vocal group that worked on harmony with the local postman, and graduated to local amateur contests and jobs in nearby restaurants. The Quartette kept George busy, too busy to pay much attention to school. Although he officially attended school for several years, most of his time was spent rehearsing and taking in the show-business atmosphere wherever he could find it. As a young man, he set out to make entertaining his profession, and broke into vaudeville, doing anything and everything in order to get a week's pay. He was the "Company" of "Fry and Company," Williams of "Brown and Williams," Glide of "Goldie, Fields, and Glide," Links of "Burns and Links," and several dozen other names as the occasion saw fit. Burns accepted jobs with dog acts, dancing acts, skating acts, singing acts—in fact, any act that would have him. He changed his name weekly to suit the whims of booking agents, and also to fool theater managers who hadn't liked him under his old names.

Gracie Allen was born in San Francisco in 1906. Her father was an entertainer named Edward Allen, and she, too, had the show-business bug at an early age. Gracie worked with her sisters in an early vaudeville act which was later incorporated into "Larry Reilly and Company." A string of bad breaks kept her from achieving any real success, and she was considering a career as a secretary when a show-business friend introduced her to an ambitious young man named George Burns. Burns, at that time, was splitting up with his partner, Billy Lorraine, to do the only kind of routine he had not yet tried: a talking act. George liked Gracie and decided she would be a good foil for him in his new act.

Their first show was in Newark, New Jesery. The duo rehearsed for this opening until they knew the material perfectly. Gracie was the straight man, and George the comic, but, as George later recalled. "They laughed at all her questions and at none of my answers." Proud, but not so proud that he didn't want a successful act, George switched roles with Gracie, and the team clicked. Gracie's warmth and God-given gift of timing made her a hit with every audience. As they traveled around and tested out new material, they sharpened Gracie's character until the scatterbrained female who delighted audiences for the next thirty years emerged. Her charm was in her sincerity. The craziest things would come out of her mixed-up mind, but to her they made perfect sense. George knew when they had a good thing going, and he resigned himself to remaining the straight man of the act. Before long he was the funniest, sharpest straight man in show business.

The team's first routine, "Dizzy," was very successful, and got the team good bookings on a steady basis. Then George bought a new routine, "Lambchops," written by comedy veteran Al Boasberg. They worked it into their act gradually, but by the time they were playing before some influential bookers, it was first-rate material. George always credited the routine with getting them their first engagement at the vaudeville mecca, the Palace. After that Palace stint, Burns and Allen were headliners, and never again had to worry about uncertain delivery or untried material. They gathered fans wherever they went, and found to their amazement that material that hadn't gone over when they were struggling now was greeted with hearty laughter by audiences who were "with" them all the way. To top off their professional good fortune, George and Gracie were married in 1925.

In 1929, the team was about to sail for England when a last-minute offer arrived to do a one-reel movie short at Warner Brothers' New York studio. They accepted the offer; the money was too good to resist. They performed their act much as they did on the stage, collected their salary, and sailed the next day. Burns and Allen were as big a hit in England as they were in America, and received an offer from the BBC to do a radio series while they were there. They made their radio debut with a 26-week program over the BBC in 1930, and took to the medium with ease. This experience came in handy upon their return to the States, when they were sought for guest appearances on many top radio shows. Something else happened while they were in England: Paramount Pictures started hiring top Broadway and vaudeville stars to do one-reel and two-reel shorts for them. Rudy Vallee, Jack Benny, Eddie Cantor, and many other headliners appeared in the Paramount shorts. When George and Gracie returned from abroad, the studio signed them for a series of one-reelers that established the comedy duo in motion pictures.

George wrote most of the Paramount shorts, which ran nine or ten minutes each. They were filmed quickly in the Paramount studios in Astoria, Long Island, and featured New York-based actors in supporting roles. Such people as

Gracie is WALKING THE BABY in the Paramount short of the same name. Greeting her are Chester Clute and George Burns.

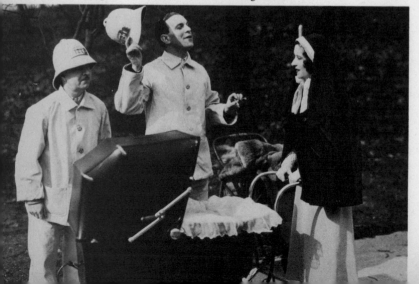

Barton MacLane, Chester Clute and Donald MacBride, all of whom were to become top Hollywood character actors, were drafted for the Burns and Allen series. The one-reelers were ideal vehicles for the comedy team, for they were working much as they did in vaudeville, with brief, amusing vignettes that required no plot or "production" to put them over. The situations were naturals for the verbal exchanges the two specialized in: George as a patient, Gracie as his nurse; George as a man in a barbershop, Gracie as his manicurist; George as a sailor on leave, Gracie as a taxi dancer in a dance hall, and so on. This was pure, undiluted Burns and Allen, and their fans loved it. As with many other entertainers, the shorts also served to make the team familiar to people around the country who had not seen their act on the stage.

Radio also contributed to George and Gracie's growing popularity. After some initial guest appearances, they became regulars on the weekly Guy Lombardo show, where they remained for two years. When Lombardo was signed by another network, Burns and Allen remained in the same time slot and starred in their own show. By 1932 they were prominent enough to rate featured roles in Paramount's all-star feature THE BIG BROADCAST, which starred Bing Crosby, Stu Erwin and Leila Hyams, and featured a host of top radio stars (Kate Smith, The Mills Brothers, Cab Calloway, Arthur Tracy, etc.). George (billed as George N. Burns) appears as the owner of radio station WADX, which will disband unless he can convince Bing Crosby to mend his ways and show up on time for every program. It's actually a straight role, and only after several reels does he come into contact with his new receptionist, Gracie. As he worries about the station, Gracie starts to babble about her younger brother, who is playing on the Sing Sing baseball team, and another brother who is on the San Quentin team ("He's just working his way through," she explains). When George expresses surprise at this situation, Gracie replies, "Well, you can just imagine how my father feels, sitting in a strait-jacket in the stands!"

The following year, George and Gracie were called back to the studio to do another feature, again with a top-name cast, INTERNATIONAL HOUSE. The difference was that this time, despite the many guest stars, the comedy duo dominated the first half of the film virtually by themselves, and only bowed out to allow W. C. Fields the run of the second half. In INTERNATIONAL HOUSE, George is the house physi-

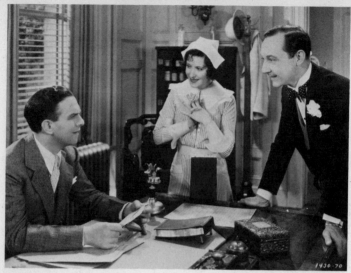

George and Franklin Pangborn do their best to make sense out of Gracie in
INTERNATIONAL HOUSE.

cian in a posh Oriental hotel, and Gracie is his nurse-
receptionist. In one scene, hotel manager Franklin Pangborn
drops in on the doctor's office, and the two men conduct a
hilarious question-and-answer session with Gracie. Here it is,
in part:

Burns: I've got a good mind to get a different nurse.
Pangborn: No no, doctor, don't do that—this one is
                different enough.
Burns: Well then, you talk to her.
Pangborn: (To Gracie) You know, you're very smart.
                To what do you attribute your smartness?
Allen: Three things. First, my very good memory, and
             the other two things, I forgot.
Burns: Look, let me talk to her. (To Gracie) What the
             manager would like to know is, did you ever go
             to school?
Allen: Oh yes, I did.
Burns: Well, what school did you go to?
Allen: I'm not allowed to tell.
Burns: You're not allowed to tell?
Allen: The school pays me twenty-five dollars a week
             not to tell.
Burns: (To Pangborn) You take her.

Pangborn: This one is on the house. You know, something must have happened to you when you were a baby.

Allen: No, nothing happened to me, but something happened to my brother when he was a baby.

Pangborn: Oh, your brother?

Allen: Yes. My father took him for a stroll in the carriage, but when my father came back he had a different baby and a different carriage.

Pangborn: Different baby and a different carriage? What did your mother say?

Allen: Oh, she didn't say anything, because it was a better carriage!

This keeps up for quite some time, utilizing the best material the team ever had, including some jokes that became part of their classic repertoire (Gracie tells George her brother had his appendix out, which left a terrible scar on his neck. "Appendicitis is on the stomach," protests George. Gracie agrees, but her brother was so ticklish that they had to operate upon his neck). When W. C. Fields comes into the film, he quickly encounters Gracie, who irritates him with some of her ridiculous chatter. He turns to a companion, grating his teeth, and mutters, "What's the penalty for murder in China?"

Sheriff W.C. Fields suspects Charlie Ruggles and Mary Boland of being thieves; George and Gracie are no help whatsoever in SIX OF A KIND.

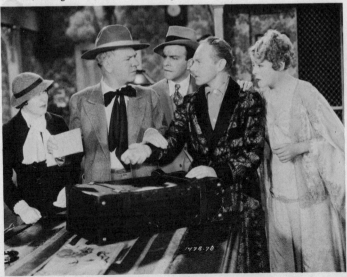

After INTERNATIONAL HOUSE, Paramount decided that
George and Gracie were too good to be "wasted" in shorts
and signed them to a feature-film contract. They appeared
first in COLLEGE HUMOR, a typical, enjoyable musical comedy with Bing Crosby, Jack Oakie and Richard Arlen, and a
host of good tunes like "Learn to Croon" and "Down the
Old Ox Road." The usual pattern in films like this, in which
Burns and Allen were featured, was to have George and
Gracie break into the story at regular intervals and go through
some of their usual dialogue. They were always fun, but this
formula wore thin from repeated use. SIX OF A KIND avoided
this by making the team part of the actual plot: A couple
(Charlie Ruggles and Mary Boland) about to leave on vacation
are cajoled into sharing expenses with another couple (Burns
and Allen) who proceed to drive them crazy. When they end
up in a strange, one-horse town, they encounter the local
sheriff—W. C. Fields—and his boisterous chickadee, Alison
Skipworth, who runs the local hotel. The comedy duo did not
look as if they had been arbitrarily inserted into this film; on
the other hand, the net effect was not good for another
reason: they were made to be so obnoxious the viewer lost
sympathy and interest within ten minutes of their introduction. Most of the time, Gracie's stupidity hurts no one; she
merely confuses things, and distracts people with her illogi-

A meeting of minds in COLLEGE HOLIDAY: George, Gracie, Jack Benny and
Etienne Girardot.

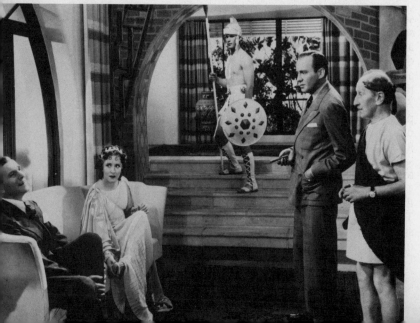

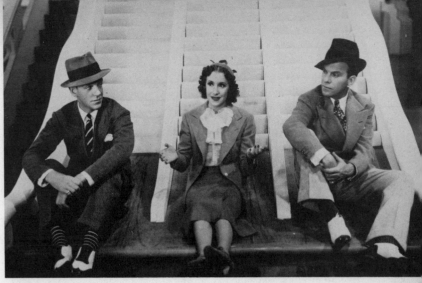

Astaire, Burns and Allen; not a likely trio on paper, but dynamite on film in
DAMSEL IN DISTRESS.

cal dialogue. In this film, however, she causes Charlie Ruggles
to fall off a cliff, and as he is dangling over a deep canyon,
holding onto a thin branch on the side of the cliff, she makes
jokes and tries to take his picture. Thus, before the film is
half over, Gracie becomes an annoying, unsympathetic character, and it is left to W. C. Fields, with his classic poolroom
routine, to salvage the film.

WE'RE NOT DRESSING was much better, a musical updating
of Barrie's *Admirable Crichton* with Carole Lombard and her
society friends shipwrecked on a lonely island, forced to
submit to the orders of lowly shipmate Bing Crosby. George
and Gracie are anthropologists on the island, with Gracie
doing her best to upset all of George's plans. There is an
amusing scene where Gracie starts talking about salt-water
taffy and George makes a play on words by calling her "daffy."
After this refreshing film, Paramount decided to put their
prize comedy team into a series of lesser pictures that did no
one, certainly not Burns and Allen, any good. MANY HAPPY
RETURNS, LOVE IN BLOOM, and HERE COMES COOKIE were
slickly made, but unimportant, films with little to offer, even
to devoted fans of George and Gracie.

Meanwhile, Burns and Allen were doing quite well with
their successful radio show, a consistent audience pleaser.
Their program was initiated with a monumental publicity
stunt of Gracie searching for her "lost brother." The gag not
only received prime coverage on their own show, but took
Gracie onto many other CBS programs, including daytime

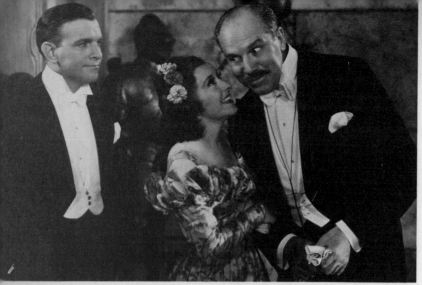

Gracie woos Montagu Love in a scene from DAMSEL IN DISTRESS.

George and Gracie keep up quite nicely with Fred Astaire in this dance routine from DAMSEL IN DISTRESS.

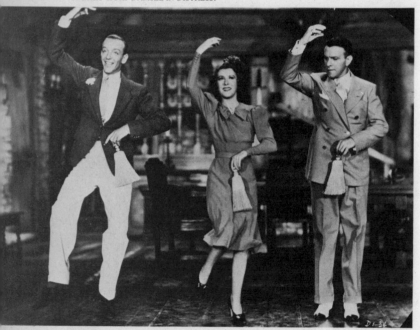

soap operas and other unrelated shows, where she would suddenly pop in to ask if her brother had been there. The stunt came to an end when she was signed for a guest appearance on Rudy Vallee's program on NBC and the network refused to carry over the rival network's publicity gimmick. The brother routine became one of Hollywood's legendary stunts, topped only by Gracie's campaign for the Presidency several years later. A cross-country train took Gracie from town to town, where she would make nonsensical speeches about American policies. As might be expected, election day saw several hundred write-in votes for Gracie on ballots around the country.

Back at Paramount things were at a standstill. Burns and Allen were always well featured in hodgepodges like THE BIG BROADCAST OF 1936 and THE BIG BROADCAST OF 1937, but it was very difficult to work up excitement for these standard appearances. It took a loan-out to RKO in 1937 to prove that Paramount had been wasting the team's potential for several years. RKO borrowed Burns and Allen for A DAMSEL IN DISTRESS, Fred Astaire's first film without Ginger Rogers in four years. Many industryites were worried about Astaire appearing without his usual partner, but the situation was met and conquered with the greatest of ease. Joan Fontaine had but to look pretty in her inconsequential scenes: Astaire had top-notch tunes like "A Foggy Day" and "Nice Work If You Can Get It," and then there were George and

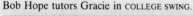

Bob Hope tutors Gracie in COLLEGE SWING.

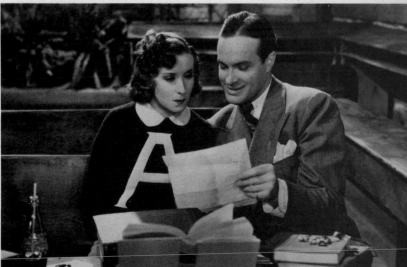

Gracie as Astaire's cronies. They provided a perfect balance to the music and romantic interludes of the film with their usual patter. In their opening scene, Gracie asks George what day it is. He tells her to look at the date on the newspaper sitting on her desk. Gracie tells him that would do no good—it's yesterday's paper. The highlight of the film is a fantastic song-and-dance production number that starts with a rhythmic repetition of the phrase "I've just begun to Live," and develops into an energetic dance routine with Burns and Allen proving themselves worthy colleagues of Mr. Astaire. George Burns recalled in later years that the whisk-broom dance, as he called it, had been a staple in a friend's vaudeville act for years. They contacted him and rehearsed the routine until they had it down pat, then went and showed it to Astaire, who loved the idea. The switch was that George and Gracie had to teach it to *him*. Both teachers and pupil came through with flying colors in the delightful scene that resulted. Without a doubt, it was Burns and Allen's shining moment on film.

When the team returned to Paramount, the studio fashioned an above-average vehicle for them, COLLEGE SWING, and even gave Gracie a chance to sing one straight song with Edward Everett Horton. The story revolves around Gracie, whose female ancestors have been flunking school for two hundred years. A pact signed two centuries ago provides that, if any girl in her family can pass through this college

Gracie looks as if she's about to tell George about one of her nutty relatives in this shot from COLLEGE SWING.

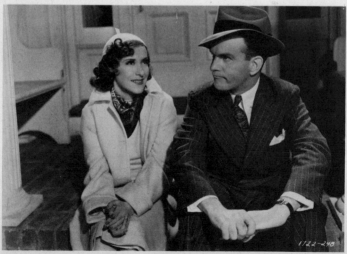

within the 200-year limit, the ownership of the school will be turned over to her. The film picks up the story in 1938, the 200th year, as Gracie hires wisecracking Bob Hope to tutor her so she can pass her final exam. The film is breezy and full of fine people like Hope and Martha Raye, and serves as a good showcase for Burns and Allen. Nevertheless, COL-LEGE SWING was the last film they made for Paramount. The following year they supported Eleanor Powell and Robert Young in HONOLULU at MGM, an innocuous and not espe-cially outstanding musical. That was their last film together.

In the late 1930's mystery author S. S. Van Dine wrote a special entry in his Philo Vance detective series called *The Gracie Allen Murder Case.* It was an offbeat, very entertain-ing mystery, with refreshing, humorous overtones. Para-mount decided to film it in 1939, but made a few changes, notably one eliminating George Burns from the story. It was Gracie's first solo film, but into the next decade she contin-ued to work on her own in such films as MR. AND MRS. NORTH, another mystery-comedy, and TWO GIRLS AND A SAILOR, in what was little more than a guest appearance.

By 1942, it was distressingly apparent that the ratings of the Burns and Allen radio show were not what they used to be. The team lost a long-time sponsor, and received another offer for a weekly show at much less money, out of which

Gracie feigns distraction while George works with his long-time writers John P. Medbury, Harvey Helm, and Willy Burns (who was also George's brother and manager).

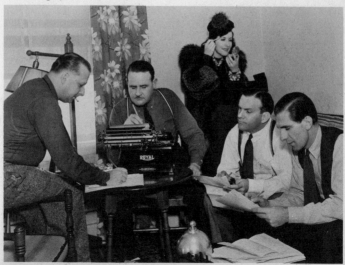

they had to hire writers, musicians and guest stars. They accepted, and made an important change that kept them up to date and rejuvenated their whole career: they changed their characters from boy and girl to husband and wife. George reasoned, accurately, that the public could no longer accept them as two young lovebirds, when it was well known that they were long-time married and the parents of two young children. The change was made, and the team's radio show remained a top airwaves attraction for many years. In 1949, Burns and Allen returned to England for the first time in eighteen years, playing the London Palladium. The response was overwhelming, with the team doing sure-fire material like Gracie's famous "Concerto for Index Finger."

When the couple returned to the U.S., they faced a new challenge: television. Other radio stalwarts held out into the early 1950's before taking a fling at the new medium, but Burns and Allen staked their claim in the fall of 1950 with a live show every other week. The response was excellent, and they were set for the rest of the decade. From the start the show created a charm all its own with such ideas as having George perform as a sort of Greek chorus, watching Gracie's antics from the sidelines and turning to the audience every once in a while to deliver a monologue. A carryover from

Gracie is taken by surprise by four imposters in HONOLULU; they are the vocal group the Kings Men (Rad Robinson, Ken Darby, Jon Dodson, Bud Linn).

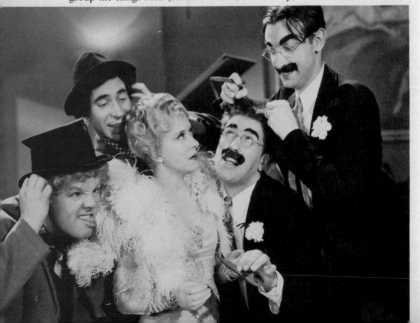

radio was to have the announcer, Bill Goodwin, work into the plot of the show. The program was a hit; two years later, George decided to start filming the show on a weekly basis. The format remained the same; Harry Von Zell replaced Bill Goodwin, Bea Benadaret continued to appear as neighbor Blanche Morton, and Fred Clark replaced Hal March as her husband Harry Morton. He in turn was replaced by Larry Keating, who held the role for the longest period.

Interviewed during their TV tenure, Gracie said, "We gave up making movies because we hated to get up at 6 A.M., we hated make-up, and we hated learning lines." "So now," added George, "we get up at 5 A.M., and work seven days a week. We shoot the television show, then come home and have to start learning the new script." The show remained high in popularity year after year, and Burns and Allen, being good troupers, weren't going to give up their ordeal and disappoint an anxious audience. The show became a well-oiled machine before long, hitting the bull's-eye almost every week and never growing tiresome. George

Burns and Allen on the air: George is carried away with his lines.

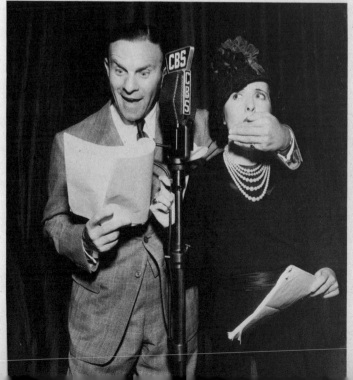

explained why the show remained popular for such a long time: "For one thing, Gracie and I aren't trying to get all the laughs. There are plenty for everybody. Ours is a relaxed show in what should be a relaxed medium. When a comedian works too hard, the audience has to work hard to follow him, and when an audience strains like that it gets indigestion. Give them a bad stomach and they don't tune in on you again . . . The format of our show is pretty simple. One character or another's got a problem. He gives it to Gracie and she runs away with it. It doesn't matter whether she ends up in the attic or across the street in a neighbor's kitchen. Gracie's got it and we let her carry it along and see what happens. I've got one rule, though. We never tell a big joke at the finish. If we've got a big point that rounds out the story, we go get it, but we don't end on it. We don't have to. The audience accepts us not as comedians but as

Gracie appeared without George in MR. AND MRS. NORTH, a mystery-comedy with Tom Conway and William Post, Jr.

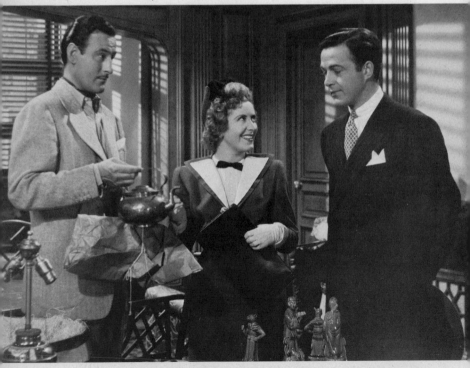

neighbors. They know all about us. We can fade out casually because we'll be back next week." The system worked like a charm, and Burns and Allen filmed an amazing total of 282 half-hour programs during their eight seasons on the air.

The program was a family affair, with son Ronnie Burns joining the cast in the mid-1950's, and George's brother, Willie Burns, participating as one of the show's four writers. The format remained the same throughout the show's history, but the jokes were kept up to date. One program took a hilarious swipe at TV westerns, with George watching a chase scene and explaining that it was an adult western— "Every Indian in that scene is over 21." In 1956 Gracie told columnist Harriet Van Horne, "Every year I think, 'Now we can retire. Now I can read a book in bed at night instead of a script.' Then George comes home and says, 'Well, they've picked up our option again, Googie,' and I know I'll have to go on reading scripts." Two years later Gracie reached the saturation point and decided to retire. The show was doing well, and could have continued indefinitely, but she had had enough, and wanted to be able to spend more time with her family. The announcement was important enough to rate a cover story in *Life*, on September 22, 1958. Six years later, on August 28, 1964, Gracie suffered a heart attack and died, with her husband at her side.

In George's words, "When Gracie retired in 1958 I started a new career for myself, which I'm doing right now. And in spite of public opinion to the contrary I still think I'm one of the great singers." That George's songs, and routines, were amusing came as no great surprise, but no one—certainly not Burns himself—could have predicted that he would embark on an acting career that would win him an Academy Award!

Many performers were considered for the film version of Neil Simon's play *The Sunshine Boys*, including Bob Hope, Red Skelton, and—at one point—George's close friend Jack Benny. Benny's death put an end to that plan, but the idea of George Burns was retained even after the producers decided to hire an actor, Walter Matthau, and not a comedian, to play the other half of a long-ago vaudeville team. Remember, except for occasional gag appearances George had been away from movies an awfully long time ("The last picture I did was in 1939, for MGM," he told me. "I must have made a good impression because here it is only thirty-six years later and they brought me back.") George turned in an excellent performance as the crusty,

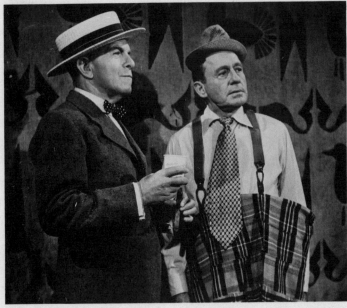

George and Jack Benny recreate some old burlesque routines on Jack's
TV show in 1963.

cranky show-biz retiree (and appeared sans toupee for the
first time in his career). Then, a few months after his eighti-
eth birthday he was voted the Oscar for Best Supporting
Actor, ushering in yet another phase of an already rich
career.

Since that time George has had the distinction of playing
the Almighty Himself in the popular movie OH, GOD! (as
well as two sequels), and brought his unpretentious charm to
even dreary vehicles like JUST YOU AND ME, KID, costarring
Brooke Shields. His best performance to date was as a feisty
senior citizen in the striking comedy-drama GOING IN STYLE,
which costarred Art Carney and Lee Strasberg.

But as far as his solo career has taken him, George Burns
has never missed an opportunity to recall his wife and
partner, Gracie Allen, and to explain that she was always
the one with the talent in their family. When we asked him,
for the first edition of *Movie Comedy Teams*, a series of
questions about his career with Gracie Allen, George provided one answer that summed everything up:

"In shorts, in features, in vaudeville, in radio, and in

television, Gracie and I loved all of it. Whatever we were doing we loved best at the time we were doing it. In short, we just loved show business." And the secret of their success was that people loved them in return.

The Burns and Allen Short Subjects

(All are one reel in length: director's name follows year.)

1. **Burns and Allen in Lambchops**—Warner Brothers—Vitaphone 1929.
2. **Fit to Be Tied**—Paramount 1930—Ray Cozine.
3. **Pulling a Bone**—Paramount 1930—Howard Bretherton.
4. **The Antique Shop**—Paramount 1931—Ray Cozine—Chester Clute, Hershall Mayall.
5. **Once Over, Light**—Paramount 1931—Howard Bretherton.
6. **One Hundred Percent Service**—Paramount 1931—Ray Cozine.
7. **Oh My Operation**—Paramount 1932—Ray Cozine.
8. **The Babbling Book**—Paramount 1932—Aubrey Scotto—Donald Meek, George Shelton, Chester Clute.
9. **Hollywood on Parade #2**—Paramount 1932—a Hollywood behind-the-scenes short with Bing Crosby, Stu Erwin, Gary Cooper and Olsen and Johnson.
10. **Let's Dance**—Paramount 1933—Aubrey Scotto—Barton MacLane.
11. **Walking the Baby**—Paramount 1933—Aubrey Scotto—Chester Clute.
12. **Hollywood on Parade #12**—Paramount 1933.
13. **Hollywood Grows Up**—Columbia 1954—Ralph Staub—A Screen Snapshots entry with Staub and Larry Simms (from the BLONDIE series) reviewing film clips from World War II, including routines by George and Gracie, and Abbott and Costello.
14. **Hollywood Fathers**—Columbia 1954—Ralph Staub—Another Screen Snapshots short, showing George playing checkers with his son Ronnie: also Joe E. Brown and Johnny Mack Brown with their sons.

The Burns and Allen Features

(Director's name follows year.)

1. **The Big Broadcast**—Paramount 1932—Frank Tuttle—
Bing Crosby, Leila Hyams, Stuart Erwin, Sharon Lynne,
George Barbier, Kate Smith, The Mills Brothers, The
Boswell Sisters, Arthur Tracy, Donald Novis, Vincent
Lopez and his Orchestra, Cab Calloway and his Orches-
tra, Norman Brokenshire, Jimmy Wallington, Don Ball,
William Brenton, Ralph Robertson, Alex Melesh, Anna
Chandler, Spec O'Donnell, Tom Carrigan, Dewey Rob-
inson, Major, Sharp and Minor, Eddie Dunn, Ernie
Adams, Oscar Smith. 80 minutes.

2. **International House**—Paramount 1933—Edward Suther-
land—W.C. Fields, Peggy Hopkins Joyce, Stuart Erwin,
Sari Maritza, Bela Lugosi, Franklin Pangborn, Edmund
Breese, Lumsden Hare, Harrison Greene, Henry Sedley,
Sterling Holloway, Lona Andre, James Wong, Ernest
Wood, Edwin Stanley, Clem Beauchamp, Norman
Ainslee, Louis Vincenot, Bo-Ling, Bo-Cing, Etta Lee,
Rudy Vallee, Cab Calloway and his orchestra, Baby
Rose Marie, Colonel Stoopnagle and Budd. 70 minutes.

3. **College Humor**—Paramount 1933—Wesley Ruggles—
Bing Crosby, Jack Oakie, Richard Arlen, Mary Carlisle,
Mary Kornman, Joseph Sauers (Joe Sawyer), Lona
Andre, Jimmy Conlin, James Donlin, James Burke,
Lumsden Hare, Churchill Ross, Robert Quirk, Jack Ken-
nedy, Howard Jones, Eddie Nugent, Grady Sutton, Toby
Wing, Dave O'Brien, Frank Jenks, Wade Boteler, Anne
Nagel, Herman Brix (Bruce Bennett). 80 minutes.

4. **Six of a Kind**—Paramount 1934—Leo McCarey—W.C.
Fields, Mary Boland, Charlie Ruggles, Alison Skipworth,
Bradley Page, Grace Bradley, William J. Kelly, James
Burke, Dick Rush, Walter Long, Leo Willis, Lew Kelly,
Alf P. James, Tammany Young, Phil Tead, George
Pearce, Verna Hillie, Florence Enright, William Augus-
tin, Kathleen Burke, Irving Bacon, Phil Dunham, Marty
Faust, Lee Phelps, Neal Burns. 65 minutes.

5. **We're Not Dressing**—Paramount 1934—Norman Taurog—
Bing Crosby, Carole Lombard, Ethel Merman, Leon
Errol, Jay Henry, Raymond (Ray) Milland, John Irwin,

Charles Morris, Ben Hendricks, Ted Oliver, Ernie Adams, Stanley Blystone, 74 minutes.

6. **Many Happy Returns**—Paramount 1934—Norman Z. McLeod—Guy Lombardo and his Orchestra, Joan Marsh, George Barbier, Raymond Milland, William Demarest, Johnny Arthur, Stanley Fields, John Kelly, Egon Brecher, Franklin Pangborn, Morgan Wallace, Kenneth Thomson, Velez and Yolanda, Larry Adler, John Taylor, Clark Rutledge, Jack Mulhall, Sidney Bracey, Kent Taylor. 66 minutes.

7. **Love in Bloom**—Paramount 1935—Elliott Nugent—Joe Morrison, Dixie Lee, J. C. Nugent, Lee Kohlmar, Richard Carle, Mary Foy, Wade Boteler, Marian Mansfield, Julia Graham, Sam Godfrey, Jack Mulhall, Frances Raymond, Bernadene Hayes, Harry C. Bradley, Douglas Wood, William Gorsman, Douglas Blackley (Robert Kent), Benny Baker, Jolly Ethel. 77 minutes.

8. **Here Comes Cookie**—Paramount 1935—Norman Z. McLeod—George Barbier, Betty Furness, Andrew Tombes, Jack Powell, Rafael Storm, James Burke, Lee Kohlmar, Milla Davenport, Harry Holman, Frank Darien, Jack Duffy, Dell Henderson, Duke York, Arthur Housman, Jack Henderson, Ed Gargan, Eddie Dunn, Richard Carle, Irving Bacon, Cal Norris and Monkey, Jester and Mole, Jack Cavanaugh and Partner, Six Olympics, Seymour and Corncob, Moro and (Frank) Yaconelli, Johnson and Dove, Big Boy Williams, Pascale Perry and Partner, Six Candreva Brothers, The Buccaneers, Sid Saylor. 65 minutes.

9. **The Big Broadcast of 1936**—Paramount 1935—Norman Taurog—Bing Crosby, Jack Oakie, Ethel Merman, Lyda Roberti, Wendy Barrie, Henry Wadsworth, C. Henry Gordon, Benny Baker, Samuel S. Hinds, Akim Tamiroff, Harold and Fayard Nicholas, Amos 'n' Andy, Ray Noble and his Band, Ina Ray Hutton and her Band, Mary Boland, Charlie Ruggles, Bill Robinson, Willie, West, and McGinty, The Vienna Boys Choir, Sir Guy Standing, Gail Patrick, David Holt, Virginia Weidler. 97 minutes.

10. **The Big Broadcast of 1937**—Paramount 1936—Mitchell Leisen—Jack Benny, Bob Burns, Martha Raye, Shirley Ross, Raymond Milland, Frank Forest, Benny Fields, Sam (Schlepperman) Hearn, Stan Kavanaugh, Benny Goodman and his Orchestra, Virginia Weidler, David Holt, Billy Lee, Leopold Stokowski and his symphony

Orchestra, Louis Da Pron, Eleanore Whitney, Larry Adler, Irving Bacon, Ernest Cossart, Billy Bletcher, Frank Jenks, Nora Cecil, Leonid Kinskey, Gino Corrado, Priscilla Lawson, Jack Mulhall, Terry Ray (Ellen Drew), Murray Alper, Eddie Dunn, Matt McHugh. 102 minutes.

11. **College Holiday**—Paramount 1936—Frank Tuttle—Jack Benny, Martha Raye, Mary Boland, Etienne Girardot, Marsha Hunt, Leif Erikson, Eleanore Whitney, Johnny Downs, Olympe Bradna, Louis Da Pron, Ben Blue, Jed Prouty, Richard Carle, Margaret Seddon, Nick Lukats, Spec O'Donnell, Jack Chapin, The California Collegians, Darwin Rudd, Kenneth Hunter, Nora Cecil, Kay Griffith, Priscilla Lawson, Terry Ray (Ellen Drew), Gail Sheridan, Snowflake, Barlowe Borland, Charles Arnt, Edward J. Le Saint, Harry Hayden, Marjorie Moore (Marjorie Reynolds). 87 minutes.

12. **A Damsel in Distress**—RKO 1937—George Stevens— Fred Astaire, Joan Fontaine, Reginald Gardiner, Ray Noble, Constance Collier, Montagu Love, Harry Watson, Jan Duggan, Mary Gordon, Fred Kelsey. 101 minutes.

13. **College Swing**—Paramount 1938—Raoul Walsh—Martha Raye, Bob Hope, Edward Everett Horton, Florence George, Ben Blue, Betty Grable, Jackie Coogan, John Payne, Cecil Cunningham, Robert Cummings, Skinnay Ennis, The Slate Brothers, Charles Trowbridge, Bob Mitchell and St. Brendan's Choristers, Jerry Colonna, Jerry Bergen, Tully Marshall, Edward J. Le Saint, Barlowe Borland, The Playboys, Richard Denning, John Hubbard, Wilfred Lucas, Nelson McDowell. 86 minutes.

14. **Honolulu**—MGM 1939—Eddie Buzzell—Eleanor Powell, Robert Young, Rita Johnson, Clarence Kilb, Willie Fung, Ruth Hussey, Cliff Clark, Edward Gargan, Eddie (Rochester) Anderson, Hal K. Dawson, Edgar Dearing, Jo Ann Sayers, Sig Ruman, Tom Neal, Mary Treen, Russell Hicks, Claire McDowell, Bert Roach, Edward Earle, Edward J. Le Saint, Bess Flowers, Betty Jaynes, Douglas McPhail. 83 minutes.

Gracie also appeared without George in the following films:

1. **The Gracie Allen Murder Case**—Paramount 1939— Alfred E. Green—Warren William (as Philo Vance), Ellen Drew, Kent Taylor, Jed Prouty, Jerome Cowan, Donald MacBride, H. B. Warner, William Demarest, Judith

Barrett, Horace MacMahon, Al Shaw, Sam Lee, Edgar Dearing, Willie Fung, Lee Moore, Richard Denning, Paul Newlan, Lillian Yarbo, James Flavin, Rube Demarest, Addison Richards, Irving Bacon, Monty Collins. 74 minutes.

2. **Mr. and Mrs. North**—MGM 1941—Robert Sinclair— William Post. Jr. (and Gracie as Mr. and Mrs. North), Paul Kelly, Tom Conway, Virginia Grey, Felix Bressart, Stuart Crawford, Rose Hobart, Porter Hall, Millard Mitchell, Jerome Cowan, Keye Luke, Lucien Littlefield, Fortunio Bonanova, Stanley Andrews, Sam McDaniel, Gladys Blake, Barbara Bedford, Inez Cooper, James Flavin, Tim Ryan, Hillary Brooke. 67 minutes.

3. **Two Girls and a Sailor**—MGM 1944—Richard Thorpe— Gloria De Haven, June Allyson, Van Johnson, Tom Drake, Jimmy Durante, Henry Stephenson, Henry O'Neill, Ben Blue, Frank Sully, Donald Meek, Carlos Ramirez, Jose and Amparo Iturbi, Albert Coates, Frank Jenks, Lena Horne, Harry James and his Band with Helen Forrest, Xavier Cugat and his Band with Lina Romay, Virginia O'Brien, The Wilde Twins, Eilene Janssen, Gigi Perreau, Doodles Weaver, Joe Yule, Kay Williams, Ava Gardner, Buster Keaton. 124 minutes.

THE THREE STOOGES

"The public, upon which the screen depends for its existence, appears . . . to be divided roughly into two groups, one composed of persons who laugh at the Three Stooges and the other made up of those who wonder why." That statement appeared in a 1937 issue of *The Motion Picture Herald*, and is just as valid today. But examine, if you will, the facts: the Three Stooges were together for nearly fifty years. Their durability as a team is virtually unparalleled in show business history, and there can be only one reason for it: a great many people *did* find them funny.

The Stooges never had any pretensions to greatness or genius; they were just talented, hardworking clowns who knew their business. And they were unique, in looks and personalities. Over the years, as their contemporaries retired

The Stooges, rehearsing at home, drive Curly's wife crazy.

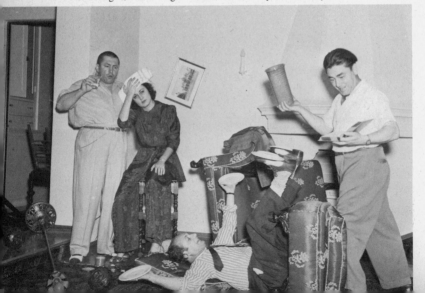

or passed on, the Stooges became the torchbearers of slapstick comedy, carrying their comic expertise into the 1970s and introducing their tried-and-true routines to the TV generation. Now the Stooges too are gone, but the team is literally more popular than ever! Their straightforward approach to knockabout nonsense has made them latter-day comic heroes. After half a century, the Three Stooges have finally come into their own.

Moe Howard, born in Brooklyn, New York, in 1905, was simply not a scholarly type of boy. He ran away from home and made his performing debut on a Mississippi riverboat in 1914. The riverboat circuit was a hectic but interesting introduction to show business for the young man, who soon abandoned the floating showcases for the life of an actor, with traveling drama troupes that performed such venerable plays as *Ten Nights in a Barroom*. He even did Shakespeare as he traveled around the country in the company of such other young actors as the McHugh family (Frank became one of movies' busiest character actors; his brother Matt later showed up in several Three Stooges comedies). After World War I, Moe and his older brother Shemp (born Samuel in 1901), formed a black-face vaudeville act that led to more traveling and eventually a job with up-and-coming comedian Ted Healy (1923). Moe recalls that originally he

Joan Crawford doesn't look too happy to have the Three Stooges accompanying her audition for stage manager Ted Healy in DANCING LADY.

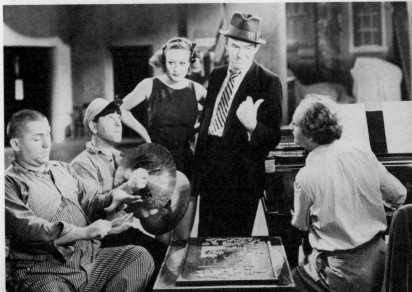

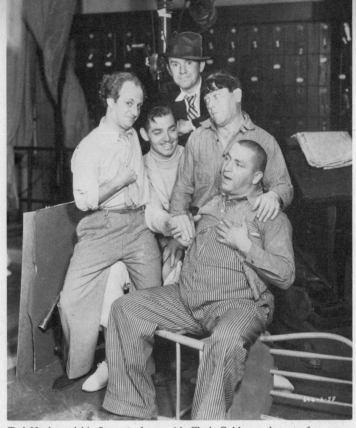

Ted Healy and his Stooges clown with Clark Gable on the set of DANCING
LADY.

and Shemp joined Healy on a temporary basis, but got along
so well that Healy made them permanent stooges. In 1928,
they were joined by another vaudevillian, Larry Fine, who
was born in Philadelphia in 1911. Like the Howards, he was
bitten with stage fever at an early age. His first job was in a
carbon copy of Gus Edwards' popular schoolroom act, playing
the sissy. Eventually, he graduated to an act called Haney
Sisters and Fine, which enabled Larry to play the violin, and
also introduced him to his future wife (one of the sisters).

Ted Healy and his Stooges (as they were then billed) did
quite well in vaudeville, and after hitting the big time they
were featured in several Broadway revues, including *Earl
Carroll's Vanities*. When talkies swept Hollywood, Healy
was one of many vaudevillians who were called to the West
Coast. He made his debut in a 1930 Fox film, SOUP TO NUTS,
a wacky comedy feature written by cartoonist-inventor Rube
Goldberg. Healy was billed solo, but some of the advertising

for the film carried the tag "Ted Healy and his Racketeers."
The Racketeers were Moe, Shemp, Larry and Fred Sanborn,
playing part-time firemen who help Healy to break up a
swanky party. After SOUP TO NUTS, Healy and his confreres
returned to New York and more vaudeville engagements,
until 1933, when MGM expressed interest in the act. When
Ted Healy and his Stooges returned to the West Coast, it
was minus Shemp, who had gone off on his own. Replacing
him was Moe's younger brother Jerry, better known as Curly,
born in Brooklyn in 1911. Under contract to MGM, Healy
and the Stooges starred in their own shorts, and had supporting roles in a handful of feature films. The shorts, several of them in color, are a pretty sorry lot; in some cases,
the Stooges merely string together leftover footage from
MGM musicals (though PLANE NUTS at least gives us an idea
of what the team's vaudeville act with Healy must have been
like). They are seen to best advantage in DANCING LADY, a

The Three Stooges scan the horizon in THE THREE TROUBLEDOERS.

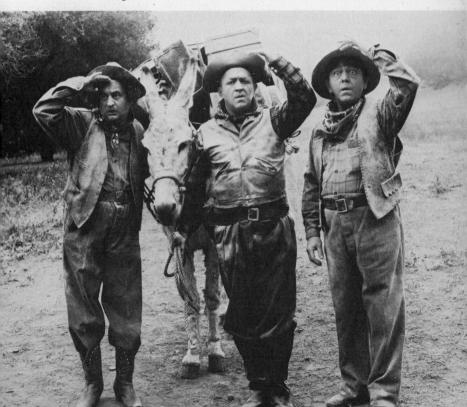

feature starring Clark Gable and Joan Crawford. Healy appeared as Gable's right-hand man in this entertaining backstage musical, and had many of the script's sharpest lines. The Stooges have some very funny moments, too, and are often seen in the background, slapping each other or getting tangled in the scenery as the camera follows one of the stars around the theater. A key scene has them acting as rehearsal musicians for an audition Joan Crawford is giving. Gable has assigned them to the task so the audition will go as badly as possible. To reassure the nervous Miss Crawford, Moe brags, "Why, I'm the best musician in the country." "Yeah," snaps Curly, "but how are you in the city?"

Not long after DANCING LADY was released, the Stooges decided to go out on their own. They did some more work with Healy at MGM, then were given the opportunity to star in a short subject for Columbia. The short, WOMAN HATERS, was one of several miscellaneous comedy subjects Columbia was releasing at the time, before their comedy department was firmly established. WOMAN HATERS does star the Stooges, but unlike their other films, they do not appear as a team. Marjorie White gets top billing, with Larry cast as "Jim," Moe as "Tom" and Jerry (Curly) as "Jack." The entire short is done in rhyme, which is none too inventive and quickly becomes tiresome. The result is a very weak two-reeler, despite the presence of such familiar comedy faces as Monty Collins, Bud Jamison, Jack Norton and Tiny Sandford (Walter Brennan also appears in the film, as a train conductor). Their second short for Columbia, PUNCH DRUNKS, is somewhat better, with a good scene in the boxing arena; the story for the short is credited to "Howard, Fine, and Howard," which explains the improvement over their first two-reel attempt. It was their third film, MEN IN BLACK, a spoof of the then-current feature MEN IN WHITE, that really got the Stooges started. While the *Motion Picture Herald* thought the short was only "fair," the two-reeler was nominated for an Academy Award, the only time a Stooges short was so honored. Jules White, who produced the short and organized Columbia's short-subjects department, recently recalled, "Boy was that reviewer wrong. It opened here at the Carthay Circle Theatre, the biggest and best in L.A. MEN IN BLACK not only went over *big*, it got the Three Stooges their contract with Columbia." This reaction is difficult to explain today, for MEN IN BLACK now looks stilted and contrived; the Stooges seem to be restrained, and the short isn't nearly as good as the team's later hospital spoofs, such as DIZZY DOCTORS, FROM NURSE TO WORSE and CALLING ALL CURS.

Be that as it may, the Stooges were pacted by Columbia for eight shorts a year (leaving them ample time to continue to tour the country doing personal appearances). What they needed most was a good director—instead of the journeymen they had on their earliest outings. This void was filled by Del Lord, a Mack Sennett veteran who had started as a driver for the Keystone Kops patrol wagon. Sennett remembered Lord fondly in later years for his ability to get the wagon, or any car, into the most outlandish positions (dangling off a cliff, for example), without damaging himself or the auto. After Sennett retired, Lord had a difficult time finding work. He free-lanced for a while, but by the mid-1930's he was forced to find a job selling used cars. When Jules White organized Columbia's shorts department, he remembered Lord's work and hired him immediately. Lord stayed at Columbia until 1949, doing first-rate comedies with Andy Clyde, El Brendel, Charley Chase and others. In 1935 he was just what the doctor ordered for the Three Stooges, and his first shorts with them—POP GOES THE EASEL, UNCIVIL WARRIORS, PARDON MY SCOTCH, THREE LITTLE BEERS—are first-rate slapstick comedies, with ingenious sight gags and

Moe, Larry and Curly, intrepid firemen, are the center of attention in this scene from the feature film START CHEERING, with Raymond Walburn, Joan Perry, Charles Starrett and Minerva Urecal taking part.

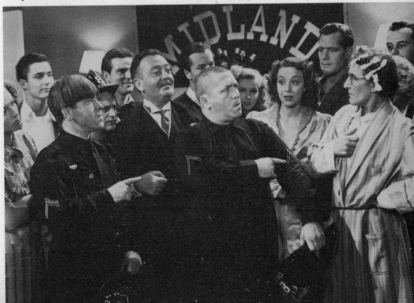

not a second of wasted footage. POP GOES THE EASEL takes place in an artist's studio, and is climaxed by a clay-throwing melee that Mack Sennett would have been proud of. In UNCIVIL WARRIORS Curly helps a pretty young girl bake a cake, and hands her a cushion instead of the pastry when she wants to apply some frosting. When the Stooges eat the finished product, they spend the next five five minutes cough-ing up feathers. PARDON MY SCOTCH is one of the Stooges' best films, with a carpentry sequence highlighting the action. And THREE LITTLE BEERS has one good sight gag after an-other, as the Stooges invade a golf course to practice for an upcoming tournament. It is special events day, and only reporters are being admitted; after a quick trip to the Men's Room, the Stooges return and go through the main gate holding their badges. Moe's reads "Press," Larry's reads "Press," and Curly's reads "Pull." Out on the course, every-thing goes wrong. Curly's ball flies into a tree branch, and unable to shake it down, he chops down the tree. Moe keeps missing his ball, and before long the whole field is covered with divots. When a gardener sees the mess, Moe snaps, "What are you complaining about? Don't you see they're

The Stooges do their best to ruffle dignified Don Beddoe in THREE SAPPY PEOPLE.

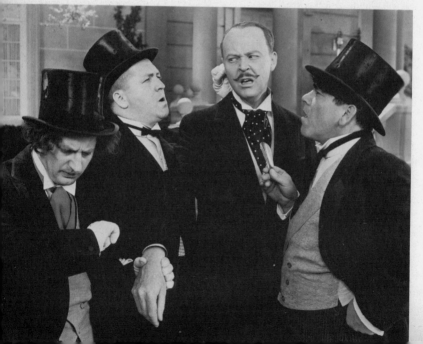

getting smaller?" The finishing touch is performed by Larry, who is about to putt when he notices something sticking up out of the ground. It is the end of a tree root; he pulls it up and within a few minutes he has ruined the entire green with this interminable weed.

By the end of 1935 the Three Stooges pattern was pretty much set, and they rolled along smoothly from that point on. In 1938 and 1939, most of their shorts were directed by Charley Chase, one of the screen's finest and most under-rated comedians, and a good director as well. Chase and the Stooges worked well together, and might have continued indefinitely. Their association was curtailed by Chase's un-timely death in 1940. Del Lord alternated with Jules White for the next few years, each turning in first-rate work. In 1945 Edward Bernds, a sound mixer on the Columbia shorts, expressed a desire to direct. His first short with the Three Stooges turned out to be the best they ever made: MICRO PHONIES. As Del Lord curtailed his output, Bernds directed more of their shorts through the 1940's, along with Jules White. Hugh McCollum, who shared producing chores with White, tried his hand at directing for a while, but after the

Curly tries to disarm Bud Jamison as tough guy John Merton prepares to move. A struggle doomed to failure, from PHONY EXPRESS.

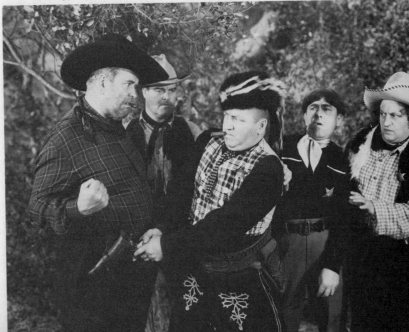

early 1950's, the Three Stooges shorts became the sole responsibility of Jules White, who continued directing them through their final short in 1959.

The Stooges were often accused of being too violent—which is, naturally, a matter of personal taste—but the truth is that their funniest films, and best routines, relied on *slapstick*, not violence . . . just as their funniest "violent" gags were the ones that were the most outlandish and unrealistic. In many of the later shorts, when the comic well was running dry, the Stooges' violence became less comic—and more painful—which certainly didn't endear them to PTA groups and the like. But Moe Howard always defended the group's modus operandi, and maintained, "We're not as sadistic as Westerns."

It is generally agreed that the best Stooges comedies were those that featured Curly as the "third Stooge." His engaging enthusiasm, agility and comic characteristics (including squeals and grunts that could mean, alternately, delight, anger and frustration) made him a perfect teammate for the stubborn directness of Moe and the blank agreeability of Larry. While there were always some clinkers, the shorts that featured Curly, made in the late 1930's and early 1940's, had a high batting average. These films also featured a marvelous stock company of supporting players. The two mainstays of Columbia's shorts were Vernon Dent and Bud Jamison. Just as people like Billy Gilbert and Charlie Hall popped up in practically all of the Hal Roach comedies of the 1930's, Dent and Jamison were in virtually all of the 30-odd two-reelers Columbia produced every year. Dent, a stocky man with a mustache, was adept at playing businessmen and officials at odds with the Stooges. Roly-poly Jamison projected a more down-to-earth image, and was usually cast as a cop or an irate neighbor.

Others who frequented the Stooges shorts included Symona Boniface, another silent-comedy veteran who specialized in Margaret Dumont-type roles. In the Stooges shorts she was forever receiving a pie in the face, or being doused with water. Christine McIntyre, an attractive blonde, was usually the heroine in Stooges comedies, although she was also adept at playing villainesses. Before Miss McIntyre was established, pert and vivacious Dorothy Appleby was often seen in the Stooges shorts. She was Columbia's all-purpose comedy foil for several years, supporting Buster Keaton, Andy Clyde and others, with a flair for comedy and extreme fortitude in the line of duty (she was often on the receiving end of pies, water and other missiles).

Being affiliated with a major studio, the Stooges shorts also featured up-and-coming actors and starlets and established character actors quite often. Among the people who turned up in Stooges shorts were: Walter Brennan (WOMAN HATERS, RESTLESS KNIGHTS), Lucille Ball (THREE LITTLE PIGSKINS), Billy Gilbert (MEN IN BLACK, PARDON MY SCOTCH), Clara Kimball Young (ANTS IN THE PANTRY), Jack Norton (RHYTHM AND WEEP), Benny Rubin (HOOFS AND GOOFS, SPACE SHIP SAPPY), Jock Mahoney (OUT WEST, FUELING AROUND, others), Bruce Bennett (BEER BARREL PALOOKAS, HOW HIGH IS UP, others), and Tom Kennedy (LOOSE LOOT, SPOOKS). Young contract player Lloyd Bridges even made a brief appearance in THEY STOOGE TO CONGA.

Many fine shorts were made with Curly and these supporting players during the 1930's and 40's, but several stand out: HEALTHY, WEALTHY AND DUMB starts as Curly wins a $50,000 radio contest. The boys, feeling extravagant, move into the Hotel Costa Plente, where three gold-digging girls go after them without much success. Finally, a telegram arrives from the radio station itemizing the tax deductions on Curly's jackpot, which leaves him with a total of $4.85. IN THE SWEET PIE AND PIE begins with the Stooges as convicts about to be executed. Three girls in need of husbands "in name

Curly sings "The Voice of Spring" as Moe and Larry provide accompaniment in the team's best short, MICRO-PHONIES.

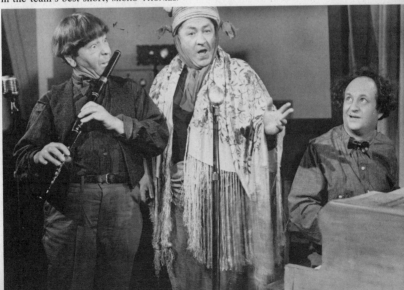

only" marry them, knowing they are about to be hanged. A pardon comes from the governor at the last minute and the girls are stuck with their unruly husbands. They plot to embarrass them by planning a society party, hoping that they will walk out. The wind-up is a hilarious pie-throwing battle which turns the party into a shambles. The most familiar Stooges theme involves a professor who tries to turn the rowdies into gentlemen. The first film to use this idea was HOI POLLOI. The idea was reworked, with better results, in HALF-WITS HOLIDAY, which ends with a masterfully staged pie fight. One of HALF-WITS HOLIDAY's funniest lines, knowing what is to come, is a throwaway, in the opening scene at the party. Symona Boniface mentions to another guest, "I'm allergic to pastry, you know." Later, Moe has to get rid of a pie quickly, and throws it up onto the ceiling. Just then, Symona approaches and insists on talking to him. Watching the pie dangling above him, Moe tries to get away. "Why young man," the lady persists, "you act as if the Sword of Damocles were hanging above you." "Lady, you must be psychic," says Moe as he runs off. She looks up and the pie plummets down and lands on her face, starting the mammoth slapstick sequence. The pie footage was so good, it was used as stock footage several times in later films like SCHEMING, SCHEMERS and THE PEST MAN WINS. HALF-WITS HOLIDAY was remade, almost scene for scene, with Joe Besser, as PIES AND GUYS, with lovely starlet Greta Thyssen getting her career started with a pie in the face. The scene was also used in STOP! LOOK! AND LAUGH!, the Three Stooges feature-film compilation of 1960.

Often the titles of the Stooges films are better than the films themselves, such as VIOLENT IS THE WORD FOR CURLY, a neat switch on VALIANT IS THE WORD FOR CARRIE, a popular 1938 film. A-PLUMBING WE WILL GO casts the boys as would-be plumbers in an elaborate mansion. They cross pipes and wires, confusing all the household appliances. The best gag comes when a wealthy matron demonstrates her new television, which is broadcasting from Niagara Falls. Suddenly a great torrent of water emerges from the set, drenching the guests. The Stooges' all-time best short was MICRO PHONIES, in which the boys are mistaken for a prima donna (Curly) and her two accompanists when they mime to a record at a radio station. They are hired for a party, and during some byplay, their record is broken. Luckily, the real singer, Christine McIntyre, does the singing for them. Their facial expressions and gestures while mouthing "The Voice

of Spring" are priceless, and a confrontation with pompous
singer Gino Corrado is also quite funny.

Other films stand out in the hundred-odd films the Stooges
made with Curly. DUTIFUL BUT DUMB casts them as Click
Clack and Cluck, photographers who go to a mythical kingdom (Vulgaria) on an assignment and end up before the
firing line. For a last wish, Curly asks if he can have a
smoke. The commandant agrees, and Curly produces a four-
foot cigar which lasts until the next morning; by that time,
the soldiers on the firing line are asleep and the Stooges
manage to escape. FROM NURSE TO WORSE has them going to
Doctor D. Lerious (Vernon Dent) with Curly pretending to
be a mad dog in order to collect insurance money. The scheme
backfires when the doctor wants to operate, and a wild chase
follows in and out of the hospital. DIZZY DOCTORS also takes
place in a hospital, where Moe, Larry and Curly are trying
to sell a new miracle product, "Brighto," which does everything from cleaning cars (it removes the paint entirely) to
removing spots on clothing (it dissolves the fabric). In BUSY
BUDDIES they run a short-order restaurant, with Curly as the
ingenious chef (to make chicken soup he pours boiling water
over a chicken and lets the liquid run over into a bowl).
When customers complain, Curly replies indignantly, "Are
you casting asparagus on my cooking?"

AN ACHE IN EVERY STAKE is one of the most beautifully

The Three Stooges *au naturel*, more or less, with Shemp Howard replacing
Curly as the "third stooge."

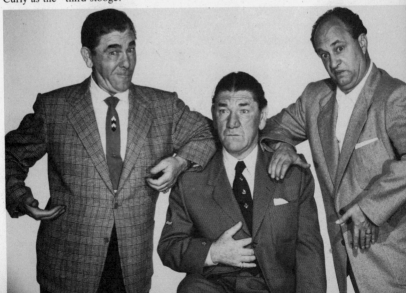

paced Stooges comedies, with not one wasted frame as the boys encounter some tricky problems in delivering ice to a hilltop home—the ice melts by the time Curly can run up the tremendous flight of steps!

Moe Howard's favorite of all the shorts he did with the Stooges was YOU NAZTY SPY, in which he burlesqued Hitler, Curly played Goering, and Larry played Goebbels. They repeated these roles in an equally funny follow-up, I'LL NEVER HEIL AGAIN.

In 1946, Jerry "Curly" Howard suffered a stroke which rendered him inactive; he died in 1952. A 1947 short, HOLD THAT LION, featured a special surprise, an unbilled cameo by Curly, seen only briefly as a fellow train passenger. He was replaced in the act by his older brother, Shemp. Shemp had been with the team in vaudeville, but had gone out on his own and met success in short subjects for Vitaphone and Columbia, and in a host of feature films, notably THE BANK DICK with W. C. Fields, in which he played the bartender. Shemp was a fine comic, but his shorts with the Stooges couldn't match those with Curly. Curly added a dimension of unreality to the act that was impossible to replace (try to

Larry, Moe and Shemp display their wares in a scene from SPOOKS, which was filmed in 3-D.

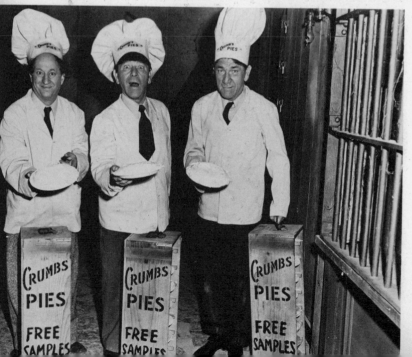

imagine the Marx Brothers without Harpo!). What's more, Shemp arrived at a time when the short-subject department at Columbia was starting its slow decline. Most of the silent-comedy veterans who used to write and direct were gone—and with them went the freewheeling Mack Sennett spirit. The shorts moved indoors, for the most part (even when exteriors were called for), and this was just one indication of a general cutback in expense. A liberal amount of stock footage from earlier films began to turn up in the "new" two-reelers; major sight gags were lifted intact from shorts that had originally featured Curly. The number of remakes grew with each passing year, and by the early 1950s even Shemp's originals were being redone. (Remember, the films weren't yet playing on TV, where nearly identical films might turn up back to back.) Shemp delivered his fair share of laughs throughout his nine-year run with the Stooges—and the *only* thing one could say against this experienced comic was that he wasn't "another Curly."

The Stooges did experiment with new ideas from time to time in the late 1940s and early 50s. Often these ideas didn't work out, but the results were interesting. CUCKOO ON THE CHOOCHOO takes place in an abandoned railroad car with Shemp, Larry and Moe working independently, not as a team; the material is weak, however, and the short doesn't come off. HE COOKED HIS GOOSE tries eschewing the usual slapstick for marital farce, with Larry two-timing Moe's wife

Moe Howard lost count of how many pies were thrown in the Stooges' films. Here's one, with Shemp the target; from BEDLAM IN PARADISE.

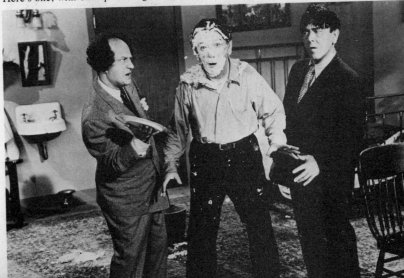

and Shemp's fiancée at the same time. One of the most successful of these oddball shorts is THREE DARK HORSES, which goes into the area of political satire with most amusing results. Released during the 1952 presidential campaign, the film satirizes political campaigns and conventions, with the Stooges being hired as delegates by scheming politico Kenneth MacDonald, who pays them to vote for his man. Moe reads a hilarious double-talk nomination speech, and when the Stooges accept a bigger bribe from the rival candidate, Moe promises to make Larry Secretary of Offense and Shemp Secretary of the Inferior.

Some changes were made in the Stooges stock company at this time. Bud Jamison died in 1944, but Vernon Dent continued to appear with the Stooges through the early 1950's. New "regulars" included Emil Sitka, adept at playing goggle-eyed scientists and miscellaneous antagonists; Phil Van Zandt, an all-purpose character actor best seen in roles as officials or henchmen; Kenneth MacDonald, a marvelously slimy villain with a fine theatrical voice who usually ended up being pelted with tomatoes, pies or other objects; and Gene Roth, a burly, distinguished man who usually played millionaires, professors and the like. Christine McIntyre re-

Lou Leonard and Maxine Gates are formidable opponents in this marital scrap from HUSBANDS BEWARE.

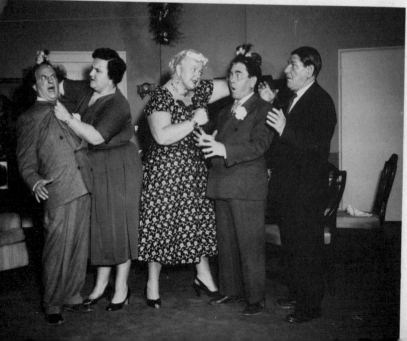

mained with the Stooges through the early 1950's as well, usually playing damsels in distress, and somehow never getting involved in any of the slapstick scenes.

In 1952 the Stooges participated in their most ambitious experiment. As producer-director Jules White recalled, "I made the first 3-D comedies to hit the screen—and thought we had a whole new life ahead of us. Boy, did I goof." White wasn't alone, of course; several major movie moguls made the same miscalculation of 3-D's short-lived appeal. But those two shorts—SPOOKS and PARDON MY BACKFIRE— have earned the Stooges a place in every subsequent 3-D revival. The comic value of these two-reelers is strictly second-rate, but the actual 3-D effects are quite good: the use of forced perspective in the construction of the stooges' bed in BACKFIRE is ingenious, and SPOOKS has one of the most effective 3-D gimmicks ever filmed—a lingering shot of a mad doctor coming toward the camera with a long, *long* hypodermic needle! The idea of throwing pies at the camera didn't work quite as well.

While many of the comedies with Shemp were weak, a number were quite good, and these shorts stand out: HULA LA LA, where the boys journey into the jungle to teach the natives some dance steps for a movie that's going on location there. The funniest gags involve a Buddha-like statue with

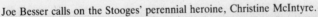
Joe Besser calls on the Stooges' perennial heroine, Christine McIntyre.

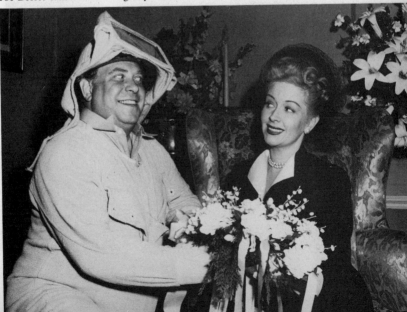

four hands (one resting against the face in a sighing gesture) which slaps anyone who tries to take the box of grenades it is guarding. HUSBANDS BEWARE has Shemp as a vocal coach with one absolutely horrible student whom he advises to "gargle with old razor blades." OUT WEST is an amusing Western spoof with hero Jacques O'Mahoney (later known as Jock Mahoney) going to get the cavalry to save the Stooges and his girl (Christine McIntyre). "I hope we're not too late," he tells an officer. "Never in the history of motion pictures has the United States Cavalry been late," the officer replies. Along with the aforementioned SCHEMING SCHEMERS, SCRAMBLED BRAINS is among the best work the Stooges ever did, with Shemp being taken home from the hospital, where he has suffered hallucinations. In one of his worst visions, he thinks his ugly nurse (Babe London) is actually a beautiful, shapely blonde. Moe and Larry take him home to recuperate, and have him play the piano to calm his nerves. This doesn't work, for every time he starts to play, he envisions a third hand playing along with him! Later, through several mishaps, the Stooges end up in a crowded phone booth, along with Vernon Dent and a bag of groceries. The results are disastrous, with Dent threatening to kill them if he ever sees them again. Shemp then goes to marry Babe

Moe threatens Larry and Joe, but it's Connie Cezan who gets the cake in the face in RUSTY ROMEOS.

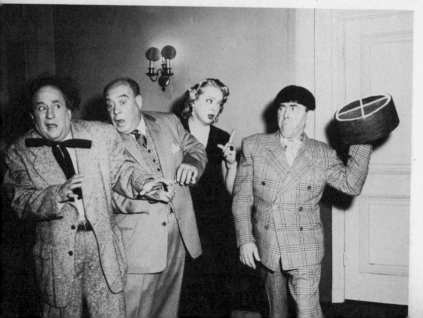

London, and just before the ceremony her father arrives. Of course, it's Dent, and the Stooges leave on the run.

In 1955, Shemp Howard died, and for the second time in a decade, the Three Stooges faced a crisis of survival. Columbia Pictures rejected the idea of "The Two Stooges," so instead, to fulfill that year's quota of shorts for Columbia, Moe and Larry performed with a stand-in (Joe Palma). Their scenes were then edited with stock footage from earlier comedies with Shemp in order to create four "new" Stooge comedies.

By this time, the Hollywood short-subject was virtually dead, and the low-budget antics of the Stooges seemed almost anachronistic (even Moe recognized the problem, remarking, "imagine us in stereophonic sound"). But Columbia wanted to continue making Three Stooges comedies, so in 1956, veteran second-banana Joe Besser (who'd worked with Olsen and Johnson and Abbott and Costello) was signed to complete the trio. His delightful comic presence helped carry a lot of weak material. One particularly funny scene in SPACE SHIP SAPPY has the boys trapped in a rocket about to crash. Besser's eyes widen and he says frantically, "I don't want to die . . . *I can't die* . . . I haven't seen THE EDDY DUCHIN STORY yet!"

The Besser shorts are at best amusing, but none of them have the sparkle of the Stooges shorts of the 1930's and 40's.

The Nine Stooges? Larry, Joe and Moe pose with their look-alikes on the set of A MERRY MIX-UP.

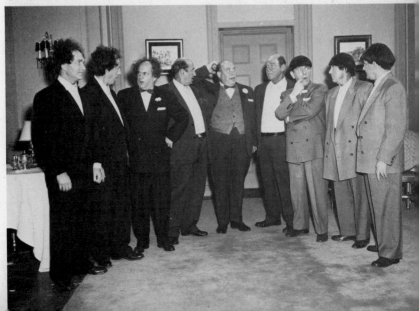

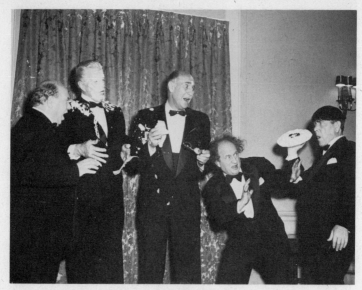

Gene Roth has been plastered, and Milton Frome is next in line on this scene from PIES AND GUYS.

The Stooges strike a pose with Greta Thyssen on the set of SAPPY BULL-FIGHTERS.

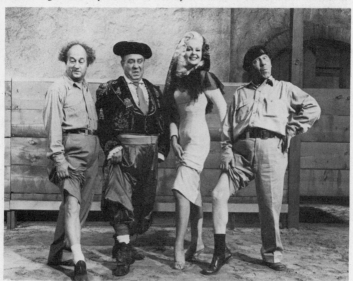

A MERRY MIX UP has the interesting premise of each Stooge appearing in triplicate, but the story line is contrived and the mistaken identity idea doesn't produce many laughs. Several of the Besser shorts have science-fiction premises (OUTER SPACE JITTERS, SPACE SHIP SAPPY, etc.), and some of the sets are rather impressive, but once again they fail to create much more than mild amusement. One of the better shorts in this series is RUSTY ROMEOS, a remake (with stock footage) of CORNY CASANOVAS, with Moe, Larry, and Joe all engaged to the same girl (Connie Cezan), who gleefully accepts their engagement rings and then plans to run off. Joe takes care of her in the end, and Miss Cezan receives a cake in the face for her trouble. One asset of several Besser shorts is a beautiful young girl named Greta Thyssen. She is much prettier than the unemployed starlets featured in most Stooges shorts of the 1950's, and a lot more enthusiastic. She also earns her money in the three shorts in which she appears, getting a pie in the face in PIES AND GUYS and having Moe shove a gooey cake in her face in QUIZ WHIZ. The identical casts and costumes of these two films seem to indicate that they were shot at the same time. Producer-director Jules White has admitted that, with the use of stock footage, some of the later shorts were filmed in *one day*. By this time, production of the shorts was a family affair at Columbia, with Jules' brother Jack White doing the scripts, and his son Harold White editing the films.

Larry takes flight, unnoticed by Moe and Curly-Joe DeRita, in the "new" Stooges' first feature-length film, HAVE ROCKET, WILL TRAVEL.

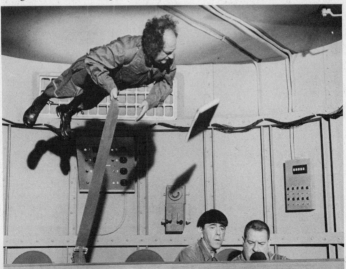

But by the late 1950's the market for shorts was limited, and it didn't pay for the studio to maintain a heavy schedule of one- and two-reelers. The Stooges outlasted everyone else at Columbia, but their contract expired at the end of 1957 and it was not renewed. They had shot enough film for Columbia to release new shorts well into 1959. Jules White left Columbia the following year, and the short-subject department was disbanded. Once the contract ran out, the Stooges were unemployed. Moe Howard's friend and former director, Edward Bernds, got him a supporting role in a low-budget science-fiction film, SPACE MASTER X-7, but the Stooges received very few offers. They were about to embark on a personal-appearance tour when Joe Besser decided to leave the act; his wife was ill at the time, and he did not like the idea of traveling without her. After this move, there was serious talk of breaking up the act when, in January of 1958, Screen Gems, Columbia Pictures' television division, packaged 78 Stooges shorts for television, and found markets in 75 cities. They were an immediate success around the country, where youngsters who had never seen the Stooges before "discovered" the slapstick team. Within a year, 156 stations were carrying the two-reelers,

The Three Stooges stand by for action in their cameo role from IT'S A MAD. MAD. MAD. MAD WORLD.

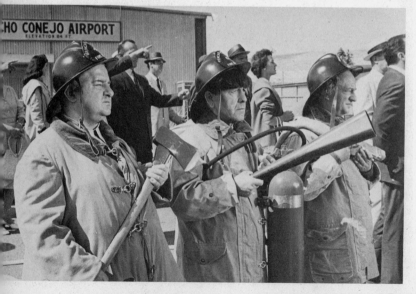

and the demand was so great that Screen Gems released all
190 comedies to the TV market. The Stooges received no
residuals from these showings, but because of them they
were back in the limelight. In January 1959, a Pittsburgh
entrepreneur booked the Stooges into his nightclub, with
special early shows for children, and was amazed at the
capacity crowds that showed up. This continued for several
months, until they were in great demand for other personal
appearances as well as guest shots on many TV shows. To
replace Joe Besser, the Stooges had hired Joe De Rita, a
rotund ex-burlesque comedian who had made several shorts
for Columbia in the 1950's. He was nicknamed Curly Joe, and
he adapted to the Stooges nonsense with the greatest of ease.

The Stooges' renewed popularity resulted in Columbia
signing them to star in a new feature-length film (up until
this time, the team's appearances in features had consisted
mostly of comic relief). The result was HAVE ROCKET, WILL
TRAVEL, an entertaining light-comedy vehicle with a topical
outer-space theme. It was vastly superior to the Stooges' last
shorts, and proved itself at the box office, leading to a string
of low-budget comedy features: THE THREE STOOGES MEET

The front page has been printed on Moe's face, and he isn't too keen on the
idea. From THE OUTLAWS IS COMING.

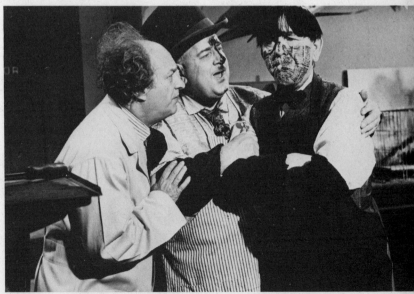

HERCULES, THE THREE STOOGES IN ORBIT, THE THREE STOOGES GO AROUND THE WORLD IN A DAZE, and THE OUTLAWS IS COMING. The Stooges were still agile enough to perform quite well, though the violence quotient was definitely reduced, and the humor was aimed more specifically at a kiddie audience. Writer Elwood Ullman and director Edward Bernds, who worked with the Stooges in their heyday, returned to the fold for these 1960s endeavors, while Moe's son-in-law, Norman Maurer (who guided the team's career from the time of their comeback) took the director's reins for the final two features. Columbia also released a feature-length compilation film, STOP! LOOK! AND LAUGH! in 1961.

That same year, the Stooges were recruited by 20th Century–Fox for what can only be called a Technicolor mistake, SNOW WHITE AND THE THREE STOOGES. It was the studio's attempt to revive the glory days of Sonja Henie and her ice-skating musicals, with Olympic champion Carol Heiss in the leading role—but this vapid retelling of the Snow White fairy tale held little appeal for kids, who came to see the Stooges and saw very little of them. What's more, their scenes were mostly sentimental and uncharacteristic.

The team fared much better on television, where they appeared as guest stars on a number of variety shows, doing sure-fire routines like the Majarajah sketch (performed to perfection in the 1941 feature film TIME OUT FOR RHYTHM) and "Stand-In," which they introduced on Broadway in *The George White Scandals of 1939*. They also filmed forty live-action wraparound segments for a series of 160 animated cartoons shown on TV as THE NEW THREE STOOGES.

In their later years, the Stooges stood as symbols of a bygone era. To some TV and movie executives, they were has-beens. To children, and longtime fans, they were a one-of-a-kind trio of living caricatures whose slapstick antics and vaudeville/burlesque routines were light-years away from the "typical" TV comedy of the 1960s.

Inevitably, age took its toll on the team. In January of 1970, Larry Fine suffered a stroke while the Stooges were filming a comic travelogue for TV called KOOK'S TOUR. He was partially paralyzed and wheelchair-bound for the rest of his life, though he recovered sufficiently to enjoy visits from fans, and even managed to make personal appearances at a number of schools in Southern California, where he reminisced about his career for audiences of young admirers.

Moe Howard attempted to keep the act alive when the possibility of doing another independent feature film arose in 1971; his plan was to cast longtime Stooges supporting player Emil Sitka in Larry's place, but the project fell through. Late in 1974, producer Sam Sherman set his mind on putting the Stooges into an exploitation feature called THE JET SET (later titled BLAZING STEWARDESSES)—and even figured a way to include Larry Fine, by writing scenes that he would play alone, talking to Moe and Curly-Joe on the telephone.

Larry Fine died on January 24, 1975, and that, it seemed, was the end of the act. But Moe persevered, and persuaded producer Sherman to retain the Three Stooges in his film, with Emil Sitka as the third member. Sherman agreed. But filming of the low-budget feature was postponed, and on May 4, 1975, Moe Howard succumbed to lung cancer.

The Ritz Brothers took the Stooges' place in BLAZING STEWARDESSES, but no one has been able to take the Stooges' place in show business. In the wake of the team's mushrooming renaissance in the 1980s, Moe's son-in-law Norman Maurer has not only initiated a new wave of licensed merchandise but convinced Columbia Pictures to try reviving the act. In 1984 the studio announced that it would launch a nationwide talent search for three newcomers to portray Larry, Moe, and Curly as 003 Stooges in a James Bond feature-film spoof.

Whatever the outcome of this project may be, it's not

The boys are apologetic, but Dean Martin is annoyed with the Stooges' inefficiency in FOUR FOR TEXAS.

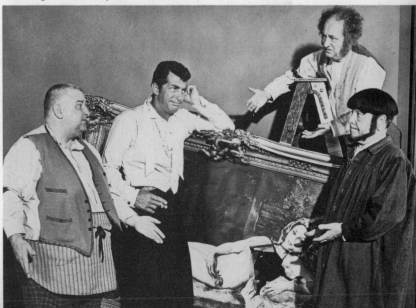

likely that anyone will succeed in "re-creating" the Three Stooges except by sheer imitation; they were unique.

And, as we survey the current movie scene, and see today's filmmakers trying to recapture—or relearn—the fundamentals of getting laughs, the Stooges' shorts, so effortless, so uncomplicated, so unpretentious, seem better and better in comparison. Time has been kind to the Three Stooges.

The Feature Films of the Three Stooges

1. **Soup to Nuts**—Fox 1930—Benjamin Stoloff—Ted Healy, Frances McCoy, Stanley Smith, Lucile Browne, Charles Winninger, Hallam Cooley, Florence Roberts, Clifford Dempsey, George Chandler, George Bickel, William H. Tooker, Heinie Conklin, Fred Sanborn, Mack Swain, Billy Barty, Roscoe Ates, Rube Goldberg (as himself). 65 minutes.

2. **Turn Back the Clock**—MGM 1933—Edgar Selwyn—Lee Tracy, Mae Clarke, Otto Kruger, George Barbier, Peggy Shannon, C. Henry Gordon, Clara Blandick, Ted Healy. 80 minutes.

3. **Meet the Baron**—MGM 1933—Walter Lang—Jack Pearl, Jimmy Durante, ZaSu Pitts, Edna May Oliver, Ted Healy, Ben Bard, Henry Kolker, William B. Davidson, Robert Greig, Rolfe Sedan, Leo White, Mary Gordon, Richard Tucker, June Brewster, The Metro-Goldwyn-Mayer Girls. 68 minutes.

4. **Dancing Lady**—MGM 1933—Robert Z. Leonard—Joan Crawford, Clark Gable, Franchot Tone, May Robson, Winnie Lightner, Fred Astaire, Robert Benchley, Ted Healy, Gloria Foy, Art Jarrett, Grant Mitchell, Maynard Holmes, Sterling Holloway, Nelson Eddy, Eve Arden, Lynn Bari. 82 minutes.

5. **Myrt and Marge**—Universal 1934—Al Boasberg—Myrtle Vail, Donna Damerel, Ted Healy, Eddie Foy, Jr., Grace Hayes, Trixie Friganza, Thomas Jackson, Ray Hedges, J. Farrell Macdonald, Bonnie Bonnell. 65 minutes.

6. **Fugitive Lovers**—MGM 1934—Richard Boleslavsky—Robert Montgomery, Madge Evans, Ted Healy, Nat

Pendleton, C. Henry Gordon, Ruth Selwyn, DeWitt
Jennings, Edward Hearn, Syd Saylor, Robert Homans,
Richard Cramer, Wade Boteler, Snowflake, Walter
Long, Al Hill, Milton Kibbee, Walter Brennan, Edward Gargan. 84 minutes.

7. **Hollywood Party**—MGM 1934—no director credited
(sequences actually directed by Allan Dwan, Richard
Boleslavsky, Edmund Goulding, Russell Mack, George
Stevens, Sam Wood, Charles Reisner)—Stan Laurel,
Oliver Hardy, Jimmy Durante, Charles Butterworth,
Polly Moran, Lupe Velez, Frances Williams, Jack Pearl,
Eddie Quillan, June Clyde, George Givot, Richard
Carle, Ben Bard, Tom Kennedy, Ted Healy, Mickey
Mouse. 70 minutes.

8. **The Captain Hates the Sea**—Columbia 1934—Lewis
Milestone—John Gilbert, Victor McLaglen, Walter
Connolly, Alison Skipworth, Wynne Gibson, Helen
Vinson, Fred Keating, Tala Birell, Leon Errol, Walter
Catlett, Claude Gillingwater, Emily Fitzroy, Geneva
Mitchell, John Wray, Donald Meek, Luis Alberni, Akim
Tamiroff, Arthur Treacher, Inez Courtney. 92 minutes.

9. **Start Cheering**—Columbia 1938—Albert S. Rogell—
Jimmy Durante, Walter Connolly, Joan Perry, Charles
Starrett, Professor Quiz, Edward Earle, Gertrude
Niesen, Raymond Walburn, Broderick Crawford, Hal
LeRoy, Ernest Truex, Virginia Dale, Chaz Chase, Jimmy
Wallington, Romo Vincent, Gene Morgan, Louise Stanley, Arthur Hoyt, Howard Hickman, Minerva Urecal,
Arthur Loft, Nick Lukats, Louis Prima and his Band,
Johnny Green and his Orchestra. 78 minutes.

10. **Time Out for Rhythm**—Columbia 1941—Sidney Salkow—
Ann Miller, Rudy Vallee, Rosemary Lane, Allen Jenkins,
Joan Merrill, Richard Lane, Brenda and Cobina, Six Hits
and a Miss, Eddie Durant's Rhumba Orchestra, Glen
Gray and Orchestra, Stanley Andrews. 74 minutes.

11. **My Sister Eileen**—Columbia 1942—Alexander Hall—
Rosalind Russell, Brian Aherne, Janet Blair, George
Tobias, Allyn Joslyn, Elizabeth Patterson, Grant Mitchell, Richard Quine, June Havoc, Donald MacBride,
Gordon Jones, Jeff Donnell, Clyde Fillmore, Minna
Phillips, Frank Sully, Charles La Torre. 96 minutes.

12. **Rockin' in the Rockies**—Columbia 1945—Vernon
Keays—Mary Beth Hughes, Jay Kirby, Tim Ryan,
Gladys Blake, Vernon Dent, Spade Cooley and his
Band. 63 minutes.

13. **Swing Parade of 1946**—Monogram 1946—Phil Karlson—Gale Storm, Phil Regan, Edward Brophy, Mary Treen, John Eldredge, Russell Hicks, Leon Belasco, Windy Cook, Connee Boswell, Louis Jordan, Will Osborne. 73 minutes.

14. **Gold Raiders**—United Artists 1951—Edward Bernds—George O'Brien, Sheila Ryan, Clem Bevans, Lyle Talbot, Fuzzy Knight, Monte Blue, John Merton, Al Baffert, Hugh Hooker, Bill Ward, Dick Crockett, Roy Canada. 56 minutes.

15. **Have Rocket, Will Travel**—Columbia 1959—David Lowell Rich—Jerome Cowan, Anna Lisa, Bob Colbert, Marjorie Bennett, Nadine Ducas, Don Lamond, Robert J. Stevenson, Dal McKennon. 76 minutes.

16. **Stop! Look! and Laugh!**—Columbia 1960—Jules White (new scenes)—Paul Winchell and dummies. Marquis Chimps, Joe Bolton; compilation including scenes from GOOFS AND SADDLES, VIOLENT IS THE WORD FOR CURLY, HOW HIGH IS UP?, SOCK-A-BYE BABY, WHAT'S THE MATADOR, MICRO PHONIES, and HALF-WITS HOLIDAY. 78 minutes.

17. **Snow White and the Three Stooges**—20th Century-Fox 1961—Walter Lang—Carol Heiss, Edson Stroll, Patricia Medina, Guy Rolfe, Michael David, Buddy Baer, Edgar Barrier, Peter Coe, Lisa Mitchell, Chuck Lacy, Owen McGivney, Sam Flint, Blossom Rock. Color—107 minutes.

18. **The Three Stooges Meet Hercules**—Columbia 1962—Edward Bernds—Vicki Trickett, Quinn Redeker, George N. Neise, Samson Burke, Mike McKeever, Emil Sitka, Hal Smith, John Cliff, Lewis Charles, Barbara Hines, Terry Huntington, Diana Piper, Gregg Martell, Gene Roth, Edward Foster, Cecil Elliott, Rusty Westcott. 89 minutes.

19. **The Three Stooges in Orbit**—Columbia 1962—Edward Bernds—Carol Christensen, Edson Stroll, Emil Sitka, George N. Neise, Rayford Barnes, Norman Leavitt, Nestor Paiva, Peter Dawson, Peter Brocco, Don Lamond, Thomas Glynn, Maurice Manson, Jean Charney, Duane Ament, Bill Dyer, Roy Engel, Jane Wald, Cheerio Meredith. 87 minutes.

20. **The Three Stooges Go Around the World in a Daze**—Columbia 1963—Norman Maurer—Jay Sheffield, Joan Freeman, Walter Burke, Emil Sitka, Peter Foster, Maurice Dallimore, Richard Devon. 94 minutes.

21. **It's a Mad Mad Mad Mad World**—United Artists 1963—Stanley Kramer—Spencer Tracy, Milton Berle, Sid Caesar, Buddy Hackett, Ethel Merman, Mickey Rooney, Dick Shawn, Phil Silvers, Terry-Thomas, Jonathan Winters, Edie Adams, Dorothy Provine, Eddie "Rochester" Anderson, Jim Backus, Ben Blue, Alan Carney, Barrie Chase, William Demarest, Peter Falk, Paul Ford, Leo Gorcey, Edward Everett Horton, Buster Keaton, Don Knotts, Carl Reiner, Joe E. Brown, Andy Devine, Sterling Holloway, Marvin Kaplan, Charles Lane, Charles McGraw, ZaSu Pitts, Madlyn Rhue, Arnold Stang, Jesse White, Lloyd Corrigan, Stan Freberg, Jimmy Durante, Jack Benny, Jerry Lewis. Color-Cinerama—192 minutes.

22. **Four for Texas**—Warner Brothers 1963—Robert Aldrich—Frank Sinatra, Dean Martin, Anita Ekberg, Ursula Andress, Charles Bronson, Victor Buono, Jack Elam, Richard Jaeckel, Fritz Feld, Mike Mazurki, Wesley Addy, Marjorie Bennett, Percy Helton, Jonathan Hale, Jack Lambert, Paul Langton, Jesslyn Fax, Teddy Buckner and his All Stars, Arthur Godfrey. Color–124 minutes.

23. **The Outlaws Is Coming**—Columbia 1965—Norman Maurer—Adam West, Nancy Kovack, Mort Mills, Don Lamond, Emil Sitka, Rex Holman, Henry Gibson, Murray Alper, Tiny Brauer, Joe Bolton, Bill Camfield, Hal Fryar, Johnny Ginger, Wayne Mack, Ed T. McDonnell, Bruce Sedley, Paul Shannon, Sally Starr. 89 minutes.

Moe Howard appeared, without the Stooges, in small roles in three films: SPACE MASTER X-7 (1958), DON'T WORRY, WE'LL THINK OF A TITLE (1966), and DR. DEATH: SEEKER OF SOULS (1973). He also served as associate producer on the 1959 Columbia feature SENIOR PROM.

Moe and Curly appeared briefly, without billing, in clown makeup in the 1933 MGM feature BROADWAY TO HOLLYWOOD, and were featured in the 1934 MGM short JAILBIRDS OF PARADISE. Curly also appeared in a short-subject without Moe and Larry at MGM called ROAST BEEF AND MOVIES in 1934.

The Three Stooges shot footage for a 1943 Columbia feature, GOOD LUCK, MR. YATES, but it was cut from the film and reused in the short subject GENTS WITHOUT CENTS. The Stooges did *not* appear in the 1934 feature GIFT OF GAB, as listed in the original edition of this book; confusion arises from the fact that a trio of performers who never worked together before (or since) received billing as the Three Stooges!

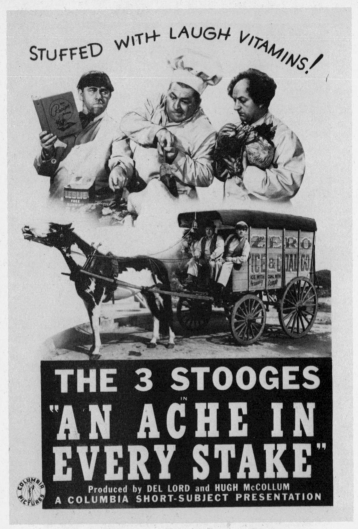

The Three Stooges Shorts

(Director's name follows year; all films two reels in length unless otherwise noted.)

With Ted Healy, for MGM
1. **Nertsery Rhymes**—1933—Jack Cummings—Bonnie Bonnell. Shot in two-color Technicolor and designed as

a framework for musical numbers left over from MGM's unreleased musical feature *The March of Time*.

2. **Beer and Pretzels**—1933—Jack Cummings—Bonnie Bonnell, Ed Brophy.

3. **Hello Pop!**—1933—Jack Cummings—Henry Armetta, Bonnie Bonnell, The Albertina Rasch Girls. Another Technicolor short incorporating leftover musical footage, including one number from the 1930 feature *It's a Great Life*.

4. **Plane Nuts**—1933—Jack Cummings—Bonnie Bonnell. This short incorporates a Busby Berkeley number, "Dance Until the Dawn," from the MGM feature *Flying High*.

5. **The Big Idea**—1934—William Crowley—Bonnie Bonnell, Muriel Evans, the Three Radio Rogues. Another short designed to make use of leftover MGM musical footage.

Guest Appearances with Ted Healy

1. **Hollywood on Parade**—Paramount 1933—no director credited—Healy and the Stooges with Bonnie Bonnell appear in this loosely structured behind-the-scenes short, set in a barroom with songwriters Mack Gordon and Harry Revel, Ben Turpin, Rudy Vallee, Benny Rubin, John Boles, Mr. and Mrs. Jimmy Durante, Florence Desmond. One reel.

2. **Screen Snapshots**—Columbia 1933—Ralph Staub—off-screen cut-ups at a nightclub with such participants as Jack Holt, Anita Page, Una Merkel, and Chico Marx. One reel.

The Columbia Shorts
Featuring Curly Howard

1. **Woman Haters**—1934—Archie Gottler—Marjorie White, Monty Collins, Bud Jamison, Snowflake, Jack Norton, Stanley "Tiny" Sandford, George Gray, Walter Brennan, A.R. Haysel, Don Roberts, Les Goodwin, Charles Richman, Gilbert Emery.

2. **Punch Drunks**—1934—Lou Breslow—Dorothy Granger, Arthur Housman, William Irving, Jack "Tiny" Lipson, Billy Bletcher, Al Hill, Chuck Callahan, Larry McGrath.

3. **Men in Black**—1934—Raymond McCarey—Del Henderson, Jeanie Roberts, Ruth Hiatt, Billy Gilbert, Little Billy, Bud Jamison, Hank Mann, Bobby Callahan, Phyllis Crane, Arthur West, Joe Mills, Irene Coleman,

3. Carmen Andre, Helen Splane, Kay Hughes, Eve Reynolds, Eve Kimberly, Lucile Watson, Billie Stockton, Betty Andre, Arthur Rankin, Neal Burns, Joe Fine, Charles Dorety, Charles King. Nominated for an Academy Award.
4. **Three Little Pigskins**—1934—Raymond McCarey—Lucille Ball, Gertie Green, Phyllis Crane, Walter Long, Joseph Young, William Irving, Joe Levine, Alex Hirschfield, Billy Wolfstone, Robert "Bobby" Burns, Jimmie Phillips, Johnny Kascier, Milton Douglas, Harry Bowen, Lynton Brent.
5. **Horses' Collars**—1935—Clyde Bruckman—Dorothea Kent, Fred Kohler, Leo Willis, Fred Kelsey, Allyn Drake, Slim Whittaker, Nelson McDowell, Milton Dogulas, Johnny Kascier, Bert Young, Ed Brandenberg, Bobby Callahn, June Gittelson, Alice Dahl, Nancy Caswell.
6. **Restless Knights**—1935—Charles Lamont—Geneva Mitchell, Walter Brennan, George Baxter, Chris Franke, James Howard, Bud O'Neill, Stanley Blystone, Ernie Young, Billy Franey, Jack Duffy, Lynton Brent, Bob Burns, William Irving, Joe Perry, Al Thompson, Bert Young, Dutch Hendrian, Marie Wells, Eadie Adams, Corinne Williams, Dorothy King, Patty Brice, Wheaton Chambers.
7. **Pop Goes the Easel**—1935—Del Lord—Robert "Bobby" Burns, Jack Duffy, Ellinor Van Der Veer, Phyllis Fine, Joan Howard, Phyllis Crane, William Irving, Al Thompson.
8. **Uncivil Warriors**—1935—Del Lord—Theodore Lorch, Lew Davis, Marvin Loback, Billy Engle, Ford West, Si Jenks, Bud Jamison, Phyllis Crane, Celeste Edwards, Lou Archer, James C. Morton, Charles Dorety, Heinie Conklin, Hubert Diltz, Charles Cross, George Gray, Jack Rand, Harry Keaton.
9. **Pardon My Scotch**—1935—Del Lord—Nat Carr, James C. Morton, Billy Gilbert, Grace Goodall, Barlowe Borland, Scotty Dunsmuir, Gladys Gale, Wilson Benge, Alec Craig, Al Thompson, Johnny Kascier, Symona Boniface, Pauline High, Billy Bletcher, Ettore Compana, Nena Compana.
10. **Hoi Polloi**—1935—Del Lord—Harry Holmes, Robert Graves, Bud Jamison, Grace Goodall, Betty McMahon, Phyllis Crane, Geneva Mitchell, Kathryn Kitty McHugh, James C. Morton, William Irving, Arthur Rankin, Rob-

ert McKenzie, Celeste Edwards, Harriet DeBussman, Mary Dees, Blanche Payson, George B. French, Gail Arnold, Don Roberts, Billy Mann.

11. **Three Little Beers**—1935—Del Lord—Bud Jamison, Nanette Crawford, Eve Reynolds, Frank Terry, Harry Semels, Jack "Tiny" Lipson, Eddie Laughton, George Gray, William Irving.

12. **Ants in the Pantry**—1936—Preston Black (Jack White) —Clara Kimball Young, Harrison Greene, Bud Jamison, Isabelle LaMal, Vesey O'Davoren, Douglas Gerrard, Anne O'Neal, James C. Morton, Arthur Rowlands, Bert Young, Lou Davis, Ron Wilson, Robert "Bobby" Burns, Lynton Brent, Arthur Thalasso, Phyllis Crane, Al Thompson, Helen Martinez, Charles Dorety, Hilda Title, Elaine Waters, Althea Henley, Idalyn Dupre, Stella LeSaint, Flo Promise, Gay Waters.

13. **Movie Maniacs**—1936—Del Lord—Bud Jamison, Lois Lindsey, Althea Henley, Kenneth Harlan, Mildred Harris, Harry Semels, Antrim Short, Jack Kenney, Charles Dorety, Elaine Waters, Bert Young, Hilda Title, Eddie Laughton.

14. **Half-Shot Shooters**—1936—Preston Black (Jack White) —Stanley Blystone, Vernon Dent, Harry Semels, Johnny Kascier, Eddie Laughton, Bert Young, Lynton Brent, Heinie Conklin, Al Thompson.

15. **Disorder in the Court**—1936—Preston Black (Jack White)—Susan Kaaren, Dan Brady, Tiny Jones, Bill O'Brien, Bud Jamison, Harry Semels, Edward LeSaint, Hank Bell, James C. Morton, Nick Baskovitch, Arthur Thalasso, Ed Mull, Eddie Laughton, Al Thompson.

16. **A Pain in the Pullman**—1936—Preston Black (Jack White)—Bud Jamison, James C. Morton, Eddie Laughton, Loretta Andrews, Ethelreda Leopold, Gale Arnold, Ray Turner, Mary Lou Dix, Hilda Title, Phyllis Crane, Eddie Laughton, Robert "Bobby" Burns.

17. **False Alarms**—1936—Del Lord—Stanley Blystone, June Gittelson, Johnny Grey, Eddie Laughton, George Gray.

18. **Whoops I'm an Indian**—1936—Del Lord—Bud Jamison, Elaine Waters, Beatrice Blinn, Robert McKenzie, Al Thompson, Eddie Laughton, William Irving.

19. **Slippery Silks**—1936—Preston Black (Jack White) —Vernon Dent, Robert Williams, Symona Boniface, Elaine Waters, Beatrice Blinn, Martha Tibbetts, Beatrice Curtis, Mary Lou Dix, Gale Arnold, Loretta Andrew, Gertrude Messinger, Hilda Title, June Gittle-

son, William Irving, Eddie Laughton, Jack "Tiny" Lipson, Bert Young.

20. **Grips, Grunts and Groans**—1937—Preston Black (Jack White)—Harrison Greene, Casey Columbo, Herb Stagman, Chuck Callahan, Blackie Whiteford, Elaine Waters, Cy Schindell, Tony Chavez, Budd Fine, Sam Lufkin, William Irving, Harry Wilson, Al Thompson, Eva McKenzie.

21. **Dizzy Doctors**— 1937—Del Lord—June Gittelson, Eva Murray, Ione Leslie, Vernon Dent, Louise Carver, Ella McKenzie, Bud Jamison, Cy Schindell, Wilfred Lucas, Eric Bunn, Frank Mills, Harley Wood, A. R. Haysel, Betty MacMahon, William Irving, Frank Austin, Robert "Bobby" Burns, Bert Young.

22. **Three Dumb Clucks**—1937—Del Lord—Lynton Brent, Frank Austin, Lucille Lund, Eddie Laughton, Al Thompson.

23. **Back to the Woods**—1937—Bud Jamison, Vernon Dent, Theodore Lorch, Bert Young, Ethelreda Leopold, Bert Young, Cy Schindell.

24. **Goofs and Saddles**—1937—Del Lord—Ted Lorch, Hank Mann, Stanley Blystone, Sam Lufkin, Hank Bell, Ethan Laidlaw, George Gray, Joe Palma, Eddie Laughton.

25. **Ca$h and Carry**—1937—Del Lord—Sonny Bupp, Al Richardson, Harlene Wood, Lester Dorr, Eddie Laughton, Cy Schindell.

26. **Playing the Ponies**—1937—Charles Lamont—William Irving, Jack "Tiny" Lipson, Billy Bletcher.

27. **The Sitter-Downers**—1937—Del Lord—Marcia Healy, Betty Mack, June Gittelson, James C. Morton, Robert McKenzie, Jack Long, Berty Young.

28. **Termites of 1938**—1938—Del Lord—Dorothy Granger, Bud Jamison, Bess Flowers.

29. **Wee Wee Monsieur**—1938—Del Lord—Bud Jamison, Vernon Dent, John Lester Johnson, Harry Semels, Ethelreda Leopold.

30. **Tassels in the Air**—1938—Charley Chase—Bess Flowers, Vernon Dent, Bud Jamison, Vic Travers.

31. **Flat Foot Stooges**—1938—Charley Chase—Chester Conklin, Dick Curtis, Lola Jensen, Heinie Conklin.

32. **Healthy, Wealthy and Dumb**—1938—Del Lord—Lucille Lund, Jean Carmen, Erlene Heath, James C. Morton, Bud Jamison, Robert "Bobby" Burns.

33. **Violent Is the Word for Curly**—1938—Charley Chase—

Gladys Gale, Marjorie Dean, Bud Jamison, Eddie Fetherstone, John T. Murray, Pat Gleason.

34. **Three Missing Links**—1938—Jules White—Monty Collins, Jane Hamilton, James C. Morton.

35. **Mutts to You**—1938—Charley Chase—Bess Flowers, Lane Chandler, Vernon Dent, Bud Jamison.

36. **Three Little Sew and Sews**—1939—Del Lord—Harry Semels, Phyllis Barry, James C. Morton, Bud Jamison, Vernon Dent, Ned Glass, Cy Schindell, John Tyrell.

37. **We Want Our Mummy**—1939—Del Lord—Bud Jamison, James C. Morton, Dick Curtis, Robert Williams, Ted Lorch, Eddie Laughton, John Tyrell.

38. **A-Ducking They Did Go**—1939—Del Lord—Lynton Brent, Vernon Dent, Bud Jamison, Vic Travers, Cy Schindell, Wheaton Chambers, Vic Travers.

39. **Yes, We Have No Bonanza**—1939—Del Lord—Dick Curtis, Lynton Brent, Vernon Dent, Suzanne Kaaren, Jean Carmen, Lola Jensen.

40. **Saved by the Belle**—1939—Charley Chase—Carmen LaRoux, Leroy Mason, Gino Corrado, Vernon Dent, Al Thompson

41. **Calling All Curs**—1939—Jules White—Lynton Brent, Cy Schindell, Beatrice Curtis, Beatrice Blinn, Dorothy Moore, Robin Raymond, Ethelreda Leopold.

42. **Oily to Bed, Oily to Rise**—1939—Jules White—Dick Curtis, Richard Fiske, Eddie Laughton, Eva McKenzie, Vic Travers, Lorna Gray (Adrian Booth), Dorothy Moore, Linda Winters (Dorothy Comingore).

43. **Three Sappy People**—1939—Jules White—Lorna Gray (Adrian Booth), Don Beddoe, Bud Jamison, Ann Doran, Richard Fiske, Eddie Laughton, Vic Travers.

44. **You Nazty Spy**—1940—Jules White—Dick Curtis, Don Beddoe, Richard Fiske, Florine Dickson, Little Billy, John Tyrell, Joe Murphy, Lorna Gray (Adrian Booth), Bert Young, Eddie Laughton, Al Thompson.

45. **Rockin' Through the Rockies**—1940—Jules White—Linda Winters (Dorothy Comingore), Dorothy Appleby, Lorna Gray (Adrian Booth), Kathryn Sheldon, Bert Young, Dick Curtis.

46. **A-Plumbing We Will Go**—1940—Del Lord—Symona Boniface, Bud Jamison, Bess Flowers, Eddie Laughton, Monty Collins, John Tyrell, Dudley Dickerson, Al Thompson.

47. **Nutty But Nice**—1940—Jules White—Vernon Dent, Eddie Garcia, John Tyrell, Ned Glass, Bert Young, Lynton

Brent, John Kascier, Ethelreda Leopold, Al Seymour
(Cy Schindell)

48. **How High Is Up?**—1940—Del Lord—Bruce Bennett,
Vernon Dent, Edmund Cobb.

49. **From Nurse to Worse**—1940—Jules White—Lynton
Brent, Vernon Dent, Dorothy Appleby, Babe Kane,
John Tyrell, Al Seymour (Cy Schindell), Joe Palma,
Poppie Wilde, Charlie Phillips, Blanche Payson, Johnny
Kascier, Dudley Dickerson, Al Thompson.

50. **No Census, No Feeling**—1940—Del Lord—Symona Boniface, Ellinor Van Der Veer, Vernon Dent, Bruce Bennett, Max Davidson, Bert Young, Frank Austin, John
Tyrell.

51. **Cookoo Cavaliers**—1940—Jules White—Dorothy Appleby, Jack O'Shea, Bob O'Connor, Lynton Brent, Blanche
Payson, Anita Garvin.

52. **Boobs in Arms**—1940—Jules White—Richard Fiske,
Evelyn Young, Eddie Laughton, John Kascier, Lynton
Brent, Cy Schindell, John Tyrell.

53. **So Long, Mr. Chumps**—1941—Jules White—Vernon
Dent, Robert Williams, Dorothy Appleby, Bert Young,
Eddie Laughton, Bruce Bennett.

54. **Dutiful But Dumb**—1941—Del Lord—Vernon Dent,
Bud Jamison, Bruce Bennett, Chester Conklin, Fred
Kelsey, Eddie Laughton, Harry Semels, Bert Young.

55. **All the World's a Stooge**—1941—Del Lord—Lelah
Tyler, Emory Parnell, Bud Jamison, Symona Boniface,
Olaf Hytten, Richard Fiske, John Tyrell, Gwen Seager,
Poppie Wilde, Ethelreda Leopold.

56. **I'll Never Heil Again**—1941—Jules White—Mary Ains-
lee, Johnny Kascier, Vernon Dent, Bud Jamison, Don
Barclay, Jack "Tiny" Lipson, Bert Young, Robert
"Bobby" Burns, Al Thompson.

57. **An Ache in Every Stake**—1941—Del Lord—Vernon
Dent, Bud Jamison, Gino Corrado, Bess Flowers,
Symona Boniface, Vic Travers, Blanche Payson.

58. **In the Sweet Pie and Pie**—1941—Jules White—Dorothy
Appleby, Mary Ainslee, Ethelreda Leopold, Richard
Fiske, John Tyrell, Eddie Laughton, Bert Young, Lynton
Brent, Al Thompson, John Kascier, Vernon Dent, Vic
Travers; in stock footage, Geneva Mitchell.

59. **Some More of Samoa**—1941—Del Lord—Louise Carver,
Monty Collins, Symona Boniface, Duke York, Mary
Ainslee, John Tyrell.

60. **Loco Boy Makes Good**—1942—Jules White—Dorothy

Appleby, Vernon Dent, Bud Jamison, Robert Williams, Eddie Laughton, John Tyrell, Ellinor Van Der Veer, Al Thompson, Bert Young, Robert "Bobby" Burns, Symona Boniface, Heinie Conklin, Lynton Brent, Vic Travers.

61. **Cactus Makes Perfect**—1942—Del Lord—Monty Collins, Vernon Dent, Ernie Adams, Eddie Laughton.

62. **What's the Matador?**—1942—Jules White—Suzanne Kaaren, Harry Burns, Dorothy Appleby, Eddie Laughton, Don Zelaya, Bert Young, Cy Schindell, John Tyrell.

63. **Matri-Phony**—1942—Harry Edwards—Vernon Dent, Marjorie Deanne, Cy Schindell, Monty Collins.

64. **Three Smart Saps**—1942—Jules White—Julie Duncan, Julie Gibson, Ruth Skinner, Bud Jamison, John Tyrell, Sally Cairns, Eddie Laughton, Vic Travers, Frank Coleman, Frank Terry, Lynton Brent, Barbara Slater.

65. **Even as I.O.U.**—1942—Del Lord—Ruth Skinner, Stanley Blystone, Wheaton Chambers, Vernon Dent, Bud Jamison, Billy Bletcher, Heinie Conklin, Jack Gardner, Bert Young.

66. **Sock-A-Bye Baby**—1942—Jules White—Julie Gibson, Clarence Straight, Bud Jamison, Baby Joyce Gardner, Dudley Dickerson.

67. **They Stooge to Conga**—1943—Del Lord—Vernon Dent, Dudley Dickerson, Lloyd Bridges, Eddie Laughton, John Tyrell.

68. **Dizzy Detectives**—1943—Jules White—John Tyrell, Bud Jamison, Dick Jensen, Lynton Brent.

69. **Spook Louder**—1943—Del Lord—Stanley Blystone, Lew Kelly, Symona Boniface, Ted Lorch, Charles Middleton.

70. **Back from the Front**—1943—Jules White—Vernon Dent, Bud Jamison, Stanley Blystone, Heinie Conklin, George Gray, Jack "Tiny" Lipson, Al Thompson, John Kascier, Harry Semels.

71. **Three Little Twirps**—1943—Harry Edwards—Chester Conklin, Heinie Conklin, Stanley Blystone, Bud Jamison, Duke York, Al Thompson.

72. **Higher Than a Kite**—1943—Del Lord—Dick Curtis, Vernon Dent, Duke York, Robert "Bobby" Burns.

73. **I Can Hardly Wait**—1943—Jules White—Bud Jamison, Adele St. Mara, Al Thompson.

74. **Dizzy Pilots**—1943—Jules White—Richard Fiske, Harry Semels.

75. **Phony Express**—1943—Del Lord—Shirley Patterson, Chester Conklin, Snub Pollard, Bud Jamison, Sally

Cleaves, Gwen Seager, John Merton, Joel Friedkin, Al Thompson, Vic Travers.

76. **A Gem of a Jam**—1943—Del Lord—Fred Kelsey, Dudley Dickerson, John Tyrell, Al Thompson.

77. **Crash Goes the Hash**—1944—Jules White—Vernon Dent, Bud Jamison, Dick Curtis, Symona Boniface, Wally Rose, Johnny Kascier, John Tyrell, Judy Malcolm, Beatrice Blinn, Ida Mae Johnson, Vic Travers, Elise Grover.

78. **Busy Buddies**—1944—Del Lord—Vernon Dent, Fred Kelsey, Eddie Laughton, John Tyrell, Vic Travers.

79. **The Yoke's on Me**—1944—Jules White—Bob McKenzie, Emmett Lynn, Eva McKenzie, Al Thompson, Vic Travers.

80. **Idle Roomers**—1944—Del Lord—Christine McIntyre, Duke York, Vernon Dent, Joanne Frank, Esther Howard, Eddie Laughton.

81. **Gents Without Cents**—1944—Jules White—Lindsay, Laverne, and Betty, John Tyrell, Robert "Bobby" Burns, Lynton Brent, Judy Malcolm.

82. **No Dough, Boys**—1944—Jules White—Vernon Dent, Christine McIntyre, Brian O'Hara, Kelly Flint, Judy Malcolm, John Tyrell.

83. **Three Pests in a Mess**—1945—Del Lord—Vernon Dent, Vic Travers, Snub Pollard, Christine McIntyre, Brian O'Hara, Heinie Conklin, John Tyrell, Hugh McCollum.

84. **Booby Dupes**—1945—Del Lord—Vernon Dent, Rebel Randall, Dorothy Vernon, John Tyrell, Snub Pollard, Wanda Perry, Geene Courtney, Lola Gogan.

85. **Idiots Deluxe**—1945—Jules White—Vernon Dent, Paul Kruger, Gwen Seager, Al Thompson.

86. **If a Body Meets a Body**—1945—Jules White—Ted Lorch, Fred Kelsey, Joe Palma, Al Thompson, John Tyrell.

87. **Micro-Phonies**—1945—Edward Bernds—Christine McIntyre, Symona Boniface, Gino Corrado, Sam Flint, Fred Kelsey, Chester Conklin, Bess Flowers, Lynton Brent, Ted Lorch, Heinie Conklin, John Tyrell.

88. **Beer Barrel Polecats**—1946—Jules White—Robert Williams, Vernon Dent, Joe Palma, Al Thompson; Bruce Bennett and Emory Parnell in stock footage.

89. **A Bird in the Head**—1946—Edward Bernds—Vernon Dent, Robert Williams, Frank Lackteen, Art Miles.

90. **Uncivil Warbirds**—1946—Jules White—Faye Williams, Eleanor Counts, Marilyn Johnson, Robert Williams,

Maury Dexter, Ted Lorch, Al Rosen, Joe Palma, Cy Schindell, Blackie Whiteford, Robert "Bobby" Burns, John Kascier, Vic Travers.

91. **Three Troubledoers**—1946—Edward Bernds—Christine McIntyre, Dick Curtis, Ethan Laidlaw, Blackie Whiteford, Hank Bell, Budd Fine, Steve Clarke, Joe Garcia, Vic Travers, Judy Malcolm.

92. **Monkey Businessmen**—1946—Edward Bernds—Kenneth Macdonald, Fred Kelsey, Snub Pollard, Jean Donahue (Jean Willes), Cy Schindell, Rocky Woods, Wade Crosby.

93. **Three Loan Wolves**—1946—Jules White—Beverly Warren, Harold Brauer, Wally Rose, Joe Palma, Jackie Jackson.

94. **G.I. Wanna Home**—1946—Jules White—Judy Malcolm, Ethelreda Leopold, Doris Houck, Symona Boniface, Al Thompson.

95. **Rhythm and Weep**—1946—Jules White—Jack Norton, Gloria Patrice, Ruth Godfrey, Nita Bieber.

96. **Three Little Pirates**—1946—Edward Bernds—Christine McIntyre, Vernon Dent, Dorothy DeHaven, Jack Parker, Larry McGrath, Robert Stevens, Ethan Laidlaw, Joe Palma, Al Thompson.

97. **Half-Wits' Holiday**—1947—Jules White—Vernon Dent, Barbara Slater, Ted Lorch, Emil Sitka, Symona Boniface, Helen Dickson, Vic Travers, Al Thompson.

Featuring Shemp Howard

98. **Fright Night**—1947—Edward Bernds—Harold Brauer, Dick Wessel, Cy Schindell, Claire Carleton, Sammy Stein, Tommy Klingston, Dave Harper, Stanley Blystone, Heinie Conklin.

99. **Out West**—1947—Edward Bernds—Jack Norman, Jacques (Jock) O'Mahoney, Christine McIntyre, Vernon Dent, Stanley Blystone, George Cheesebro, Frank Ellis, Heinie Conklin.

100. **Hold that Lion**—1947—Jules White—Kenneth Macdonald, Emil Sitka, Dudley Dickerson, Heinie Conklin, Vic Travers; cameo appearance by Curly Howard.

101. **Brideless Groom**—1947—Edward Bernds—Dee Green, Christine McIntyre, Emil Sitka, John Kascier.

102. **Sing a Song of Six Pants**—1947—Jules White—Dee Green, Harold Brauer, Virginia Hunter, Vernon Dent, Phil Arnold, Cy Schindell, Johnny Kascier, Bing Connelly.

103. **All Gummed Up**—1947—Jules White—Christine McIntyre, Emil Sitka, Al Thompson, Vic Travers, Al Thompson, Cy Schindell.

104. **Shivering Sherlocks**—1948—Del Lord—Christine McIntyre, Kenneth MacDonald, Frank Lackteen, Duke York, Vernon Dent, Stanley Blystone, Cy Schindell.
105. **Pardon My Clutch**—1948—Edward Bernds—Matt McHugh, Emil Sitka, Alyn Lockwood, Doria Revier, Wanda Perry, Stanley Blystone, George Lloyd.
106. **Squareheads of the Round Table**—1948—Edward Bernds—Phil Van Zandt, Vernon Dent, Jacques (Jock) O'Mahoney, Christine McIntyre, Harold Brauer, Joe Garcia, Douglas Coppin.
107. **Fiddlers Three**—1948—Jules White—Vernon Dent, Phil Van Zandt, Virginia Hunter, Sherry O'Neil, Joe Palma, Cy Shindell, Al Thompson.
108. **The Hot Scots**—1948—Edward Bernds—Herbert Evans, Christine McIntyre, Ted Lorch, Charles Knight.
109. **Heavenly Daze**—1948—Jules White—Vernon Dent, Sam McDaniel, Vic Travers, Symona Boniface, Marti Shelton, Judy Malcolm.
110. **I'm a Monkey's Uncle**—1948—Jules White—Dee Green, Virginia Hunter, Nancy Saunders.
111. **Mummy's Dummies**—1948—Edward Bernds—Dee Green, Phil Van Zandt, Ralph Dunn, Vernon Dent, Suzanne Ridgeway, Virginia Ellsworth, Wanda Perry.
112. **A Crime on Their Hands**—1948—Edward Bernds—Kenneth MacDonald, Christine McIntyre, Charles C. Wilson, Lester Allen, Cy Schindell, Heinie Conklin, George Lloyd.
113. **The Ghost Talks**—1949—Jules White—Phil Arnold, Nancy Saunders.
114. **Who Done It?**—1949—Edward Bernds—Christine McIntyre, Emil Sitka, Dudley Dickerson, Duke York, Ralph Dunn, Charles Knight.
115. **Hocus Pocus**—1949—Jules White—Mary Ainslee, Vernon Dent, Jimmy Lloyd, David Bond, Ned Glass.
116. **Fuelin' Around**—1949—Edward Bernds—Jacques (Jock) O'Mahoney, Christine McIntyre, Emil Sitka, Vernon Dent, Phil Van Zandt, Harold Brauer, Andre Pola.
117. **Malice in the Palace**—1949—Jules White—George Lewis, Frank Lackteen, Vernon Dent, Joe Palma.
118. **Vagabond Loafers**—1949—Edward Bernds—Christine McIntyre, Kenneth MacDonald, Symona Boniface, Emil Sitka, Dudley Dickerson, Herbert Evans, Barbara Slater.
119. **Dunked in the Deep**—1949—Jules White—Gene Stutenroth (Roth).
120. **Punchy Cowpunchers**—1950—Edward Bernds—Jacques

(Jock) O'Mahoney, Christine McIntyre, Kenneth Mac-Donald, George Chesebro, Bob Cason, Ted Mapes, Stanley Price, Dick Wessel, Emil Sitka, Heinie Conklin.

121. **Hugs and Mugs**—1950—Jules White—Christine McIntyre, Nanette Bourdeaux, Kathleen O'Malley, Joe Palma, Wally Rose, Pat Moran, Emil Sitka.

122. **Dopey Dicks**—1950—Edward Bernds—Christine McIntyre, Stanley Price, Phil Van Zandt.

123. **Love at First Bite**—1950—Jules White—Christine McIntyre, Yvette Reynard, Marie Monteil, Al Thompson.

124. **Self-Made Maids**—1950—Jules White—The Stooges played their own leading ladies in this film.

125. **Three Hams on Rye**—1950—Jules White—Nanette Bordeaux, Emil Sitka, Christine McIntyre, Mildred Olsen, Judy Malcolm, Ned Glass.

126. **Studio Stoops**—1950—Edward Bernds—Kenneth Mac-Donald, Charles Jordan, Christine McIntyre, Vernon Dent, Joe Palma, Stanley Price.

127. **Slaphappy Sleuths**—1950—Jules White—Stanley Blystone, Emil Sitka, Gene Roth, Nanette Bordeaux, Joe Palma.

128. **A Snitch in Time**—1950—Edward Bernds—Jean Willes, Henry Kulky, John Merton, Bob Cason.

129. **Three Arabian Nuts**—1951—Edward Bernds—Vernon Dent, Phil Van Zandt, Dick Curtis, Wesley Bly.

130. **Baby Sitters' Jitters**—1951—Jules White—Lynn Davis, David Windsor, Margie Liszt, Myron Healey.

131. **Don't Throw That Knife**—1951—Jules White—Dick Curtis, Jean Willes.

132. **Scrambled Brains**—1951—Jules White—Babe London, Vernon Dent, Royce Milne, Emil Sitka.

133. **Merry Mavericks**—1951—Edward Bernds—Don Harvey, Marily Martin, Paul Campbell, Emil Sitka, George Chesebro; in stock footage, Vic Travers, Al Thompson.

134. **The Tooth Will Out**—1951—Edward Bernds—Margie Liszt, Vernon Dent, Emil Sitka, Dick Curtis, Slim Gaut.

135. **Hula-La-La**—1951—Hugh McCollum—Jean Willes, Kenneth MacDonald, Emil Sitka, Maxine Doviat, Lei Aloha, Joy Windsor.

136. **Pest Man Wins**—1951—Jules White—Margie Liszt, Nanette Bordeaux, Emil Sitka, Vernon Dent, Helen Dickson; in stock footage, Symona Boniface, Eddie Laughton, Vic Travers, Al Thompson, Heinie Conklin.

137. **A Missed Fortune**—1952—Jules White—Nanette Bordeaux, Suzanne Ridgeway, Vivian Mason, Vernon Dent, Stanley Blystone.

138. **Listen, Judge**—1952—Edward Bernds—Kitty McHugh, Vernon Dent, Mary Emory, John Hamilton, Gil Perkins, Chick Collins, Emil Sitka, Phil Arnold.
139. **Corny Casanovas**—1952—Jules White—Connie Cezan.
140. **He Cooked His Goose**—1952—Jules White—Mary Ainslee, Angela Stevens, Thelia Darin.
141. **Gents in a Jam**—1952—Edward Bernds—Emil Sitka, Kitty McHugh, Mickey Simpson, Dani Sue Nolan.
142. **Three Dark Horses**—1952—Jules White—Kenneth MacDonald, Ben Welden.
143. **Cuckoo on a Choo Choo**—1952—Jules White—Patricia Wright, Victoria Horne, Reggie Dvorack.
144. **Up in Daisy's Penthouse**—1953—Jules White—Connie Cezan, John Merton, Jack Kenny, Suzanne Ridgeway.
145. **Booty and the Beast**—1953—Jules White—Kenneth MacDonald, Vernon Dent; in stock footage, Vic Travers, Heinie Conklin, Dudley Dickerson, Curly Howard.
146. **Loose Loot**—1953—Jules White—Kenneth MacDonald, Tom Kennedy, Nanette Bordeaux, Suzanne Ridgeway; in stock footage, Emil Sitka.
147. **Tricky Dicks**—1953—Jules White—Benny Rubin, Connie Cezan, Ferris Taylor, Phil Arnold, Murray Alper, Suzanne Ridgeway.
148. **Spooks**—1953—Jules White—Phil Van Zandt, Tom Kennedy, Norma Randall. Released in 3-D.
149. **Pardon My Backfire**—1953—Jules White—Benny Rubin, Frank Sully, Phil Arnold, Barbara Bartay, Fred Kelsey, Ruth Godfrey, Angela Stevens, Thelia Darin. Released in 3-D.
150. **Rip, Sew and Stitch**—1953—Jules White—in stock footage Vernon Dent, Phil Arnold, Harold Brauer.
151. **Bubble Trouble**—1953—Jules White—Emil Sitka; in stock footage, Christine McIntyre.
152. **Goof on the Roof**—1953—Jules White—Frank Mitchell, Maxine Gates.
153. **Income Tax Sappy**—1954—Jules White—Benny Rubin, Vernon Dent, Joe Palma, Marjorie Liszt, Nannette Bordeaux.
154. **Musty Musketeers**—1954—Jules White—Vernon Dent, Phil Van Zandt, Ruth Godfrey White, Norma Randall, Diana Darrin, Joe Palma, Heinie Conklin; in stock footage, Virginia Hunter, Sherry O'Neill.
155. **Pals and Gals**—1954—Jules White—Christine McIntyre, George Chesebro, Heinie Conklin, Ruth Godfrey, Norma Randall, Stanley Blystone, Joe Palma; in stock footage, Vernon Dent, Norman Willis, Frank Ellis.

156. **Knutzy Knights**—1954—Jules White—Ruth Godfrey, Joe Palma; in stock footage, Jacques O'Mahoney, Christine McIntyre, Phil Van Zandt, Vernon Dent.

157. **Shot in the Frontier**—1954—Jules White—Emil Sitka, Ruth Godfrey White, Theila Darin, Vivian Mason, Kenneth MacDonald, Emmett Lynn, Babe London, Joe Palma.

158. **Scotched in Scotland**—1954—Jules White—Phil Van Zandt, Christine McIntyre, George Pembroke; in stock footage, Charles Knight, Ted Lorch, Herbert Evans.

159. **Fling in the Ring**—1955—Jules White—Frank Sully, Cy Schindell, Joe Palma; in stock footage, Dick Wessel, Claire Carleton, Harold Brauer, Tommy Kingston.

160. **Of Cash and Hash**—1955—Jules White—Christine McIntyre, Frank Lackteen, Kenneth MacDonald, Stanley Blystone; in stock footage, Christine McIntyre, Cy Schindell.

161. **Gypped in the Penthouse**—1955—Jules White—Jean Willes, Emil Sitka, Al Thompson.

162. **Bedlam in Paradise**—1955—Jules White—Phil Van Zandt, Sylvia Lewis; in stock footage, Marti Shelton, Judy Malcolm, Veron Dent, Symona Boniface, Vic Travers.

163. **Stone Age Romeos**—1955—Jules White—Emil Sitka, Dee Green, Nancy Saunders, Virginia Hunter, Joe Palma, Cy Schindell, Bill Wallace, Barbara Bartay.

164. **Wham Bam Slam**—1955—Jules White—Alyn Lockwood; in stock footage, Doris Revier, Wanda Perry, Matt McHugh.

165. **Hot Ice**—1955—Jules White—Kenneth MacDonald, Lester Allen, Barbara Bartay, Budd Fine, Blackie Whiteford; in stock footage, Christine McIntyre, Charles C. Wilson, Heinie Conklin, Cy Schindell.

166. **Blunder Boys**—1955—Jules White—Benny Rubin, Angela Stevens, Kenneth MacDonald, Barbara Bartay, Bonnie Menjum, Barbara Donaldson, Marjorie Jackson, June Lebow, Al Thompson, Johnny Kascier.

167. **Husbands Beware**—1956—Jules White—Emil Sitka, Maxine Gates, Lou Leonard; in stock footage, Christine McIntyre, Dee Green, Nancy Saunders, Doris Colleen, Johnny Kascier.

168. **Creeps**—1956—Jules White—voice of Phil Arnold.

169. **Flagpole Jitters**—1956—Jules White—Frank Sully, Beverly Thomas, Barbara Bartay, Bonnie Menjum, Don Harvey, David Bond, Dick Alexander; in stock footage, Mary Ainslee, Ned Glass.

170. **For Crimin' Out Loud**—1956—Jules White—Barbara Bartay, Emil Sitka, Charles Knight, Ralph Dunn; in stock footage, Christine McIntyre, Duke York.
171. **Rumpus in a Harem**—1956—Jules White—George Lewis, Harriette Tarler, Diana Darrin, Helen Jay, Ruth Godfrey White, Suzanne Ridgeway, Frank Lackteen; Joe Palma doubling for Shemp; in stock footage, Vernon Dent.
172. **Hot Stuff**—1956—Jules White—Connie Cezan, Phil Van Zandt, Gene Roth, Evelyn Lovequist, Andre Pola; Joe Palma double for Shemp; in stock footage, Vernon Dent, Christine McIntyre, Jacques O'Mahoney, Emil Sitka, Harold Brauer.
173. **Scheming Schemers**—1956—Jules White—Kenneth Mac-Donald, Emil Sitka; Joe Palma doubling for Shemp; in stock footage, Christine McIntyre, Symona Boniface, Emil Sitka, Dudley Dickerson, Herbert Evans, Helen Dickson, Vic Travers, Al Thompson.
174. **Commotion on the Ocean**—1956—Jules White—Gene Roth, Emil Sitka, Harriette Tarler; Joe Palma doubling for Shemp; in stock footage, Charles Wilson.

Featuring Joe Besser
175. **Hoofs and Goofs**—1957—Jules White—Benny Rubin, Harriette Tarler, Tony the Wonder Horse.
176. **Muscle Up a Little Closer**—1957—Jules White—Maxine Gates, Ruth Godfrey White, Matt Murphy, Harriette Tarler.
177. **A Merry Mix-Up**—1957—Jules White—Nanette Bordeaux, Jeanne Carmen, Ruth Godfrey White, Suzanne Ridgeway, Hariette Tarler, Diana Darrin, Frank Sully.
178. **Space Ship Sappy**—1957—Jules White—Benny Rubin, Doreen Woodbury, Lorraine Crawford, Harriette Tarler, Marilyn Hanold, Emil Sitka.
179. **Guns A-Poppin'**—1957—Jules White—Frank Sully, Joe Palma; in stock footage, Vernon Dent.
180. **Horsing Around**—1957—Jules White—Emil Sitka, Harriette Tarler, Tony the Wonder Horse.
181. **Rusty Romeos**—1957—Jules White—Connie Cezan.
182. **Outer-Space Jitters**—1957—Jules White—Emil Sitka, Gene Roth, Phil Van Zandt, Joe Palma, Dan Blocker, Diana Darrin, Harriette Tarler, Arline Hunter.
183. **Quiz Whizz**—1958—Jules White—Milton Frome, Gene Roth, Greta Thyssen, Bill Brauer, Emil Sitka.
184. **Fifi Blows Her Top**—1958—Jules White—Vanda Dupree,

Phil Van Zandt, Harriette Tarler, Wanda D'Ottoni; in stock footage, Christine McIntyre, Yvette Reynard, Al Thompson.

185. **Pies and Guys**—1958—Jules White—Gene Roth, Milton Frome, Greta Thyseen, Helen Dickson, John Kascier, Harriette Tarler, Emil Sitka; in stock footage, Symona Boniface, Helen Dickson, Vic Travers, Al Thompson, Barbara Slater.

186. **Sweet and Hot**—1958—Jules White—Muriel Landers.

187. **Flying Saucer Daffy**—1958—Jules White—Gail Bonny, Emil Sitka, Harriette Tarler, Bek Nelson, Diana Darrin, Joe Palma.

188. **Oil's Well That Ends Well**—1958—Jules White—no supporting cast.

189. **Triple Crossed**—1959—Jules White—Angela Stevens, Connie Cezan; in stock footage, Diana Darrin, Mary Ainslee.

190. **Sappy Bullfighters**—1959—Jules White—Greta Thyssen, George Lewis; in stock footage, Eddie Laughton, Cy Schindell.

Miscelleaneous Short Subjects
Featuring Curly

1. **Screen Snapshots #6**—Columbia 1935—Ralph Staub—Ken Murray shares footage of an annual charity baseball game in which top comedians and leading men participate. One reel.

2. **Screen Snapshots #9**—Columbia 1939—Ralph Staub—The Stooges are seen at a horse show, along with Clark Gable, Carole Lombard, Jean Parker, William Boyd, Allan Jones, Irene Harvey, Robert Taylor, Bing Crosby, Joe E. Brown, Virginia Bruce, Allan Jones, and Robert Young. One reel.

Featuring Joe De Rita

1. **The Three Stooges Scrapbook**—Columbia 1963—Sidney Miller—Don Lamond, Norman Maurer. An unsold TV pilot released to theaters instead. Color—8 minutes.

2. **Star Spangled Salesman**—U.S. Treasury Department—Norman Maurer—Carl Reiner, Carol Burnett, Milton Berle, Howard Morris, John Banner, Werner Klemperer, Rafer Johnson, Tim Conway, Harry Morgan, Jack Webb. A promotional short for U.S. Savings Bonds. Color—17 minutes.

THE RITZ BROTHERS

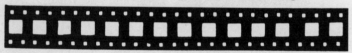

Either you love them or you hate them. Ever since 1925 the bombastic Ritz Brothers have elicited this kind of strong audience response. Film critic Pauline Kael rates the antics of Harry Ritz alongside those of Marcel Marceau. Mel Brooks has called Harry the funniest man alive. Sid Caesar and other funnymen have expressed their debt to Harry and his brothers. Apparently there are just as many, among the press and the public, who've never found the Ritz trio amusing. But majority rules, in show business and in life. The Ritz Brothers entertained audiences for six decades—and kept 'em laughing long and loud enough to remain headliners all that time.

The brothers were born in Newark, New Jersey, the sons of Max J. Joachim, a haberdasher who soon moved his growing family to Brooklyn. Al, the oldest, was born in 1903; Jimmy followed in 1906 and Harry in 1908. The clan also included another brother, George, and a sister, Gertrude. The brothers always cited their father as their original inspiration. Max Joachim ws a happy, loving man who had come to this country from Austria and tried several businesses before settling in the hat trade. He was always clowning with his boys, and they inherited his contagious sense of fun. The brothers went through high school in Brooklyn, but all of them were stagestruck early in life. Al, the oldest, won an amateur contest at the age of ten. He started as a dancer, and Harry and Jimmy followed the same route several years later. The three went their separate ways after high school graduation, each struggling to make a living as a single on the local vaudeville circuits.

There are many versions of how the three boys came together; one has it that Al suggested the move. Another claims that the fourth Ritz brother, George, proposed the idea. George did become their first manager, securing them their earliest bookings and setting them on the road to

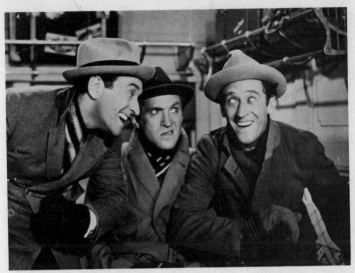

Al (left) and Jimmy (right) are enthusiastic about something in ONE IN A MILLION. but Harry doesn't seem so sure.

success. Another controversy arises over how the name "Ritz" was chosen, although the story the brothers always tell asserts that the name was taken from a passing laundry truck when an agent told them they would have to change their monicker. The Ritz Brothers opened at the College Inn at Coney Island in 1925, a night-spot that also housed a young musician-entertainer named Jimmy Durante. The act was called "The Collegians," and Al, Jimmy and Harry wore big red bow ties, large straw hats, and oversized pants. The emphasis was on precision dancing, but the routine encompassed music and comedy as well. With this auspicious debut under their belt, George got the Collegians booked into Fox's Folly Theater in Brooklyn at $25 a week. The boys were, oddly enough, an immediate hit, and before long they were commanding $400 a week with a four-week guarantee. They played the choicest vaudeville houses in New York— Loew's State and the Palace among them—before catching the eye of showman Earl Carroll.

Carroll kept the Ritz Brothers employed for several years, in various editions of his *Vanities* as well as in his first non-revue musical in many years, *The Florida Girl*. The boys were given a featured spot, and were listed in the cast of characters as Al Socrates, Jimmy Plato and Harry Aris-

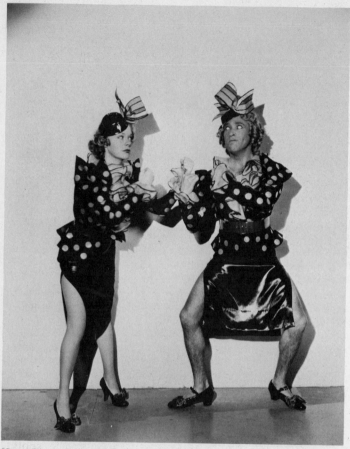

Harry Ritz prepares to settle his differences with Alice Faye in a posed shot from ON THE AVENUE. That outfit doesn't look good on *either* of them.

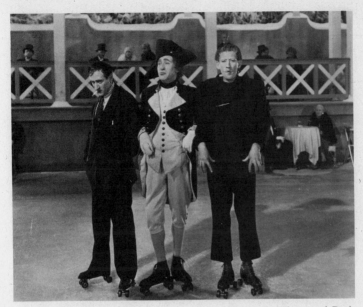

The Ritz Brothers pay tribute to Peter Lorre, Charles Laughton and Boris Karloff—on skates—in ONE IN A MILLION.

totle. They interpolated their "collegian" act verbatim, and went over quite well with the Broadway audiences. The critics who bothered to comment were divided in their opinions of the newcomers, saying, as so many others were to do in later years, that it was all a matter of personal taste. The Ritz Brothers had it made, and continued to appear in Carroll productions such as *The Casino Vanities* and *The Continental Vanities*, returning to prime vaudeville spots when Broadway wasn't keeping them busy. In 1934 they made a short-subject in the New York studios of Educational Pictures, a comedy firm that specialized in making cheap shorts with upcoming talent and faded stars. Their talent roster in the 1930's included Danny Kaye, Imogene Coca and Milton Berle, from the former group, and Buster Keaton and Harry Langdon, from the latter. The Ritzes' short, HOTEL ANCHOVY, was produced and directed by veteran comedy maker Al Christie, with Harry as the manager, Al as the house detective, and Jimmy as the bellboy in Doris Hill's failing seaside resort. The short may not be hilarious but it's energetic, and shows the brothers to good advantage.

The two-reeler received good distribution, and was seen
by director Sidney Lanfield. He liked the Ritz Brothers, and
persuaded 20th Century-Fox, for whom he was working, to
sign the boys to an exclusive contract. They were brought to
Hollywood, and spotlighted in a top-grade musical comedy
directed by Lanfield, SING, BABY, SING, starring Alice Faye
and Adolphe Menjou. The film had a strong plot—a spoof
of the Elaine Barrie-John Barrymore romance—and fine
songs like the title tune and "You Turned the Tables on
Me." In addition to these assets, Fox decided to use SING,
BABY, SING as a showcase for their new contract comedians.
They were given the opening scene, doing an operatic rendition of "The Music Goes Round" in a nightclub, several solo
spots throughout the film, and a special credit at the end
which explained that Fox was presenting the Ritz boys for
the first time. In an unusual move, after the "The End"
title, the Ritz Brothers came on screen *again* to take a final
bow. In addition to all this hoopla, the Ritzes came on
strong with some of the best material they ever had: takeoffs
of Ted Lewis and Harry Richman, a Dr. Jekyll and Mr.

The Ritz Brothers and friend in the finale of YOU CAN'T HAVE EVERYTHING.

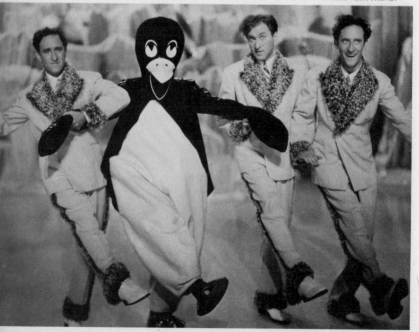

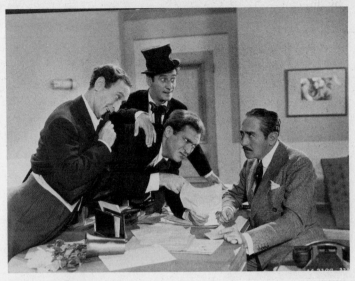

The Ritzes drive a hard bargain with producer Adolphe Menjou in THE GOLDWYN FOLLIES.

Hyde sketch, and several musical numbers. The film was a big success and brought the brothers into Hollywood in style. It also didn't hurt the blossoming career of Alice Faye, and gave a newcomer named Tony Martin a solo number as well.

From that point on, Fox kept the Ritz Brothers busy in a rapid succession of musicals—mostly with Alice Faye—and several well-made comedy vehicles. They seemed intrusive in ON THE AVENUE, which was doing fine with Dick Powell, Madeleine Carroll, Alice Faye and an Irving Berlin score, but they tried their best with a version of "Let's go Slumming" featuring Harry in drag, and a very funny rendition of "Ortchi-Tchorniya," which served to break up Dick Powell's Broadway debut. In YOU CAN'T HAVE EVERYTHING, they were back in their metier—a nightclub setting—where they always seemed to have an extra spark. The other feature numbers, including one called "Long Underwear," were supposed to be the brothers' big comedy numbers, but the sequence in a Greenwich Village nightclub presented them at their best, with a mock audience that really seemed to be enjoying the brothers' antics. ONE IN A MILLION also showed them to good advantage, especially in a number performed on skates (the film's star was Sonja Henie) in which the brothers mimicked three movie heavies: Peter Lorre, Charles Laughton (as Captain Bligh) and Boris Karloff (as Frankenstein).

LIFE BEGINS AT COLLEGE (1937) proved that the Ritz Brothers could support a film by themselves, and didn't have to rely on Alice Faye to see them through ninety minutes. COLLEGE had plenty of subplots, to be sure, but the brothers were given actual roles for the first time, and carried the film quite well. They also did several musical specialties, including an excellent "Spirit of '76" takeoff, and capped the film with a hilarious football sequence that served as a rousing climax. The running gag is that their college team has been doing so well, the coach can afford to put the three nitwits into the game. He does so only when the team has such a marked lead that their inept antics can't hurt the score.

In 1938, Samuel Goldwyn borrowed the brothers from Fox for his Technicolor extravaganza, THE GOLDWYN FOLLIES. The FOLLIES turned out to be one of the producer's biggest bombs, with an incredibly jumbled cast sinking in a sea of clichés and uninspired musical numbers. The Ritzes managed to survive in their few scenes, as animal trainers who try to attract producer Adolphe Menjou ("When you think of animals, think of us," they propose) but end up as actors in his film. Their major number, "Serenade to a Fish," is one of the film's few highpoints, with the boys as would-be Italian gondoliers who sink into the Venetian canal when a friendly whale douses them and capsizes their boat.

Back at Fox, things were beginning to change for the Ritz Brothers. Their films were no longer top-drawer musicals of the caliber of SING, BABY, SING. They were making minor efforts like STRAIGHT, PLACE, AND SHOW instead, and the boys weren't happy about it. These films weren't all that bad—in fact, KENTUCKY MOONSHINE included a hilarious Snow White spoof that remained in their nightclub act for several decades—but the brothers felt that they weren't being treated right. While Darryl F. Zanuck had been supervising their "A" musicals, their latest efforts were in the "B" category, which was under the jurisdiction of Sol M. Wurtzel. The brothers decided to grin and bear it for a while, but after a preview of one of their films, Harry declared, "Things have gone from bad to Wurtzel." The situation was temporarily smoothed over with a film that turned out to be the team's best: THE THREE MUSKETEERS.

THE THREE MUSKETEERS remains today a vivid, entertaining musical comedy. Despite a tendency to dismiss it as a Ritz Brothers vehicle, the film is remarkably faithful to

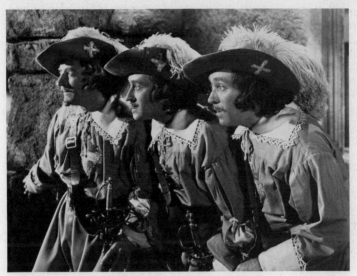

Athos, Porthos and Aramis never had it so good; the Ritz Brothers in their best film, THE THREE MUSKETEERS.

Harry, Don Ameche and Jimmy have their eye on something in this scene from THE THREE MUSKETEERS.

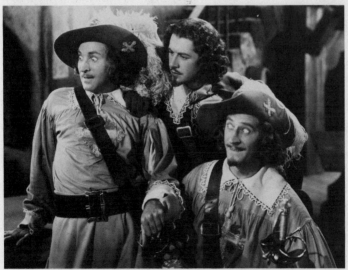

Dumas' classic story. Contrary to popular belief, the brothers do not play the title characters; instead, they masquerade as the musketeers, who are bound and gagged early in the film and are unable to move about. Don Ameche plays the naive but sincere D'Artagnan, and sings several pleasant songs; Gloria Stuart is a lovely and regal Queen; Pauline Moore is an antiseptic but adequate heroine; and Binnie Barnes displays both beauty and a willingness to "take it" in the name of comedy, as Lady DeWinter. In one scene, the Ritzes are sent to retrieve a message which villainess DeWinter has hidden in the bodice of her dress. They shake her up and literally turn her upside down to obtain the precious note, which will save their queen and prove their worth as swashbuckling musketeers. THREE MUSKETEERS was hardly Fox's most important release of 1939, yet great care was taken with its production. The director was Allan Dwan, who had made Douglas Fairbanks' 1922 ROBIN HOOD one of the great swashbucklers of all time. The cast was filled with expert character actors such as Lionel Atwill, John Carradine, Joseph Schildkraut and Douglass Dumbrille. The costumes

The brothers Ritz look upward for clues in the murder-mystery THE GORILLA; the film's star is standing behind them.

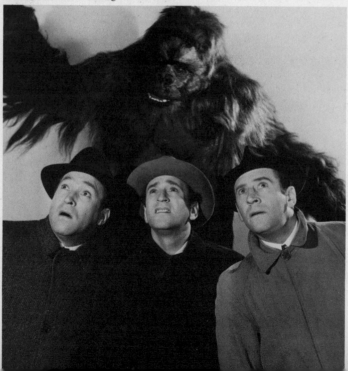

and sets (particularly the castle) gave the film the feel of a gargantuan production when in fact it was an economical, slickly produced picture.

As THREE MUSKETEERS was being released, the Ritz Brothers clashed with 20th Century-Fox over their next assignment, a film version of the stage success *The Gorilla*, which had been bought and adapted for them. Fox claimed to have spent $175,000 in preparation for the film, but when shooting time arrived, The Ritzes decided that they did not want to appear in another "B" picture for the studio and walked out. They were immediately suspended, and Fox filed suit for $150,000 damages. The walkout received full press coverage, and was quite a dramatic move for a vaudeville team with no profound artistic ambitions. Suspensions were frequent during the Hollywood studio system's reign but most of them involved actors and actresses who were anxious to further their careers in prestigious roles. Several weeks after the Ritz walkout, *The New York Times* carried a story that all was forgiven on both sides and the brothers were returning to work. Jimmy Ritz explained with a straight face, "We are very, very happy to be back, and Mr. Zanuck is very, very happy to have us back. The whole thing was just a misunderstanding. You know what I mean?" Harry added, "I want to tell you this is a great corporation we're working for. They're right and we're right. You know what I mean?" No one really did know what Harry meant at the time, but the true outcome of the brouhaha became evident several months later when Fox dropped the three comics from its roster.

THE GORILLA, which caused all the noise, was very obvious stuff, yet it is one of the films for which most people remember the Ritz Brothers. Based on a 1925 Ralph Spence play, the story was somewhat changed to allow the brothers to play detectives investigating a series of murders committed by a man in a gorilla suit. None of the critics was impressed, with most of the compliments going to Patsy Kelly, who, as usual, made the most of her supporting role. The brothers' last film for Fox, completed and released in 1939, was PACK UP YOUR TROUBLES, a World War I opus starring Jane Withers. The brothers had their big chance at the beginning of the picture, doing an amusing routine for a booking agent, but after that, they became embroiled in a so-so plot that spent most of its time with little Janie and did the brothers little good. After the completion of the film, they packed their own bags and left 20th Century-Fox.

The following year, the Ritzes made their first film for

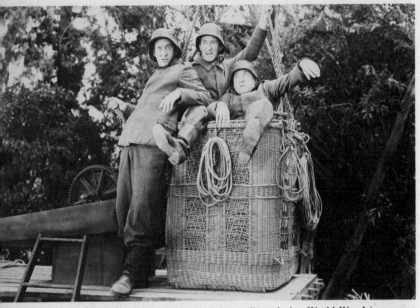

The Ritz Brothers land behind enemy lines during World War I in PACK UP YOUR TROUBLES.

The boys are at the wrong end of a knife-throwing act in ARGENTINE NIGHTS.

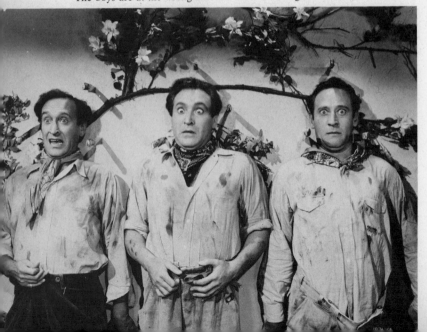

Universal Pictures, ARGENTINE NIGHTS, which paired them with another popular trio: the Andrew Sisters (Maxine, Patty and LaVerne). The girls were in good voice at this time, but they were never much in the acting department; the bulk of the comedy burden was handled by Harry, Jimmy and Al. One scene that attracted most moviegoers at the time had the three brothers devouring a huge hero sandwich, with one brother at one end, another at the other end, and the third one in the middle. They also did some song-and-dance numbers, along with the Andrews girls and an all-girl orchestra on which the flimsy plot was hinged. In a climactic scene the brothers disguised as the Andrews Sisters, in Carmen Miranda-like costumes, with predictable results. ARGENTINE NIGHTS was the last film the team made for several years. They returned to New York and kept busy with personal appearances, nightclubs and radio. Their string of movies had boosted their popularity to an all-time high, and they were in great demand all over the country.

In 1942 they returned to Universal with a three-picture pact. It is difficult to see what the Ritz Brothers and Universal saw in each other at this time. On the Ritzes' part, they had rebelled at Fox because of the "B pictures they were

The Ritz Brothers' films of the 1940's always had meaningful titles. This scene is from HI'YA CHUM.

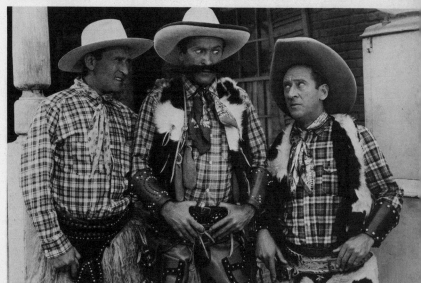

doing, yet the type of "B" Universal offered them made the minor Fox efforts look like colossal endeavors. As for Universal, they already had two teams under contract—Abbott and Costello, and Olsen and Johnson—and why they needed a third is a mystery. With all three teams on the lot at the same time, plus the usual quota of Universal Westerns, horror pictures and cheap musicals, the studio was far from being the best, but was most certainly the noisiest lot in Hollywood.

The Ritz Brothers' first film under this new agreement was BEHND THE EIGHT BALL (1942), a 60-minute extravaganza co-starring Universal contractees Carol Bruce, Dick Foran and Grace McDonald. With five musical numbers in the hour-long film, there wasn't much time for plot, but what there was involved a comic whodunit, with William Demarest doing service as a local police detective. The following year brought another quickie (this one running sixty-*one* minutes) called HI'YA CHUM, co-starring Jane Frazee and Robert Paige, the musical lovers who had intruded on HELLZAPOPPIN several years earlier. Still, the Ritzes had a way of punching over even mediocre material, such as a ballet parody that underscored their special gift for combining song and dance with comedy. The story had the boys buying a restaurant in a California boom town, and one usually restrained critic deemed the results "horrible." Later, in 1943, Universal released their final film: NEVER A DULL MOMENT. Whenever Hollywood decides to use this all-purpose title for a movie, it seems that the film is duller than usual. In the Ritz Brothers' case, their energetic antics kept the film from being dull, but at the same time, they could not keep the film from being anything but limp.

That marked the end of the brothers' career in movies. But the brief tenure at Universal had served its purpose: to keep their name in the public eye. From that point on, the Ritzes spent their time doing what they felt they did best, live performance, primarily in nightclubs. They played top spots in New York, Las Vegas, Miami, and other cities for the balance of their careers.

In 1952 the team made its television debut on NBC's *All Star Revue* to tremendous response, and returned that fall with another hour-long program. But Harry, Jimmy, and Al had no love for TV and shied away from the medium for a number of years. After a five-year hiatus, they returned as guests on a Ginger Rogers special and received such enthusiastic response that they announced plans to launch a series of their own, a weekly filmed series of comic fairy tales.

"Comedy is in pretty bad shape, and TV could use a few laughs," Harry explained to an interviewer, adding, "We could use the dough, too." Al added that their nightclub audiences served as a barometer for their material. "From their reactions we've learned that they like what we're doing—fresh material, but the same old Ritz Brothers."

Their filmed show never came about, but the Ritzes continued to travel the nightclub circuit, drawing tremendous crowds wherever they played. When they opened at Jack Silverman's International in New York in 1961, a reviewer noted that the place was packed, and commented, "Subtle they're not. New they're not. But funny!" The act was booked into New Orleans' Roosevelt Hotel for Christmas week in 1965. During the engagement Al, the oldest brother, suffered a heart attack and died December 22, at the age of 62. The brothers were very close, and proudly proclaimed that they had never had an argument in all their years together. Al's death was a terrible blow to Harry and Jimmy, but not long after his passing, the two remaining brothers

A moment of triumph from NEVER A DULL MOMENT. Five points to anyone who can figure out this still.

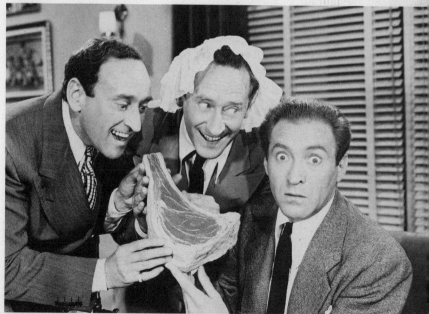

rearranged their act in order to continue working in clubs—having a spotlight take the place of Al in their famous profile precision dance.

In the late 1960s, the Ritz Brothers turned up several times on Joey Bishop's late-night TV show, doing their time-worn routines for a new generation of viewers. They also appeared as guest joke-tellers on the comedy quiz show *Can You Top This?* When Dick Cavett inagurated *his* interview program on PBS in 1977, he had his boyhood idols, Harry and Jimmy, as premiere-week guests. And Alan King recruited Harry to count from one to ten with his eyeballs (a favorite bit) for *The First Annual Comedy Awards* show on ABC.

The brothers even returned to the big screen, if fleetingly. Along with a passel of show-business veterans, they made a cameo appearance in the misfire comedy WON TON TON, THE DOG THAT SAVED HOLLYWOOD—winning one of the film's few genuine laughs with their crazy-walk exit. Longtime admirer Mel Brooks gave Harry a funny bit in his feature SILENT MOVIE. And independent producer Sam Sherman cast the brothers in his low-budget picture BLAZING STEWARDESSES, in which Harry and Jimmy ran through some of

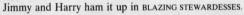

Jimmy and Harry ham it up in BLAZING STEWARDESSES.

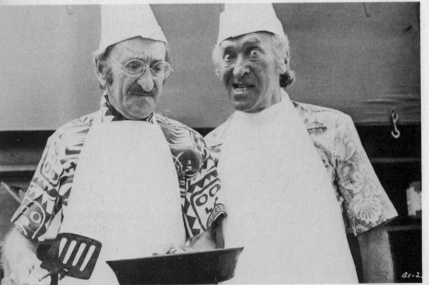

their patented shtick unencumbered by such burdens as direction or a script.

The Ritz Brothers have been inactive since, and that's a shame. They come out of a show-business tradition, combining music and comedy, that's all but gone today. It remains for their films to remind us what that brand of entertainment was all about.

The Films of the Ritz Brothers

(Director's name follows year.)

[Note: Al Ritz did extra-work in THE AVENGING TRAIL (Metro, 1918), starring Harold Lockwood, and it is reportedly for this film that he changed his name from Joachim to Ritz.]

1. **Hotel Anchovy**—Educational-Fox 1934—Al Christie—Doris Hill, Robert Middlemass, Harry Short, Eddie Roberts. 18 minutes.
2. **Broadway Highlights #6**—Paramount 1936—The Ritz Brothers are seen briefly in performance, doing a Ted Lewis impersonation. One reel.
3. **Sing, Baby, Sing**—20th Century-Fox 1936—Sidney Lanfield—Alice Faye, Adolphe Menjou, Gregory Ratoff, Ted Healy, Patsy Kelly, Michael Whalen, Montagu Love, Dixie Dunbar, Douglas Fowley, Tony Martin, Virginia Field, Paul Stanton, Paul McVey, Carol Tevis, Cully Richards, Lynn Bari. 87 minutes.
4. **One in a Million**—20th Century-Fox 1937—Sidney Lanfield—Sonja Henie, Adolphe Menjou, Don Ameche, Ned Sparks, Jean Hersholt, Arline Judge, Borrah Minevitch, Dixie Dunbar, Leah Ray, Shirley Deane, Montagu Love, Albert Conti, Julius Tannen, The Girls' Band. 95 minutes.
5. **On the Avenue**—20th Century-Fox—1937—Roy Del Ruth—Dick Powell, Madeleine Carroll, Alice Faye, George Barbier, Alan Mowbray, Cora Witherspoon, Walter Catlett, Douglas Fowley, Joan Davis, Stepin Fetchit, Sig Rumann, Billy Gilbert, E. E. Clive, Douglas Wood, John Sheehan, Paul Irving, Harry Stubbs, Ricardo Mandia, Edward Cooper, Paul Gerrits. 89 minutes.

6. **You Can't Have Everything**—20th Century-Fox 1937—Norman Taurog—Alice Faye, Don Ameche, Charles Winninger, Louise Hovick (Gypsy Rose Lee), Rubinoff, Arthur Treacher, Tony Martin, Phyllis Brooks, Wally Vernon, Tip Tap and Toe, Louis Prima, George Humbert, Jed Prouty, Dorothy Christy, Lynn Bari. 99 minutes.

7. **Life Begins at College** (retitled LIFE BEGINS IN COLLEGE for TV)—20th Century-Fox 1937—William Seiter—Joan Davis, Tony Martin, Gloria Stuart, Fred Stone, Nat Pendleton, Dick Baldwin, Joan Marsh, Jed Prouty, Maurice Cass, Marjorie Weaver, Robert Lowery, Ed Thorgerson, Lon Chaney, Jr., J. C. Nugent, Fred Kohler, Jr., Elisha Cook, Jr., Charles Wilson, Frank Sully, Norman Willis, Lynn Bari, Spec O'Donnell. 94 minutes.

8. **The Goldwyn Follies**—Samuel Goldwyn-United Artists 1938—George Marshall—Adolphe Menjou, Zorina, Andrea Leeds, Kenny Baker, Helen Jepson, Phil Baker, Ella Logan, Jerome Cowan, Nydia Westman, Charles Kullman and the American Ballet of the Metropolitan Opera, Edgar Bergen and Charlie McCarthy, Frank Shields, Joseph Crehan, Frank Mills, Alan Ladd. Color—120 minutes.

9. **Kentucky Moonshine**—20th Century-Fox 1938—David Butler—Tony Martin, Marjorie Weaver, Slim Summerville, John Carradine, Wally Vernon, Berton Churchill, Eddie Collins, Cecil Cunningham, Paul Stanton, Mary Treen, Francis Ford, Brian Sisters, Clarence Hummel Wilson, Claude Allister, Frank McGlynn, Jr., Jan Dugan, Si Jenks, Joe Twerp, Irving Bacon, Olin Howland. 85 minutes.

10. **Straight, Place, and Show**—20th Century-Fox 1938—David Butler—Richard Arlen, Ethel Merman, Phyllis Brooks, George Barbier, Sidney Blackmer, Will Stanton, Ivan Lebedeff, Gregory Gaye, Rafael Storm, Stanley Fields, Tiny Roebuck, Ben Welden, Ed Gargan, Pat McKee. 66 minutes.

11. **The Three Musketeers**—20th Century-Fox 1939—Allan Dwan—Don Ameche, Lionel Atwill, Gloria Stuart, Pauline Moore, Binnie Barnes, John Carradine, Miles Mander, Joseph Schildkraut, Moroni Olsen, Douglass Dumbrille, John King, Russell Hicks, Gregory Gaye, Lester Mathews, Georges Renavant, Montagu Shaw, Jean Parry, Fredrik Vogeding. 73 minutes.

12. **The Gorilla**—20th Century-Fox 1939—Allan Dwan—Anita Louise, Patsy Kelly, Lionel Atwill, Bela Lugosi,

Joseph Calleia, Edward Norris, Wally Vernon, Paul Harvey, Art Miles. 59 minutes.

13. **Pack Up Your Troubles**—20th Century-Fox 1939—H. Bruce Humberstone—Jane Withers, Lynn Bari, Joseph Schildkraut, Stanley Fields, Fritz Leiber, Lionel Royce, Georges Renavant, Adrienne d'Ambricourt, Leon Ames, William von Brincken, Ed Gargan, Robert Emmett Keane, Henry Victor, Billy Bevan. 75 minutes.

14. **Argentine Nights**—Universal 1940—Albert S. Rogell—The Andrews Sisters, Constance Moore, George Reeves, Peggy Moran, Anne Nagel, Kathryn Adams, Ferike Boros, Paul Porcasi. 74 minutes.

15. **Behind the Eight-Ball**—Universal 1942—Stanley Roberts —Carol Bruce, Dick Foran, Grace McDonald, Johnny Downs, William Demarest, Richard Davies, Sonny Dunham and Orchestra. 60 minutes.

16. **Hi'Ya, Chum**—Universal 1943—Harold Young—Jane Fraze, Robert Paige, June Clyde, Edmund MacDonald, Lou Lubin, Brooks Benedict, Richard Davies, Ray Miller, Paul Hurst, Earl Hodgins, Michael Vallon. 61 minutes.

17. **Screen Snapshots No. 5**—Columbia 1943—Ralph Staub—USO tour footage with Cesar Romero, Dick Ney, Gig Young, Sabu, Marlene Dietrich, Constance Moore, George Jessel, Leo Carrillo, Billy Anderson. 10 minutes.

18. **Screen Snapshots No. 8**—Columbia 1943—Ralph Staub—Gene Autry, Tyrone Power, Lou Holtz, the Marx Brothers, Annabella, Kay Kyser, Alan Mowbray. 10 minutes.

19. **Never a Dull Moment**—Universal 1943—Edward Lilley—Frances Langford, Stuart Crawford, Elizabeth Risdon, Mary Beth Hughes, George Zucco, Jack LaRue, Sammy Stein, Barbara Brown, Douglas Wood, Charles Jordan, Igor and Pogi. 60 minutes.

20. **Blazing Stewardesses**—Independent-International 1975—Al Adamson—Harry and Jimmy appeared in this film with Yvonne DeCarlo, Bob Livingston, Connie Hoffman, Regina Carrol, T. A. King, Don "Red" Barry, Geoffre Land, Sheldon Lee, Carol Bilger, Nicole Riddell. Color—89 minutes. (An additional song and dance routine by the Ritz Brothers cut for theatrical release has been restored for the homevideo version of this film.)

21. **Won Ton Ton, The Dog Who Saved Hollywood**— Paramount 1976—Michael Winner—Bruce Dern, Madeline Kahn, Art Carney, Phil Silvers, Teri Garr, Ron Leibman; Harry and Jimmy Ritz were among the many cameo guest stars including Robert Alda, Morey Amsterdam,

Richard Arlen, Billy Barty, Edgar Bergen, Milton Berle, Janet Blair, Joan Blondell, Dennis Morgan, Dorothy Lamour, Alice Faye, Ann Miller, Rhonda Fleming, Victor Mature, Zsa Zsa Gabor, Cyd Charisse, Peter Lawford, Walter Pidgeon, Henny Youngman, Romo Vincent, Virginia Mayo, Rory Calhoun, Shecky Greene, Henry Wilcoxon, Ricardo Montalban, Jackie Coogan, Johnny Weissmuller, Aldo Ray, Ethel Merman, Yvonne De Carlo, Andy Devine, Broderick Crawford, Jack La Rue, Nancy Walker, Gloria DeHaven, Louis Nye, Stepin Fetchit, Ken Murray, George Jessel, Dean Stockwell, Tab Hunter, Eli Mintz, Fritz Feld, Edward Ashley, Kres Mersky, Jane Connell, Dennis Day, Mike Mazurki, Jesse White, Carmel Myers, Jack Carter, Jack Bernardi, Barbara Nichols, Army Archerd, Fernando Lamas, Huntz Hall, Doodles Weaver, Pedro Gonzales-Gonzales, Eddie Le Veque, Ronny Graham, Eddie Foy Jr., Patricia Morison, Guy Madison, Regis Toomey, Ann Rutherford, James E. Brodhead, John Carradine, Keye Luke, Phil Leeds, Cliff Norton, Sterling Holloway, William Benedict, Dorothy Gulliver, William Demarest, Augustus von Schumacher, Color—92 minutes.

Harry Ritz made a cameo appearance by himself in Mel Brooks' SILENT MOVIE (1976).

Footage of the Ritz Brothers was used in two other feature films:

TAKE IT OR LEAVE IT, a 1944 20th Century-Fox picture which incorporated clips from various earlier Fox films, including the "Ortchi-Tchorniya" number from ON THE AVENUE; and THE SOUND OF LAUGHTER, 1963 compilation film from Mack Sennett and Educational Pictures comedies from the 1930s, including the Ritz Brothers' HOTEL ANCHOVY.

OLSEN and JOHNSON

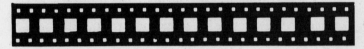

Long before mixed-media presentations, Ernie Kovacs and Rowan and Martin's *Laugh-In*, there were Olsen and Johnson. For forty-five years they made people laugh with a never-ending procession of astounding sight gags, wheezy puns and a flair for the ridiculous that has never been duplicated. Critics were seldom kind to Olsen and Johnson, even when their *Hellzapoppin* had a record-breaking run on Broadway, but the two comics didn't care. Their pleasure was in seeing audiences double up with laughter. "Anything for a laugh" was their motto, and when they said "anything," they meant it.

Their lunacy was seldom captured on film, and this is a shame, but their starring movies for Universal in the 1940's do serve to prove that there is really no such thing as an old joke, if it succeeds in amusing an audience. Their films remain fresh and funny, and one only wishes there was more of *them* in the pictures. Discounting their minor efforts from the 1930's, their major films—HELLZAPOPPIN, CRAZY HOUSE, GHOST CATCHERS, SEE MY LAWYER—often stifle their madcap minds and force them to take a back seat to such dubious luminaries as Martha O'Driscoll and Gloria Jean. One wishes they could have worked for Mack Sennett or Hal Roach, doing two-reel comedies. With Olsen and Johnson's megawatt personalities, the expertise of the writers at Sennett and Roach, and the short-and-sweet short-subject format, the results might have been truly gratifying. (In fact, RKO announced a series of Olsen and Johnson shorts in the early 1930s, but the films never came to be.) Instead, we must settle for feature films that often work at half steam, but even a small dose of Olsen and Johnson's infectiously silly brand of humor can be a breath of fresh air these days. As Ole Olsen once remarked, "We may make a mistake now and then, but you must admit that when we do, we do it with enthusiasm."

John Sigvard Olsen, better known as Ole, was the son of
Norwegian immigrants; he was born in Peru, Indiana, in
1892. His parents gave him a musical background, and Ole's
ambition was to be a concert violinist. He worked his way
through Northwestern University by playing fiddle with a
quartet in a local restaurant. Harold Ogden Johnson, known
as Chic, was born in Chicago in 1891. He also had musical
aspirations, and attended the Chicago Musical College, study-
ing classical piano. He left college and sought nightclub
work as a ragtime pianist. In 1914, the pianist in Olsen's
quartet quit, and Johnson was hired as his replacement. Or,
as Johnson put it, "He wore sidebutton yellow shoes, and he
was the first man I ever heard imitate a busy signal on the
telephone. I knew I had to have him as a partner." The two
hit it off immediately, and before long decided to abandon
the quartet and go out on their own as a musical act. The
two young, ambitious men toured in vaudeville on the
Pantages Circuit. "The two of us had a musical act—I
played the fiddle," Ole later recalled. "But we quickly learned
to gag up the act because the big money in vaudeville was
going to those who could get laughs. Later on we worked in
bits with members of the stage crews wherever we played,
then with other acts on the same bill. Finally, we decided
that the only way to work properly in this fashion was to
have people who worked just for us."

From a fairly good start of $250 a week on the Pantages,
the team jumped to the Keith-Orpheum Circuit within a few
years, and their salary skyrocketed to $2500. In 1918 they
were well-known around the country, billed on the Keith
Circuit as "likeable lads loaded with laughs." By the early
1920's Olsen and Johnson were headliners, doing essentially
the same routines they continued to use for the rest of their
lives. Their use of the blank-loaded shotgun became legendary: Chic would shoot into the rafters and a chicken would
fall to the stage. Ole would grimace and say, "Well it's a
good thing cows don't fly," at which point a cow would
plummet to the platform. They also were known for their
sight gags involving a large, portable bathtub that predated
Ernie Kovacs' tub gags by thirty years. In 1924 they appeared at a gala benefit performed for the National Vaudeville Artists Association in New York along with such acts as
Clark and McCullough, Jack Benny, Irving Berlin, Fanny
Brice, Ben Bernie, George M. Cohan, Eddie Cantor, Gus
Edwards, Ted Lewis, Eva Tanguay and Bert Wheeler.

Around this time, Olsen and Johnson established their

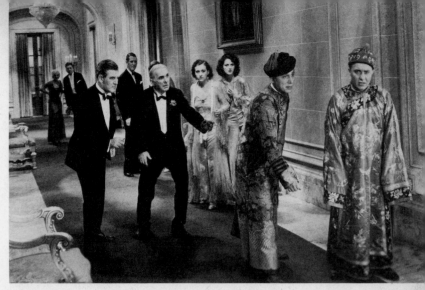

Ole and Chic seem out of place at this society event: from FIFTY MILLION FRENCHMEN.

own traveling unit show, with stooges, comics, singers, musicians, and others who accompanied them around the country. It became a family affair, with the wives and children of both Ole and Chic getting into the act. Many years later, Olsen said, "We kept expanding through the last years of vaudeville until we had a unit that enabled us to survive its collapse . . ." The team also experienced early success on radio, and later were considered pioneers of that entertainment medium. Not to leave any phase of show business untapped, the team also penned several songs, including a 1923 ditty called "Oh Gee, Oh Gosh, Oh Golly I'm in Love," which Abel Green and Joe Laurie, Jr., labeled a contender for the title of the biggest "nut song" of the year (the winner was "Yes We Have No Bananas").

Olsen and Johnson continued to travel around the country, but their greatest success was always outside the big cities. They were one of the hottest acts in the Midwest, and credited their later success and longevity to the fact that they had made so many friends during their years of touring the U.S. In 1930, with the talkie boom in full swing, Hollywood beckoned, and Olsen and Johnson appeared in their first film, for Warner Brothers, OH SAILOR BEHAVE! They were billed as the film's stars in all advertising (which tagged them "America's Funniest Clowns"), but in true musical-comedy tradition, they were actually comedy leads who had to share the focus with a pair of young lovers. The film was adapted from a successful Broadway play by Elmer Rice, but the screenplay was tailored to meet Olsen and Johnson's specifications by allowing them a good number of comic sequences, and some fairly elaborate sight gags. The film is set in Naples (on the Warner Brothers backlot) where newspaper reporter Charles King falls in love with heiress Irene Delroy. They go through a complicated series of misunderstandings and interim marriages before finally coming together at the end. Meanwhile, Ole and Chic are American sailors on leave in Venice who are assigned to find a man with a wooden leg who has robbed the Navy storehouse. Their detective work begins as they stand on a street corner and look for men who are limping. They aim a pea-shooter at a man's leg, and if he jumps, they know he isn't the one they want. Their investigation comes to an abrupt halt when they both catch the eye of a flirtatious young girl (Lotti Loder). Somewhere along the line they sing a tune they composed for the film. "The Laughing Song," which makes use of Chic's trademark, a long, hysterical laugh. In the film's climax, they hop onto a pair of water-bicycles and ride through the canals of Venice. Best of all is the pair's dialogue, quite funny and full of wild double-entendres, and another tune, "We're on the Highway to Heaven."

The picture did not cause any fireworks, because it came at a time when every studio was doing the same kind of film, importing as many stars from vaudeville and Broadway as they could handle. But Warner Brothers was pleased enough

Olsen and Johnson tease Helen Broderick in FIFTY MILLION FRENCHMEN; the heavy makeup was used for the two-color Technicolor camera.

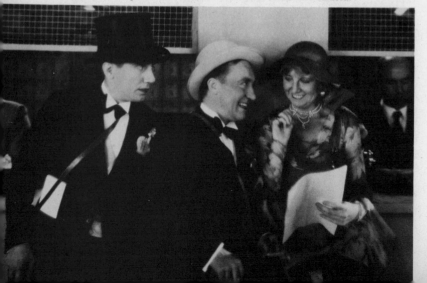

with the film's reception to have Olsen and Johnson return the following year to make two more films in quick succession. The first of the two, FIFTY MILLION FRENCHMEN, was filmed in Technicolor ("so bad that it blurs the vision and hurts the eyes," wrote *Harrison's Reports*, a film review source of the day). Set in Paris, the plot makes Olsen and Johnson subordinate to the romantic leads again. William Gaxton stars as a man who bets his rival (John Halliday) that he can win and marry the girl of his dreams (Claudia Dell) without any money or family name to help him. Halliday hires two detectives, Chic and Ole, to trail Gaxton and make sure he doesn't win his wager. While following him, the boys get to like Gaxton, and when he is thrown in jail, they come to his rescue in the film's climactic chase. To draw attention to Gaxton's frame-up, they decide to attract as many gendarmes as possible, and run all over Paris inciting the cops to chase them into the jailhouse. This is easily the film's most rousing scene, for otherwise FIFTY MILLION FRENCHMEN is pretty flat. Olsen and Johnson's best scenes come when they encounter American tourist Helen Broderick, who announces that she has come to Paris to be dishonored. They do their best, but everything they come up with, including a peepshow device, is too tame for her. Another factor that gives the film added interest today is a brief appearance by Bela Lugosi as a local fakir. Neither that nor much else in the film attracted the critics in 1931, who failed to find the film amusing, and missed the music that went with it when it was a stage play. *The Motion Picture Herald* echoed others' sentiments when it said that Olsen and Johnson were quite funny but the rest of the film was rather weak.

The team's next Warners film, released just a few months after FRENCHMEN, allowed them to carry the film on their own, co-starred with comedienne Winnie Lightner. The film was GOLD DUST GERTIE, and while it afforded the duo a chance to work as leads, with some good sight gags thrown in, it pleased only their staunchest fans. "It opens like a conventionally mediocre 2-reel comedy of the chair-throwing school," wrote *The New York Times*, "and at the point where it apparently should end, it keeps on unreeling to depressing lengths." The plot involves two bathing-suit salesmen who are trying to elude an ex-wife (Lightner) determined to collect a bundle in alimony. One of the film's few distinctions is that Ole Olsen sports a mustache for the only time on the screen.

After GOLD DUST GERTIE, Olsen and Johnson left Hollywood for greener pastures; in other words, the vaudeville circuit again, with their unit show. But their reputation was growing, and better offers started to come in. In 1933 the team made its Broadway debut when Ole and Chic were signed to replace Jack Haley and Sid Silvers in the hit musical *Take a Chance*. Members of the original cast who stayed on with them included Ethel Merman and Jack Whiting, and the score boasted such tunes as "Eadie was a Lady" and "You're an Old Smoothie." True to form, the critics disapproved of the casting change, referring to Olsen and Johnson as vaudeville comics who should have stayed there. Audiences didn't seem to mind, and the two stars enjoyed a good run with the show. Two years later they were back in New York when the Roxy Theater booked their revue, *Everything Goes*, in lieu of their usual vaudeville bill. The 75 member troupe, headed by Olsen and Johnson, played a week's engagement during the Christmas season, doing four shows a day, five on weekends. It marked the first time the Roxy had booked a musical revue to accompany their movie attraction.

Olsen and Johnson invaded Republic Pictures for COUNTRY GENTLEMEN.

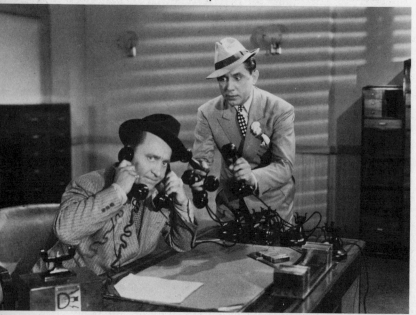

Everything Goes was a suitable title for the 15-scene revue, but when Olsen and Johnson went out of town again they returned with a better name. While in Los Angeles, they received an invitation to attend a gala festival in Phoenix, Arizona. At the same time, a neighboring town called Buckeye corraled the comedy team to appear at their annual festivities, which the town called "Helzapoppin'." Ole and Chic were attracted to the name and asked permission to use it themselves: from then on, *Hellzapoppin'* (with the extra "l") was the name of their touring show. While in Los Angeles, Olsen and Johnson initiated a radio show over station KFI. *Variety's* review reflected the general feeling about the team at that time: "Kind of a show that will make the RFD boys drop their plows and run to the nearest set. But not so in the urban centers. Olsen and Johnson radio routine is too dated for the city mob and the comics have made no effort to modernize their formula or the gags. The Olsen stock laugh is still the topper. Only thing new is the femme scream at the opening 'to be sure everyone is awake.' "

The journey to Los Angeles also resulted in two more starring films, this time for the fledging Republic Pictures. Republic was never known for its lavish budgets, and the two films revealed their shoestring backing. However, Republic always knew how to stock its supporting casts with top character actors, and these "pros" saved many a sagging picture. Olsen and Johnson's first film for the studio, released in January 1937, was COUNTRY GENTLEMEN. Ole and Chic play two fast-talking con men who sell phony gold bonds, then settle in a small town where they see a potential sucker list in the local veterans' home. They sell the vets shares in a worthless nearby oilfield, while Ole falls in love with the lovely proprietress of their hotel, Lila Lee. She begs him to go straight, and he falls under her spell. Before he can convince his partner to give up their shady dealings, the townspeople catch onto their schemes and decide that jail is the place for them. As they are about to be arrested, the supposedly dried-up oil well erupts, and the allegedly deserted goldmine turns out to be a prospering lode. The reviews on COUNTRY GENTLEMEN were generally negative, but most critics saw potential in the film that hadn't been realized. Once again it was a case of padding a good two-reel idea into a six-reel feature. The film was also criticized for making Ole a romantic lead. No one disputed the valuable contribution made by Joyce Compton as a dumb-blonde secretary, however; throughout the 1930's and early 40's, no one played dumb blondes as well as Miss Compton, and her presence was an asset to any film.

ALL OVER TOWN, the team's second vehicle for Republic, was released in September 1937, and prompted the general reaction that, next to this, COUNTRY GENTLEMEN was a gem. The low budget was more damaging to this film than to the earlier one, yet the cast was filled with valuable supporting players who gave the film most of its life. Ole and Chic more or less play themselves in this one, which has a tired story line about a girl inheriting a "jinxed" theater with a mortgage hanging over it. Olsen and Johnson help her to put on a money-making show, but wind up with a resounding flop. In desperation, they turn to a Mr. MacDougal, "The Mackeral King" (played by Laurel and Hardy perennial James Finlayson) to sponsor them on a radio program. Chic and Ole are kidnapped before the broadcast, but manage to subdue their assailants and make it to the studio in the nick of time to save the day for young Mary Howard and her boyfriend (Harry Stockwell). ALL OVER TOWN was directed by James W. Horne, formerly a director of Laurel and Hardy, who had much better material than this. The cast included such stalwarts as Finlayson, Franklin Pangborn, Stanley Fields and comedy "regulars" Gertrude Astor, Blanche Payson and Fred Kelsey, but it just didn't jell. At this point it looked as if Olsen and Johnson would be touring in vaudeville for a mighty long time.

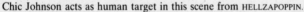

Chic Johnson acts as human target in this scene from HELLZAPOPPIN.

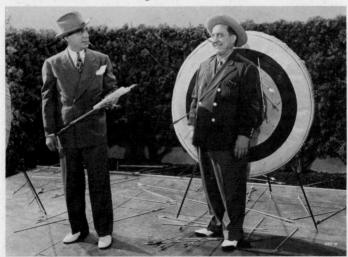

Then, one day in 1938, Broadway impressario Lee Shubert was persuaded to go to Philadelphia to catch Olsen and Johnson's *Hellzapoppin* revue while it was playing at a local theater. He went, saw the excellent audience reaction, and approached Olsen and Johnson about expanding their revue (it was then one hour long) for Broadway. He wanted the same crazy format, even the same troupe, but a longer presentation. The deal was set, and *Hellzapoppin'* was ready for Broadway by September 22, 1938, brought in at a cost of $15,000. The opening-nighters were not prepared for what they saw: the wildest conglomeration of sight gags and audience participation ever presented in a legitimate theater. The response that night was tremendous, but the next day the critics were quite harsh, and at best, tolerant. The show had two factors in its favor, despite this critical brush-off; first, Olsen and Johnson had many fans who were presold on the show, and second, Walter Winchell, then the undisputed king of the columnists, loved the show and decided to promote it. He helped to promote it into one of the longest-running shows ever to play on Broadway: a total of 1,104 performances.

It is difficult to describe *Hellzapoppin'*, because the show was different every night. One evening a musical number might appear before intermission; the next evening it could be the finale; and another performance it might not be used

An artistic moment with Mischa Auer from HELLZAPOPPIN.

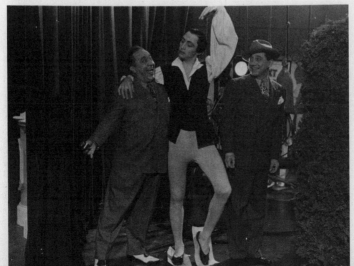

at all. The show was completely freewheeling, madcap comedy with no holds barred. Near the beginning of the show, a page would walk up and down the aisles carrying a small flower-pot, calling "Mr. Jones! Mr. Jones!!" He reappeared every so often during the show, and with each trip the plant would be bigger and bigger. When the audience left the theater at the end of the show, the man would be perched on a branch in a huge tree planted in the lobby, still yelling "Mr. Jones!" Likewise, a woman (usually Mrs. Chic Johnson) would continually stalk through the theater searching for her husband Oscar. Every night a man would come in late to a special orchestra seat and take off his overcoat. A hanger would suddenly sail down from the ceiling, the man would nonchalantly hang up his coat, and the hanger would zip back into the heavens. In a country-store sequence of the show, people sitting in the first few rows were liable to win anything from a live chicken to a "pottie-seat," as it was called. Cast members were situated throughout the audience, a constant source of frustration to the management when the theater was selling out and a dozen choice seats had to be reserved for performers. One gag had a man arguing with his wife in a box above the orchestra; after a particularly violent round of insults, he would throw her (a dummy, of course) into the aisle below. Audience members were sometimes drawn into the fun, but Olsen and Johnson were careful not to embarrass them, saving the rough jokes for cast members. One night by accident, an exception was made. Volunteers were solicited for a Coney Island funhouse scene, and a dozen people went on stage. Most were members of the cast. One gag would have a chorus girl, wearing a wide skirt, step over an air-blower which would billow her skirt into the air. In this particular performance an elderly lady from the audience had the misfortune to step over the blower, and when *her* dress was lifted, her reaction was swift and violent. She took her umbrella and started beating everyone in sight. The response was so uproarious that Olsen and Johnson decided to keep the gag in the show, using a cast member instead of an unsuspecting lady for all future performances.

The insanity extended backstage, too, as chronicled by one dazed reporter who visited the show during its second year. "The confusion that sweeps regularly through Olsen's dressing room—an unfailing source of wonder to hardbitten backstage Johnnies—would effectively eclipse so casual an item as a loose ham bone. Scores of people wander in and out every performance, including insurance agents, out-of-town mayors, vaudeville hams, anybody who mentions Indiana (Olsen's home state) to the doorman. Mr. Olsen himself wonders sometimes who they all are, but he lingers briefly over speculation of this kind. Apparently they are strangers bent chiefly on milling about and watching him dart back and forth in shorts." Practical jokes were also in order, as Ole would slip a piece of ice down the back of his sister-in-law, Ruth Faber, also in the cast, or Chic would cavort in the wings to distract the actors on stage.

During the show's run, Olsen and Johnson always made good newspaper copy, on stage and off. Olsen's restaurant on 40th Street was sort of an extension of *Hellzapoppin'*, with crazy gags greeting its customers on all sides. The critics were confounded, but Olsen and Johnson had conquered New York. Their next move was to try to reconquer Hollywood. A news item appeared in *Variety* during the show's run announcing that Olsen and Johnson were planning to make a film of *Hellzapoppin'* exactly as it appeared in the theater. "Film would be a unique experiment in that, with the exception of Olsen and Johnson, cast would have no starred or featured player headaches; no connected continuity; no romance and no exterior location scenes." Alas, none of this came to be. Instead, the two comics signed with Universal Pictures to do *Hellzapoppin'* in Hollywood. They left the cast of their Broadway hit after more than two years, with

Olsen and Johnson disagree with director Richard Lane on how to film HELLZAPOPPIN; if only they had won.

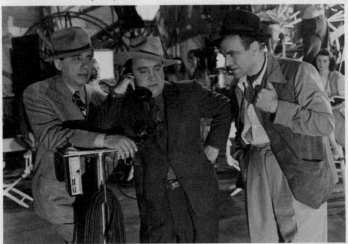

Jay C. Flippen replacing Olsen and Happy Felton replacing Johnson (there was talk of Harry Langdon taking the latter role, and an audition, but Langdon was not hired). At the same time, Joe Besser and Ole Olsen, Jr. (despite his name, Ole's *brother*) took *Hellzapoppin'* on the road. After a short vacation, Ole and Chic arrived in Hollywood to try to duplicate their stage success on film.

HELLZAPOPPIN, released in December 1941, did not duplicate the stage success. It was successful at the box office, but the HELLZAPOPPIN moviegoers saw bore little resemblance to the lunatic stage show. It was simply a matter of Universal Pictures refusing to take a chance on a pastiche of gags and songs without any plot, and remolding the idea to suit their more "normal" standards. The strange part of the film is that the opening scenes make fun of Hollywood's insistence on changing successful shows, while the rest of the film proceeds to do exactly that. HELLZAPOPPIN has some inspired moments, and does include a lot of ingenious and

Chic Johnson plays cupid for Ole Olsen and Martha Raye in a posed shot from HELLZAPOPPIN.

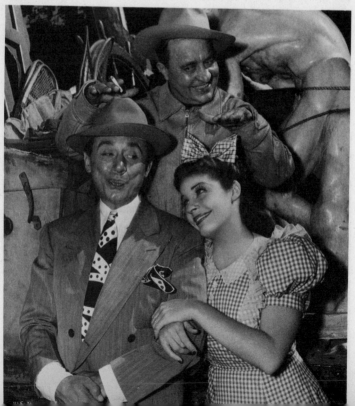

screamingly funny gags, but not enough to overcome an uninteresting love triangle and make the film the comedy classic it should have been.

The film opens in Hades, with scores of devils prancing about as a title song is sung in the background. These devils take delight in torturing their victims with a variety of odd contraptions. Just, then, in a puff of smoke, a taxicab appears with Olsen and Johnson inside. Chic steps out and comments, "That's the first taxi driver who went strictly where I told him to go." Then a devil takes care of the driver. Ole and Chic suddenly turn straight ahead and yell to the projectionist to run the film back so they can see that again. The projectionist is Shemp Howard, trying to run the film while arguing with a girl friend in his projection booth. After arguing with the boys, he agrees to run the film back and the scene is repeated. Meanwhile, a man with a potted plant runs through the scene yelling for "Mr. Jones!" and a woman traipses in front of everyone screaming "Oscar!" The devils take after Olsen and Johnson, and they run off. At this point we see that they have been on a movie set all the time. They go to talk to the film's director (Richard Lane), who has an argument with them about filming HELLZAPOPPIN. He tells them that they can't just film a bunch of crazy gags. "Every picture's got to have a love story." Chic tells him that they did the show on Broadway for two years, and they ought to know how to film it. "This is Hollywood," says Lane. "We change everything here— we've *got* to." As the three are talking, they walk through the sound stage, passing through various sets, their costumes changing as they go through each door. When they walk through an Alaskan set in heavy winter coats, they pass a sled marked "Rosebud." Finally Lane sits them down with screenwriter Elisha Cook, Jr., and tries to show them his conception of how the film should look. They "visualize" it on a piece of paper which turns into a screen. The picture fades into this story-within-a-story, and the actual film begins.

From this point, the film goes downhill and seemingly ignores the satire that has preceded it, by going ahead and adding a dreary love story to the usual quota of Olsen and Johnson gags. A lot of time is spent on the love triangle involving Robert Paige, who is trying to put on a show at his Long Island estate, Jane Frazee, and her fiancé Lewis Howard. Still more footage is devoted to man-chasing Martha Raye, who goes after money-chasing Count Mischa Auer. Olsen and Johnson take a back seat to all of this, sharing the film's genuinely funny moments with Hugh Herbert, as a screwball private eye who walks in and out of the film at odd moments. In one scene he peeks out from behind a tree, and moves his head from side to side; every time it passes behind the tree it changes hats and costumes. "Don't ask me how I do it, folks," Herbert laughs. Later, while talking to Jane Frazee, he spots something out front and without missing a beat of his conversation, says, "Oh hello Mom, I'll be home for supper . . . have meat." In one of the film's most satisfying moments, a song done by Paige and Frazee is covered by a title card that reads "Attention—If Stinky Miller is in the audience—Go home." The song continues, and a moment later another title card appears: "Stinky Miller—Your Mother Wants You." After another pause a third title reads "Stinky Miller—Go Home." At this point, the two lovers stop singing. Hugh Herbert pops out from behind a curtain and tells Stinky Miller to stop stalling and go home. Paige and Frazee which patiently while the silhouette of a boy appears at the bottom of the screen and walks up the "aisle" to go home. Then they continue their song where they left off.

Still later, Olsen and Johnson are talking to Lewis Howard when the picture starts to jump. They call up to Shemp Howard in the projection booth, but he is tangled up in film and isn't much help. Then the picture jumps out of frame, putting the heads of Ole and Howard on the bottom half of the frame and their feet on the top half. Chic has bent down to tie his shoelace, so he is crouched down in the bottom part of the frame. Olsen and Howard try to straighten the film by pushing the frame up, but they don't want to hurt Chic, down below. Finally the film is returned to normal (after Chic mutters a few words about hiring relatives to project their films) and the scene continues.

Unfortunately, such gags are far too few in HELLZAPOPPIN, particularly in the second half. The film ends with an especially weak gag that doesn't even involve Olsen and Johnson! But this was not the way the film was shot. In a 1971 interview, director H. C. Potter explained, "A lot of things that I had worked very hard on—innovations—were, after I left Universal, gone completely. I screamed and yelled bloody hell, but there was nothing I could do about it." For one thing, Potter never intended to *show* the projectionist, in order to maintain the illusion that O & J were really talking to someone in the projection booth of each theater. It was Universal's decision to film additional footage with Shemp Howard. Potter also shot a much crazier finale, featuring a premiere of the movie at Grauman's Chinese Theater—with the usher riding by on a giant flatbed, perched in a tree, hollering for Mrs. Jones, and culminating in Olsen and Johnson placing their feet in cement, only to sink completely under the surface of the bubbly goo for THE END. But apparently this was all too nutty for the Universal executives, who scrapped this material and reworked the film in order to make HELLZAPOPPIN more "acceptable" to movie audiences.

A few weeks before HELLZAPOPPIN opened in movie theaters around the country, Olsen and Johnson opened a new show on Broadway, again produced by the brothers Shubert. Its name was *Sons O' Fun*, but it bore a striking resemblance to their first Broadway hit. In effect, it was merely a revision of *Hellzapoppin'*, which itself had been officially "revised" several times during its three-year run. The two most obvious changes were additions to the cast: sizzling Carmen Miranda, whose South-of-the-border songs and dances were then in vogue, and Ella Logan, a fine young singer who would later dazzle Broadway in *Finian's Rainbow*. Also on hand to help Chic and Ole was Joe Besser, whom critic Brooks Atkinson described as "enormously funny." The critics, Atkinson included, still could not warm up to Olsen and Johnson and their brand of humor, although their reviews were more guarded this time than they were when *Hellzapoppin* first opened. *Sons O'Fun* opened on December 1, 1941, and ran nearly two years, much to the amazement of its critics, and even its backers. During the New York run, Olsen and Johnson continued to make the entertainment pages of the New York dailies with regularity; they were always cooking up something that would make good copy. In 1943 they printed the following letter and sent it to show-business people around town. It is worth reprinting here to show how far Chic and Ole carried their anything-for-a-laugh slogan. In addition, it's quite funny. The cover of the pamphlet reads "POOR OLE!" The heading of the letter reads "COMMITTEE FOR THE RELIEF AND WELFARE OF OLE OLSEN; Private and Confidential." The letter itself:

Dear, very dear Friend,

Here, at long, long last, is the glorious opportunity you and all the rest of Ole Olsen's friends have wanted!!! Here is your opportunity to do something noble and beautiful for wonderful, kind, gentle Ole Olsen . . . your friend and ours . . . a man who is the epitome of all human generosity and who has never missed an opportunity to do something for his friends, or for any unfortunate. You doubtless read (or heard about) the following item which appeared in Walter Winchell's column of April 5th, 1943:

"Hard to believe item; that Ole Olsen, who split $15,000 weekly all those years (HELLZAPOPPIN cleared over five million), is said to be the victim of unsound investments. Intimates fear he's broke."

Winchell helped to "make" Ole. Winchell now has Ole "broke." Poor Ole! What can we do? He needs help. Poor Ole! He needs your worn out shoes. He needs old clothes. He needs underwear and socks. Poor Ole! Ole must eat. He needs groceries; soft drinks to drink; Ole needs bath tubs to bathe in; cows to milk—or goats; chickens which lay eggs, or chickens which don't lay eggs—or roosters which, of course, don't. Poor Ole! Ole needs baby carriages, blankets, furniture, bed-pans. Ole must begin life anew and new things would embarrass Poor Ole! *Poor, poor Ole!* After two or three more years of SONS O' FUN, and after he goes to Hollywood to make the picture, he will need new material for a new show. He will need props, homing pigeons, merde de cheval for gags, guns, worn out electric bulbs, beans to drop on audiences, live animals, soap. (NOTHING IN RUBBER . . . OLE IS VERY PATRIOTIC), midgets, toupees, or WHATEVER your big heart dictates in this pitiful situation. Help us to keep *Poor Ole* out of the *Poor-house!!!!*

Don't send your contributions to Chic Johnson's thousand acre farm in Carmel, New York, with its hundreds of cows, thousands of chickens, etc. By no means send it to Ole's apartment house with fifty-two apartments (no vacancies), at 45th and Lexington, or to his busy restaurant and budget shop at 45 West 54th Street, or to his thirteen acre Mid-Island shopping center, or to SONS O' FUN, 46th St. Theatre (which is grossing $30,000 a week), or to his Westwood Ice Arena in Los Angeles, Calif., seating 9,000 people, or to Universal Studios where he starts shooting on his new picture in June and another in the coming February.

Please *don't* send your contribution to any of the above places as it would embarrass his customers and tenants.

So here's what we hope you will be thrilled to do, in order to prove to Mr. Winchell that a man who has friends is *never* broke. Help us to convince Mr. Winchell in this way:

1. Make up a package or crate of things.
2. Put a note inside reading FOR OLE OLSEN.
3. Address to: Walter Winchell, c/o Stork Club, 3 East 53rd Street, New York, N.Y.
4. *DO NOT* PUT YOUR RETURN ADDRESS ON IT.

In poor Ole's name, and in the name of sweet charity, our deep thanks.

                              THE COMMITTEE

P.S.—I'm sure that any donation that does not fit poor Ole—will eventually find its way to some charitable organization.

After completing their run with *Sons O' Fun* in New York, Ole and Chic went back to California to do a second film for Universal, CRAZY HOUSE. Someone at Universal thought it would be a good idea to cram the film with a score of "guest stars," ranging from Percy Kilbride to Count Basie and his Band. Except for some unnecessary specialty numbers, the idea fared pretty well, with comic experts like Billy Gilbert, Edgar Kennedy, Hans Conried, Shemp Howard and Franklin Pangborn adding their own touches to the wacky Olsen and Johnson brand of humor. The film opens as word reaches Universal Studios in Hollywood that Olsen and Johnson are coming. The studio is thrown into an uproar. Executives, actors and extras go running in all directions shouting, "Olsen and Johnson are coming!" Andy Devine rides down a Western street with his raspy voice echoing "Olsen and Johnson are coming!" Leo Carrillo clears another Western set, telling his amigos that Olsen and Johnson are coming. The scene cuts to Basil Rathbone as Sherlock Holmes; Nigel Bruce, as Dr. Watson, comes in to tell him the important news, but Holmes is already aware of the fact. "I know, Watson. Olsen and Johnson are coming." When asked how he knows, Rathbone replies, "I am Sherlock Holmes. I know everything."

Finally Ole and Chic arrive and march into the office of the studio head. Using the intercom in his reception room, Chic announces, "Universal's number one comedy team is here." "Oh, Abbott and Costello," beams the boss happily,

Shemp Howard keeps trying to sell something to Olsen and Johnson in CRAZY HOUSE; his running gag is one of the film's best.

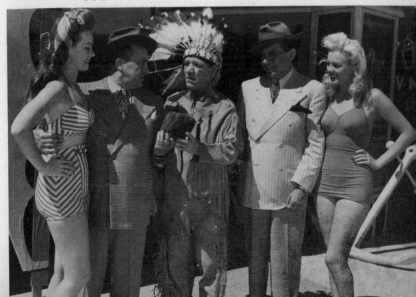

"Send them right in." When it turns out to be Olsen and Johnson, his reception is less than cordial as he explains that the studio will not tolerate them for another picture. After a heated argument, Ole and Chic come up with a plan: they'll produce their own picture and finance it themselves. They hire ambitious Patric Knowles to direct, discover car-hop Martha O'Driscoll and make her their star, and go through an endless series of pranks as they match wits with comedienne Cass Daley and her stand-in, who's a dead ringer for her. Shooting begins, with acts like the Glenn Miller Singers doing a bunch of forgettable tunes, and Shemp Howard constantly approaching the boys with screwy offers ("Want to buy an oven? It's hot"). Things move along fine until Ole and Chic discover that their supposed backer, Percy Kilbride, doesn't have any money, and their creditors, headed by Billy Gilbert, are going to confiscate their film. The boys end up in court, where they send the judge (Edgar Kennedy) into a state of utter confusion, and finally get permission to premiere their film and offer it to the studios for sale.

Chic and Ole host the gala premiere and pull crazy stunts outside the theater (their interview microphone bends when anyone tries to talk into it, and squirts water in Cass Daley's face). Inside, everything is going fine until director Knowles discovers that someone has stolen the second reel of the film. While he goes to get it, Olsen and Johnson come on stage to stall for time. They spot Allan Jones in the audience and with very little prompting he gets up to sing "The Donkey Serenade." Knowles returns with the missing reel, the film is shown, and bidding is opened to the movie executives in the audience. Chic places a hot iron under the seat of the Universal president, causing him to leap out of his seat when a buyer is solicited. Knowles ends up with Martha O'Driscoll, the creditors are happy, but then Chic opens the curtain to reveal two young lovers in a warm embrace. He takes out a rifle and shoots them. "This is one picture that isn't going to have a happy ending," he explains, as the two comics bid the audience good-bye.

CRAZY HOUSE is a fast-moving, very enjoyable film that rates as one of the team's best. The opening sequences are ingenious and quite funny, and the duo's scenes throughout the film maintain a high level of comedy and a sense of the offbeat. The film's only lulls are, of course, when the focus is on the romantic leads, and during some of the excessively long musical numbers, which in typical 1940's tradition are loud and overarranged. Cass Daley, a sort of road-company

Martha Raye, is even louder than the musical background, but she comes off better in this film than she does in some of her other appearances during this era. Credit must also go to director Eddie Cline, who managed to keep the film moving at a fast pace; Cline was never hailed as a great director, but comedy classics like MILLION DOLLAR LEGS and THE BANK DICK are pretty good credits for anyone.

Instead of waiting a year, Ole and Chic decided to do another film for Universal just a few months after CRAZY HOUSE was completed. Released in mid-1944, the new picture was GHOST CATCHERS. Although the formula was the same as usual, GHOST CATCHERS came closer to Olsen and Johnson's original conception of insane humor than any of their other films. The story has southern colonel Walter Catlett bringing his two daughters (Gloria Jean and Martha O'Driscoll) to New York so they can perform at Carnegie Hall. He unwittingly buys a haunted house from crooked real estate dealer Walter Kingsford, and he and his daughters have a terrible time sleeping through their first night in the house. Martha runs next door to get help, unaware that "next door" is Olsen and Johnson's madcap nightclub, where she is abducted and made the center of attraction before disappearing through a trap door. Finally she tells Chic and Ole her troubles, and they come with her to see if they can

Olsen and Johnson in the act of being frightened. From GHOST CATCHERS.

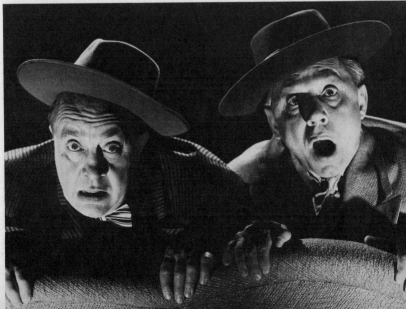

help. The house is full of strange noises: continual tap-dancing, horse hoofs, and so on. The others are scared, but Chic tells them, "Now don't get the idea that I'm afraid, because I don't believe in ghosts." Then, turning to the camera. "But then, I didn't believe in radio either!"

Through an intricate plan of recreating the past, the tap-dancing ghost (who persists in pinching Gloria Jean) is driven from the house. But the other noises continue, and Ole and Chic decide to stay overnight and investigate. As they enter their bedroom, Ole asks if Chic remembers the Abbott and Costello movie HOLD THAT GHOST. "Now that was a very unbelievable picture," he says as he criticizes the strange gags that they pulled. As he is talking, the two men are undressed by unseen hands, with their shoes and other garments flying across the room by themselves. Suddenly they start twirling in circles, and as they do their pajamas appear in place of their clothes. Only after they turn out the light do they realize what has happened.

When the noises resume, Chic and Ole climb out of bed to see what they can find. They discover two elves, with long white beards and pointed caps, who think the boys are part of their gang. They solemnly lead Ole and Chic to the basement hideout of the crooks who are causing these disturbances. As they walk along, Ole mutters, "I suppose they're taking us to Snow White." One elf turns around and grumbles disgustedly. "Everywhere we go . . . *Everywhere we go!*" When they arrive in the underground headquarters, they outwit the other gang members (Andy Devine in a horse's costume, Lon Chaney dressed as a bear, etc.,) until a silly mistake gives them away and a chase follows. The masked leader of the gang takes Chic, Ole, Catlett and his daughters and seals them up in a brick enclosure in the basement. As the last brick is put into place, the prisoners are sure they will never escape. Then they realize that one wall of their cell leads to the basement of Olsen and Johnson's nightclub. Some conveniently forgotten tools help them to break through the wall into the club. When the villains overhear their plans, they try to catch up with the culprits, and follow them into the nightclub. There, the leader of the gang is finally unmasked, and it turns out to be Leo Carrillo, the boys' manager.

Naturally, Gloria Jean is given several opportunities to sing, along with romantic lead Kirby Grant and vocalist Ella Mae Morse. Even Morton Downey shows up in one scene. But the film is genuinely inventive, with some wonderful throwaway gags and excellent special effects. Jack Norton, movies' perennial drunk, shows up in one scene as the tap-dancing ghost who's been haunting Catlett's house; other familiar faces dot the supporting cast. (An additional piece of trivia: the young drummer in Kirby Grant's orchestra, during the nightclub scenes, is Mel Torme.) Eddie Cline, who worked so well with the team on CRAZY HOUSE, also directed this vehicle, with delightful results.

After these two films, Olsen and Johnson returned to Broadway for a third musical comedy revue, *Laffing Room Only*. The material was new for this comic hodgepodge, but the format was the same successful one that had made their earlier shows long-running hits. By this time, any Olsen and Johnson show was truly a family affair. Besides Chic and Ole, there were Mrs. Johnson, continually searching for her husband Oscar, June Johnson, Chic's pretty young daughter, Marty May, June's husband, Ole Olsen, Jr., who was, as mentioned before, actually Ole's brother, and J. C. Olsen, who was Ole's son. *Laffing Room Only* brought the usual lukewarm response from the critics, and the usual legion of fans to the theater. The show enjoyed a respectable, if not overwhelming run, after which Chic and Ole departed for Hollywood to make their last film there.

The film was SEE MY LAWYER, based very loosely on a show presented on Broadway by George Abbott. The film version for Universal turned out to be the weakest of Olsen and Johnson's films for the studio, not because the comics weren't funny, but simply because they had so little to do in the film. Their other Universal vehicles had all featured guest stars and musical numbers, but this one had so many that the two stars were lost in the jumble. The story, such as it is, had the comedy duo trying to break their contract with nightclub owner Franklin Pangborn, who is doing terrific business with the boys and is unwilling to let them go. They kill two birds with one stone by insulting the nightclub patrons that evening; in doing so, they drive Pangborn to the breaking point, and at the same time create a lot of lawsuits to help three young attorneys (Noah Beery, Jr., Alan Curtis and Richard Benedict) get on their feet. Pangborn pulls a fast one by selling them the nightclub for a good price, without telling them that they are also inheriting the lawsuits. Most of the claimants were phony anyway— paid off by Chic and Ole—so they have the last laugh. One lawsuit, however, turns out to be real. Ed Brophy has filed suit for the indignity he encountered in their club, and the boys are forced to go to court. They make a shambles of the courtroom, convince the judge to move the trial to their nightclub, and win the case in a strange finale. The romantic subplot, involving dancer Grace McDonald and one of the three lawyers (she really loves Beery but Curtis gets in the way) gets lost in the shuffle, happily, but so do Olsen and Johnson.

The film is crowded with an unbelievable number of acts, including acrobats, jugglers, contortionists, dancers, the King Cole Trio, singer Yvette, a flamenco troupe and several others. This leaves Olsen and Johnson with about 15 minutes in the entire film, and only one genuinely funny scene. This is the one where they decide to insult the customers in Pangborn's nightclub, and proceed to do so by ripping the dress off a young girl, squirting seltzer in the face of a wealthy matron, taking guest Vernon Dent literally when he toasts, "Here's mud in your eye," and so on. Pangborn steps in to stop the mayhem and receives a pie in the face. It's all fairly obvious material, but it nevertheless constitutes the film's best scene. An earlier sequence where Chic and Ole drive their car into an office building has potential but falls flat, and the courtroom scene, which should have been the film's highlight, is too sloppily constructed to have any punch (the best gag comes when Brophy uses his kindly old mother, Mary Gordon, as his lawyer, and she brings in a violinist to add emotion to the testimony).

After SEE MY LAWYER, Universal apparently lost interest in the team (after all, they already had Abbott and Costello under contract) and failed to renew their pact. No other offers came up, so Olsen and Johnson bid Hollywood farewell to blaze new trails. They went back on the road with their unit revue, touring the country and stopping for special engagements like the Roxy in New York in 1947. In 1949 they kept busy by presenting a show called *Grandstand Gayeties* at the Canadian National Exposition, and serving as replacement for Milton Berle's TV show that same summer. Their TV program debuted July 5th over NBC-TV, and received an excellent review from *Variety:* "Olsen and Johnson have certainly run the gamut. The zanies have been in every branch of the amusement industry during their approximately 35 years as a team, and now they're a cinch to carve a new career for themselves on television." There was special praise for the production staff who put together the heavily gimmicked show, which cost a lofty $20,000 a week. Incredibly, the same year, the busy team opened a show at

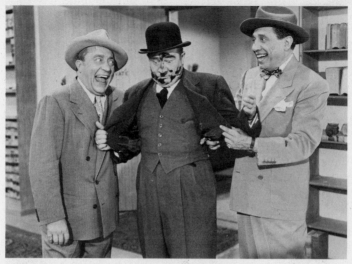

Ed Brophy has been had by those laughing boys Ole and Chic in SEE MY LAWYER.

New York's Madison Square Garden, on a limited-run basis, called *Funzapoppin*. The production, which reportedly cost $500,000 to stage, featured some two hundred performers (comedy stooges, singers, specialty acts and a chorus line), and, of course, Chic and Ole, handling the zany blackouts and sight gags.

That fall, Ole and Chic made a brief foray into television on a regular basis with a program called *Fireball Fun for All*. It didn't last very long, and the undaunted duo returned to their revue, which traveled to England and Australia. Like many other American performers, Olsen and Johnson were warmly received Down Under, and they referred to Australia as "a second home" for many years. In October 1950, the team returned to New York with their fourth and final Broadway revue. *Pardon Our French*. Almost predictably, the critics were unimpressed with the show, and with its "discovery," Denise Darcel, but the show did business for its comparatively brief run. Ole Olsen, who suffered a broken right thigh during rehearsals, was forced to turn over most of his role to Marty May, appearing briefly in a few scenes that didn't involve any strenuous work. Despite his on-stage absence, Ole continued to preside over the same sort of backstage mayhem that characterized their earlier shows. An awed reporter for the *Herald Tribune* wrote, "In dressing room No. 6 at the Broadway Theater, Olsen held court for the numerous visitors who drop backstage from the audience to say hello. Between shaking hands, mass introductions, the mail, and long-distance phone calls, the comedian managed to keep his mind off the fact that he wasn't on stage. Occasionally he was reminded of the action in the theater when sharp rifle fire echoed through the dressing room. At one point he was carrying on conversations with four English midgets, homeward bound, who had lost their tickets; an English variety artist who was wondering how to carry sixty pair of stockings, a heavy radio and other props back home, and with a contractor who is building a car wash for Olsen on Long Island. At the same time he was keeping track of the election returns for his curtain speech. Rudy Vallee dropped in for a chat, and finally a dentist and a visitor from France appeared. By this time, the cubbyhole of a dressing room, no more than four feet by eight, was getting crowded and warm. The situation was further confused by the volleys of gunfire on stage over which Olsen was shouting to be heard. According to reliable information, this sort of open court goes on every night. Olsen and Johnson have thousands of friends all over the country who feel they would be slighting the comedians if they didn't drop around and shake hands."

Throughout the 1950's, Olsen and Johnson continued to tour around the country, and often around the world, sometimes reviving *Hellzapoppin* on the straw-hat circuit, other times bringing their revue into a showcase like New York's Latin Quarter nightclub. In the summer of 1959 they staged a show called *Hellza-Splashin'* at the Aqua Amphitheater in Flushing, Long Island, later the site of the New York World's Fair. When asked why they were still going through their paces after forty-five years, Ole Olsen had a succinct and honest answer. "This work is fun. This is our life."

Eventually even Ole and Chic decided to take it easy and appeared less and less as the 1960's approached. On February 28, 1962, Chic Johnson died of a kidney ailment in a hospital in Las Vegas, Nevada, where he was vacationing with his wife. At the time, Ole Olsen was in Germany, touring U.S. army bases. He followed his partner in 1965, but his words, when he heard of Chic Johnson's death, serve as a fitting epitaph for both men. He recalled their forty-seven years together, entertaining through two world wars and never once thinking of splitting up. He recalled a toast that the two comics would give at the end of every show. "I said to the audience, 'May you live as long as you want,' and he would say 'and may you laugh as long as you live.' I guess that was sort of our motto." And a good one, too.

The Films of Olsen and Johnson

(Director's name follows year.)

1. **Oh Sailor Behave!**—Warner Brothers 1930—Archie Mayo—Irene Delroy, Charles King, Lowell Sherman, Noah Beery, Lotti Loder, Vivien Oakland, Charles Judels, Elise Bartlett, Lawrence Grant, Gino Corrado. 68 minutes.
2. **Fifty Million Frenchmen**—Warner Brothers 1931—Lloyd Bacon—William Gaxton, Helen Broderick, Lester Crawford, John Halliday, Charles Judels, Claudia Dell, Evalyn Knapp, Carmelita Geraghty, Daisy Belmore, Vera Gordon, Nat Carr, Bela Lugosi. Color—68 minutes.
3. **Gold Dust Gertie**—Warner Brothers 1931—Lloyd Bacon —Winnie Lightner, Arthur Hoyt, George Byron, Vivien Oakland, Dorothy Christy, Virginia Sale, Charles Judels. 66 minutes.
4. **Hollywood on Parade**—A-2—Paramount 1932—behind-the-scenes and informal footage of the stars, with Bing Crosby, Stuart Erwin, Burns and Allen, and Gary Cooper; O & J pull a crazy publicity stunt when they land at Lost Angeles airport. 10 minutes.
5. **Hollywood on Parade**—B-13—Paramount 1934—Marie Dressler, Dolores Del Rio, Gene Raymond, Leslie Howard, Norma Shearer, Clark Gable, Herbert Marshall, Diana Wynyard, Clive Brook, Will Rogers, Baby LeRoy, the 1934 Wampas Baby Stars. O & J are seen cavorting at the beach. 10 minutes.
6. **Country Gentlemen**—Republic 1937—Ralph Staub— Joyce Compton, Lila Lee, Pierre Watkin, Donald Kirke, Ray Corrigan, Sammy McKim, Wade Boteler, Ivan Miller, Olin Howland, Frank Sheridan, Harry Harvey, Joe Cunningham, "Prince" the dog. 66 minutes.
7. **All Over Town**—Republic 1937—James W. Horne—Mary Howard, Harry Stockwell, Franklin Pangborn, James Finlayson, Eddie Kane, Stanley Fields, D'Arcy Corrigan, Lew Kelly, John Sheehan, Earle Hodgins, Gertrude Astor, Blanche Payson, Otto Hoffman, Fred Kelsey. 62 minutes.

8. **Hellzapoppin**—Universal 1941—H. C. Potter—Martha Raye, Mischa Auer, Jane Frazee, Hugh Herbert, Robert Paige, Shemp Howard, Clarence Kolb, Nella Walker, Katherine Johnson, Lewis Howard, Richard Lane, Elisha Cook, Jr., Gus Schilling, George Chandler. 84 minutes.

9. **Crazy House**—Universal 1943—Edward Cline—Martha O'Driscoll, Patric Knowles, Cass Daley, Percy Kilbride, Leighton Noble, Thomas Gomez, Edgar Kennedy, Andrew Tombes, Ray Walker, Robert Emmett Keane, Franklin Pangborn, Chester Clute, Billy Gilbert, Richard Lane, Hans Conried, Shemp Howard, Fred Sanborn, Alan Curtis, Leo Carrillo, Allan Jones, Robert Paige, Grace McDonald, Lon Chaney, Andy Devine, The Demarcos, Marion Hutton, the Glenn Miller Singers, Chandra Kaley Dancers, Laison Brothers, the Five Hertzogs, Bobby Brooks, Ward and Van, Terry Sheldon, Harry Powers, Billy Reed, Count Basie Band, Delta Rhythm Boys. 80 minutes.

10. **Ghost Catchers**—Universal 1944—Edward L. Cline—Gloria Jean, Martha O'Driscoll, Leo Carrillo, Andy Devine, Lon Chaney, Kirby Grant, Walter Catlett, Ella Mae Morse, Morton Downey, Walter Kingsford, Tom Dugan, Edgar Dearing, Wee Willie Davis, Ralph Peters, Frank Mitchell, Tor Johnson, Bess Flowers, Jack Norton, Edward Earle, Mel Torme. 68 minutes.

11. **See My Lawyer**—Universal 1945—Edward L. Cline—Alan Curtis, Grace McDonald, Noah Beery, Jr., Franklin Pangborn, Edward S. Brophy, Richard Benedict, Lee Patrick, Gus Schilling, William B. Davidson, Stanley Clements, Mary Gordon, Ralph Peters, Ed Gargan, Vernon Dent, Ruth Roman, Bobby Barber, Cyril Ring, George Davis, Sid Saylor, George Chandler, Eddie Dunn, Leon Belasco, Tom Dugan, Marie Harmon, Gene Stutenroth (Roth), Carmen Amaya and Company, The King Cole Trio (featuring Nat "King" Cole), The Christiani Troupe, Yvette, The Six Willys, The Hudson Wonders, The Rogers Adagio Trio, The Four Teens. 67 minutes.

12. **It's a Tough Life**—Universal-International 1957—Arthur Cohen—Harry S. Truman, Jack E. Leonard, Joe E. Lewis, Hal March, Keefe Brasselle, Gloria DeHaven, Roberta Sherwood, George Jessel, Charlie Spivak, Phil Foster, Jerry Lester, Jimmy Durante. O & J make a brief poolside appearance in this travelogue which features celebrities at work and play in Miami Beach. Color—10 minutes.

ABBOTT and COSTELLO

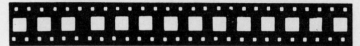

They lacked the artistry of Laurel and Hardy; they never captured the insanity of the Marx Brothers; they did not sing or dance like the Ritz Brothers. Why, then, were Abbott and Costello so popular during the 1940's and early 1950's? This question plagues film historians today, who can find no earthly reason for the team's existence. The answer is simple: They were very, very funny.

By the time Abbott and Costello were "discovered" in 1938, they had been together nearly a decade, working on their patter routines until they were letter perfect. The result was that radio and movie audiences saw the comedians at their peak. They worked like a well-oiled machine; few comedians possessed such infallible timing. Many of their wartime films date badly because of dialogue that is no longer topical, and brassy music that is no longer listenable. But their routines remain fresh and funny, and their plays on words continue to delight new generations of fans who have discovered the team on television.

Unlike Laurel and Hardy, Abbott and Costello were not film comedians; they came out of burlesque and vaudeville, where they were not required to be in character, but merely to exchange funny dialogue. Even in their Broadway show, *Streets of Paris*, they were merely two comics who wandered in and out of the revue doing various routines. When they were signed to star in movies, there was no time, nor was there any apparent need to work out definite characters for Bud Abbott and Lou Costello. The characters were fairly evident from their radio routines: Abbott was the domineering wise guy, Costello the guillible patsy. Because their personalities were not completely thought out at this time, they never really developed, and with few exceptions, the team never strove to portray realistic characters in their films. If they had any flaw, this was it. They always provided laughs, but they could never establish the bond that made

275

Laurel and Hardy so popular with audiences: they never convinced their fans that the two guys they were playing were real people, worth caring about. Scenes like the one in PARDON MY SARONG, where Bud gives Lou a gun to shoot himself, so their stranded party will have one less mouth to feed, are indicative of misfire ideas that never would have been acceptable if Bud and Lou had created believable characters for themselves.

William "Bud" Abbott was born in 1895 (often given as 1898) in either Asbury Park, Atlantic City, or Coney Island (all three have been given by the performer in official biographies). His mother was a bareback rider and his father an advance man for Ringling Brothers Circus. The Abbotts traveled quite a bit with the circus, but Bud spent most of his youth in Coney Island, and attended public school there when he was in town. Growing up in the circus atmosphere attracted him to a life of action, which he pursued in several ways during adolescence: he became a racing-car driver, but reportedly quit to please his mother, and later tried his hand at lion-taming with the circus, finally abandoning that to concentrate on a safer occupation. Bud went into the business end of show business, organizing touring shows, working in box offices, and the like. With his brother Harry he built up a theater chain that folded at the end of the 1920's when, like many other businessmen, the Abbott brothers realized that much of their money had never really existed. Bud broke into the performing side of show business in Brooklyn, where he learned the exacting art of being a straight man. The story goes that a partner was needed for Lou Costello one night, whose own straight man had failed to appear. This was one of several versions of how Abbott and Costello came together, but was the one the two comics quoted most often, and also the most believable.

The comic Bud Abbott appeared with that night was Lou Costello, born Francis Cristillo in 1906. While there is some doubt about Bud's birthplace, Lou made his home town known throughout his career. Whenever the name of a city was needed in a routine, he would use Paterson, New Jersey. Lou had a more conventional childhood than Bud, growing up in Paterson and excelling in sports at high school. On the recommendation of his baseball coach, he won a scholarship to Cornwall-on-Hudson Military School in New York, which he left before completing his education. With his athletic prowess (and without the excess weight he added later in life) he was convinced that there would be work for

him in the movies. He journeyed to Hollywood and reportedly, after working as a prop man and scenery shifter, ob-
tained work as a stunt man at MGM. This type of story is
always difficult to confirm, but it is true that even in the
1950's, when he was no longer a young man, Costello took
spectacular falls at the drop of a hat. Early biographies of
Costello state that he doubled for cowboy star Tim McCoy,
wore a gorilla suit for a chase scene with Karl Dane in
CIRCUS ROOKIES, dove out of a window doubling for Dolores
Del Rio in THE TRAIL OF '98, and engaged in a fight scene in
Polly Moran's saloon in ROSE MARIE. One article claimed he
had appeared in sixty-odd films during his stay at MGM.
When talkies came in, he left Hollywood and worked his
way into vaudeville and burlesque, soon meeting and teaming with the ex-auto racer, lion tamer, manager, and box-
office attendant, Bud Abbott.

Abbott and Costello found work in vaudeville, but as
talkies flourished, the two-a-days experienced a rapid and sad
decline. Before long, Bud and Lou were working in burlesque, along with scores of other entertainers who later
made names for themselves, from Leon Errol to Phil Silvers.
Wrote Abel Green and Joe Laurie, Jr., in their book *Show
Biz*, "All that could be said for burly in 1938 was that it was
the last spawning ground of new talent since vaudeville had
died. Burly, desperate for any kind of entertainment, opened
its arms to genuine, if untried, talent, which soon left it for
greener pastures." For most of the 1930's, Abbott and Costello
worked steadily in burlesque houses around the country,
gradually building up a reputation as they honed their routines down to marvels of rapid-fire dialogue. An engagement
at Minsky's on Times Square in New York—one of five
Minsky houses then in business—led to nonburlesque jobs
around the city, and eventually to the prestigious Loew's
State Theater. They were signed as guests on Kate Smith's
popular radio show, and scored such a hit that they became
regulars on the program. They branched out into nightclub
work, and had their first taste of stardom when they were
co-starred with Bobby Clark in a Broadway revue called
Streets of Paris, which opened in June 1939. Also in the cast
was a new Latin import named Carmen Miranda. The plotless, two-act conglomeration of songs, sketches, and comedy
patter was compared to *Hellzapoppin'* by most of the critics.
Brooks Atkinson wrote in *The New York Times*, "Costello
and Abbott [sic] are . . . pretty funny fellows in low comedy
antics," and the New York *Herald-Tribune* echoed these

sentiments, declaring, "They are the big hit of *Streets of Paris.*" All of Abbott and Costello's reviews, from the very start to their final press clippings, dwelled on the fact that their material was ancient, yet none of these critics ever denied that it was also funny. Despite this constant cry, audiences loved Bud and Lou, and didn't mind that some of the jokes they used were older than *they* were.

In 1940, with the team enjoying great popularity over the nation's airwaves, they went to Hollywood to make their first movie, ONE NIGHT IN THE TROPICS. This original screen musical boasted a score by no less than Jerome Kern, Dorothy Fields, and Oscar Hammerstein II. It was based on an Earl Derr Biggers story called "Love Insurance," and it starred Allan Jones, Nancy Kelly, and Robert Cummings. Bud and Lou were clearly in support, providing comedy relief with interpolations of such classic bits as "Jonah and the Whale," "Mustard," and "Who's on First?" The film was pleasant enough but nothing special, and it wasn't much of a success—though Abbott and Costello made a resounding hit with the people who *did* get to see it, including critics, who singled them out as the film's strongest asset.

The duo's movie career didn't really get started until 1941, when they starred in a film called BUCK PRIVATES. Universal, which had put them under contract, was one of Hollywood's

Nat Pendleton is doing all right with Bud Abbott, but Lou Costello is a very stubborn rookie in BUCK PRIVATES.

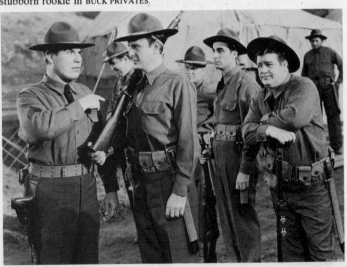

oldest movie factories, specializing in popular entertainment, ranging from horror films to Deanna Durbin musicals. They seldom spent much money on any film, producing a profitable program of "B" pictures and inexpensive star vehicles. The reported cost of BUCK PRIVATES was $90,000, but its gross was a figure many times that amount. With that one picture, the comedy team zoomed to the number three position on the *Motion Picture Herald's* poll of the year's top money-making stars at the box office. BUCK PRIVATES' success also won the team a contract at MGM to do one picture a year for three years. It is easy to see why the film was so popular in its time; it opens with newsreel footage of President Franklin D. Roosevelt announcing the country's first peacetime draft, and with the Secretary of Defense picking the first draftee. Bud and Lou, sidewalk tie salesmen, are chased by cop Nat Pendleton into what they think is a movie theater. That's what it was, but now it's an Army induction center. "What picture is playing here?" Lou asks. "You're in the Army now," replies an officer on guard. "Oh good, I haven't seen that one," Lou tells Bud. Before they know what has happened, they have enlisted and are forced to go through the rigors of induction. At this point, the film's subplot is introduced, with rich-boy Lee Bowman and his former valet Alan Curtis signing up for service, Bowman

Bud and Lou follow Joan Davis as they prowl around a haunted house in HOLD THAT GHOST.

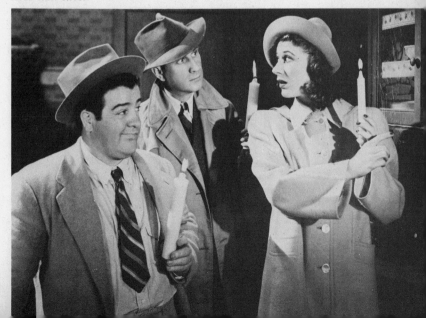

confident that his influential father will get him released within a week. By the end of the film, of course, Bowman changes from a conceited know-it-all to a dedicated serviceman; he wins the girl (Jane Frazee), and everybody lives happily ever after. This subplot shares the spotlight with Bud and Lou, and the singing Andrew Sisters; the result is an enjoyable, but episodic film. In one scene Bud asks Lou for the loan of $50. Lou has only $40, so Bud tells him that he can owe him the extra $10. This baffles Lou, who asks for his money back; Bud gives him the money, but keeps the $10 that he is "owed." This snowballs until Lou is not only broke, but in debt to Abbott. Another good sequence has Bud trying to teach Lou the fundamentals of army drilling. "Throw your chest out!" he orders. "I'm not through with it yet," Lou complains. A film highlight has Costello "volunteered" to represent his section in a boxing match on the base, and another good scene has him pretending to be a novice in shooting craps, but tossing out a stream of gambling jargon throughout the game. In fact, practically of all of the team's routines are good in this film, the only lulls coming when the story switches to the romantic leads, or presents a number like "Rock me Brother with a Solid Four."

Never ones to rest on their laurels, Universal decided to parlay their popular comedy team into a box-office bonanza by

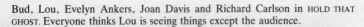

Bud, Lou, Evelyn Ankers, Joan Davis and Richard Carlson in HOLD THAT GHOST. Everyone thinks Lou is seeing things except the audience.

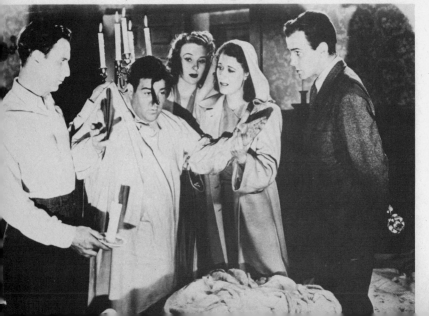

keeping them working steadily. BUCK PRIVATES was released in early 1941; by the end of the year three more Abbott and Costello vehicles were playing around the country. IN THE NAVY tried to duplicate the success of their first hit by putting the two rookies out to sea, with crooner Dick Powell playing a popular singer trying to hide his identity during his Navy stretch. The Andrews Sisters were back again to share musical honors, with Bud and Lou lost in the commotion except for several bright comedy spots (Lou multiplying 7 times 13 to get 28, trying to bed down for the night in a hammock above the ground, etc.). Their next, HOLD THAT GHOST, was one of the team's all-time best films, with Bud and Lou spending a night in a "haunted" house with other guests such as Richard Carlson, Evelyn Ankers and hilarious Joan Davis, who plays a professional radio screamer. The gags inside the house have been reused by A & C countless times, but seldom with such success: Lou, left alone in a darkened room, sputters incoherently as a candle on the table before him moves back and forth, and up and down. Every time Abbott comes in to check on him, the scene is normal, but as soon as he leaves, the candle starts going again and Lou goes into his hilarious fits of frenzy.

The A & C formula seemed to be a winning one, with KEEP 'EM FLYING and RIDE 'EM COWBOY following in quick succession. FLYING has the expected airplane sight gags, but benefits in large part from Martha Raye in a dual role. RIDE

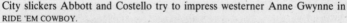

City slickers Abbott and Costello try to impress westerner Anne Gwynne in RIDE 'EM COWBOY.

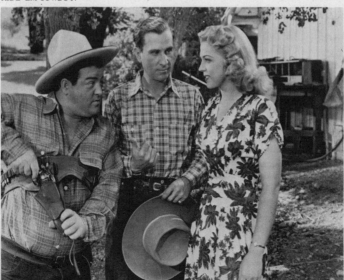

'EM COWBOY takes A & C back to the land of subplots, but gives them enough footage to make the film worthwhile for their fans. One scene that should have been hilarious, however, is ruined by clumsy presentation. The routine is an old burlesque chesnut, "Crazy House," with Lou having a bad dream that he is in a hospital where he must have peace and quiet. This is destroyed by an unending procession of crazy people marching through his room—one thinks Lou's stomach is a flower bed and starts to water it, two outlaws shoot it out in front of his bed, and so on. Presented correctly, this is a side-splitting sketch, but the film's director (Arthur Lubin) decided to abandon the traditional straightforward presentation in favor of a more filmic technique, that of showing Lou tossing in bed, with the picture periodically fading into a dream sequence of various loonies bothering him. The impact is gone, because the sequence becomes disjointed and has no continuity. The team knew this was a great routine, however, for they used it again—to better effect—on TV. Lou Costello performed it again, without Bud, on a Steve Allen show in the 1950s, and made it part of his repertoire when he played Las Vegas late in life. It's just too bad it wasn't captured for posterity in this film.

In 1942 the team fulfilled its first obligation to MGM by starring in RIO RITA, a half-hearted remake of the musical first filmed in 1929 with Wheeler and Woolsey. Bud and Lou were forced to share the footage with romantic leads John

When Bud and Lou, Chicago bus drivers, take their vehicle to California, William Demarest gets on their trail, in PARDON MY SARONG.

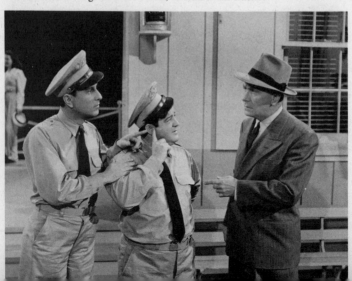

Carroll and Kathryn Grayson, and were saddled with an updated script full of saboteurs and time bombs. The resulting film is one of their lesser efforts, with a heavy-handed slapstick routine where Lou is caught in a giant washing machine—and only a hint of true A & C in verbal exchanges like the one about Mrs. Pike's Pekingese dog: Pike's Peke. Back at Universal, they were back on track with PARDON MY SARONG, to put them back in the groove. The film starts out promisingly, with Bud and Lou as Chicago bus drivers cajoled into taking a playboy yacht racer (Robert Paige) cross-country to Los Angeles, where he is scheduled to enter a competition. Process server William Demarest follows them to nail them for stealing the company bus, but loses them when their vehicle drives into the Pacific Ocean. Bud and Lou end up as crew members aboard Paige's yacht, where Virginia Bruce, the sister of a rival yachter, is also seeking refuge. Virginia sabotages the compass and unwittingly strands the party at sea, until they find an uncharted island. Here, the film slows down considerably as native girl Nan Wynn and other islanders (looking suspiciously like Universal contract starlets) do a seemingly endless series of musical numbers. The film picks up again in its final third, with jewel thief Lionel Atwill setting a trap for Lou, and sending his hencemen, led by Jack LaRue, onto a wild chase for a jewel in Lou's possession. The chase takes Lou and Bud, who has come to help him, into an island volcano, where they pre-

Detectives William Gargan and William Bendix are sure they know WHO DONE IT but they're wrong.

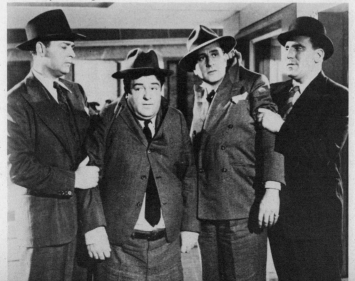

tend to be statues, through the jungle, where they swing à la Tarzan on hanging vines, and into the sea, where Lou unwittingly takes up water skiing to catch up with Atwill's motorboat. This final chase is lightning-paced, with a string of ingenious and amusing gags (Lou is being pulled by the motorboat, standing on a board, but a swordfish cuts his platform in half and transforms it into two unwieldy skis!).

WHO DONE IT? continued this string of successes with the duo as inept sodajerks (a wiseguy kid bets Lou on how much he can drink, loses the bet but gets three free sodas in the process) who become involved with murder at a radio station. Costello proves the biggest thorn in the side of investigating detective William Bendix in the amusing comedy mystery that follows, with some fine moments backstage at the radio station. IT AIN'T HAY is Damon Runyon-esque material adapted for A & C, who get involved with a horse named Teabiscuit. HIT THE ICE is fast-paced comedy with Bud and Lou as sidewalk photographers who accidentally get involved in a bank robbery with mobster Sheldon Leonard, and spend the rest of the film trying to clear themselves. In 1944 the team made the best of their three films for MGM, LOST IN A HAREM. The absurd plot has them playing prop men stranded with a traveling show in the Near East, being thrown in jail along with the show's star, Marilyn Maxwell. Prince John Conte agrees to get them out if they will help him recapture his kingdom, which has been taken

Sultan Douglass Dumbrille hypnotizes Lou, Bud and Marilyn Maxwell in LOST IN A HAREM.

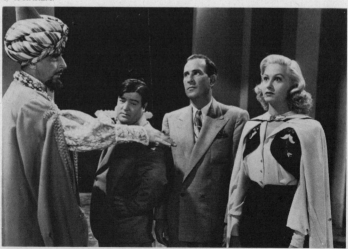

over by sultan Douglass Dumbrille. The rest of the film is rather predictable, with the script allowing for the fact that Jimmy Dorsey and his entire orchestra have also been captured by the sultan, and ordered to perform. A & C get through all of this better than most of the other cast members, but only one scene hits the bull's eye. Dumbrille, tired of their interference, hypnotizes them into thinking they are termites, and before long, they have chewed their way through most of the furniture in the room where they are being held captive.

Their next Universal film, IN SOCIETY, is noteworthy only for its final chase scene, which uses stock footage of a scene from W. C. Fields' 1941 Universal film NEVER GIVE A SUCKER AN EVEN BREAK almost in its entirety. It also has some amusing moments with Bud and Lou as plumbers doing their best to wreck an elaborate mansion. HERE COME THE CO-EDS has a sense of foreshadowing in its casting of Lon Chaney, Jr., as a villain determined to stop A & C from raising money to save the girls' school where they work. In the film's funniest scene, Lou goes into the boxing ring with "The Masked Marvel," who turns out to be the brawny Chaney. The son of the "Man of a Thousand Faces" was just a supporting player in this Abbott and Costello opus, but several years later, he was to help revitalize their career.

While their films maintained a good level of comedy, and were always slickly produced, Abbott and Costello went into

Bud and Lou in disguise from LOST IN A HAREM.

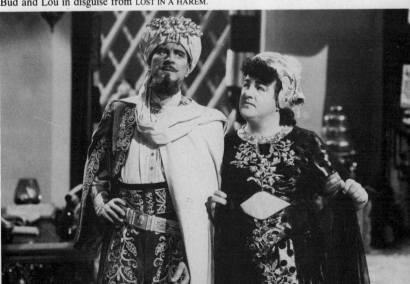

a slump during the mid-1940's. Perhaps their formula was wearing thin, or perhaps it was just oversaturation. 1944 was the first year they didn't rate among the top-ten money-makers (though this was caused in part by a lengthy illness that kept Costello from working at all). MGM cancelled their annual picture contract after a 1945 flop, ABBOTT AND COSTELLO IN HOLLYWOOD (although Metro certainly wasn't pushing that one very hard. MGM stars made guest appearances in all sorts of films, but the guest list in this one was rather meager. Customers who expected to get an inside look at Movieland, with glimpses of many luminaries, were rather disappointed). THE NAUGHTY NINETIES didn't have much going for it except some good verbal exchanges, so the writers decided to interpolate the team's classic "Who's on First" routine into the proceedings for guaranteed laughs. This marvelous piece of material was always associated with the team, and they repeated it many times on radio, in personal appearances, and on their TV series. Reportedly, President Roosevelt was a great fan of the routine, and A & C were invited to cut a gold record of it for the Baseball Hall of Fame in Cooperstown, New York. It starts with Bud Abbott explaining their baseball-team line-up: Who's on first, What's on second, I-Don't-Know's on third. At this point Lou is confused, and starts the ball rolling.

Margaret Dumont, vacationing from the Marx Brothers, has just as much trouble with Lou Costello in LITTLE GIANT.

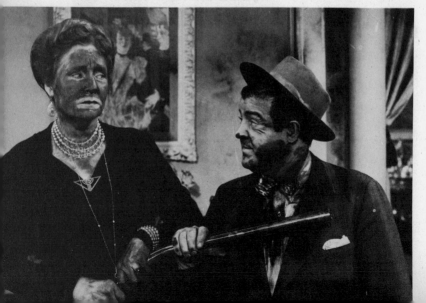

A: I say Who's on first, What's on second
I-Don't-Know's on third . . .
C: Yeah, you know the fellow's name?
A: Yes.
C: Well, who's on first?
A: Yes.
C: I mean the fellow's name.
A: Yes.
C: I mean the guy playing first.
A: Who.
C: The fellow playing first.
A: Who.
C: The first baseman.
A: Who.
C: The guy playing first.
A: Who is on first!
C: Well what are you asking *me* for?

It snowballs into a delightful mix up with Lou, in desperation, finally declaring, "Well, I don't give a damn!" "Oh, says Bud, "*he's* our shortstop!" The routine is still great, but it couldn't save NAUGHTY NINETIES from being one of the duo's weaker efforts.

After a well-publicized rift with Bud Abbott in 1945, Lou Costello expressed the desire to try something different in the duo's films, and Universal agreed that a change of pace might be good. In LITTLE GIANT Lou worked solo, with a more subdued script than usual, playing a door-to-door salesman of vacuum cleaners. He encounters Bud twice, playing twin brothers who are store managers in different cities on the road. There's no real zest in the film, which obscures one's abilities to judge Abbott and Costello as solo performers. They experimented once more, working separately in the same story, but this time the results were a delight. THE TIME OF THEIR LIVES is Abbott and Costello's most unusual film, and in many ways their best. The story opens during the Revolutionary War in the Colonies, where Lou is a dedicated watch-tinker with one prized possession, a letter of commendation from General George Washington. Lou is courting a young servant girl, but a butler in the same house (Bud Abbott) is also vying for her attention. He schemes to put Lou out of the way by locking him in a trunk in the barn outside their house. The girl is away while this is going on, and accidentally breaks in on a party of conspirators who are plotting against the Colonies; they are led by the young

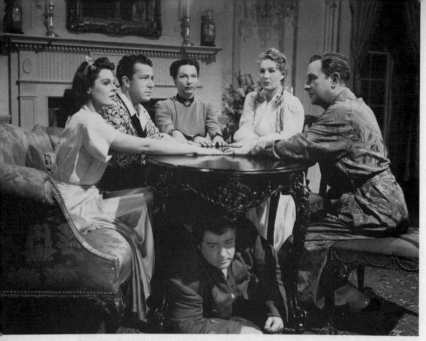

Ghostly Costello tries to communicate with Lynne Baggett, John Shelton, Gale Sondergaard, Binnie Barnes and Bud Abbott in THE TIME OF THEIR LIVES.

master of the household. The conspirators kidnap the girl so she won't be able to talk, but meanwhile the mistress of the house (Marjorie Reynolds) discovers what is going on, and rushes out to the barn to get her horse. She wants to warn the Revolutionaries that they are in danger; before she leaves she frees Costello and pleads with him to go with her. As they ride away, they are mistaken for traitors themselves and are shot, their bodies dumped into a well on the estate of her house. The soldiers post a curse on the well, dooming their traitorous souls to stay within the confines of the estate for eternity. Lou and Marjorie eventually awaken, and soon realize that they are ghosts. Their attempts to run away from the estate are thwarted by an invisible force that blocks their way.

The scene fades to modern times, with a look-alike ancestor of the Revolutionary conspirator coming up to look over his house. He has renovated the home and plans to move in with his future wife. Along with him on this trip are his sister (Binnie Barnes) and a psychiatrist friend (Bud Abbott). They are shown into the manor by eerie housekeeper Gale Sondergaard ("Didn't I see you in REBECCA?" Binnie asks). Lou and Marjorie recognize the two descendants from colonial days, and at first they seek revenge, using their invisibility to their advantage. Then they realize that if these people

can search the house and find Lou's old letter from George
Washington, it will prove that they never were traitors, and
their souls will be freed from the confinement of two centuries. They try every means possible to communicate with the
new house guests, and finally, with the help of self-proclaimed
medium Sondergaard, make their mission known. A search,
and some hard thinking, finally reveal that Lou's letter is in
the compartment of an old clock now residing in a New
York museum. Bud, driven by a strange feeling of repen-
tance that he can't explain, tries to get the clock, and when
all legal efforts fail, he steals it. There is a mad scramble to
find the combination of the two clock hands that will open
the secret compartment that holds the letter, as the police
come to arrest Abbott and reclaim the clock. At the very
last minute, the compartment is opened, the letter found,
and the two souls freed. Lou goes up to heaven to join his
true love, the servant girl, after two hundred years, and sees
her through the heavenly gates. They have a fond reunion,
and he asks to be let in, but she explains that she can't,
pointing to a sign on the gate that reads "Closed for Washington's Birthday."

THE TIME OF THEIR LIVES is a well written, charming movie
that draws fine, noncomedic performances from both Abbott and Costello. Lou has a natural acting ability, and plays

Marjorie Main introduces the boys to her unruly brood (Audrey Young is the
pretty one on the right) in THE WISTFUL WIDOW OF WAGON GAP.

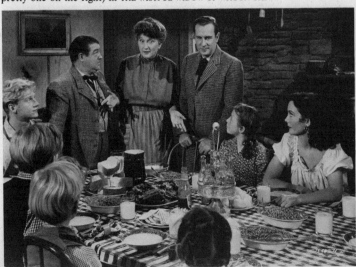

his straight scenes with sincerity; Bud is the butt of many of the invisible Costello's pranks, and registers well as the psychiatrist who after a while isn't too sure about his own mental health. The special effects are for the most part convincing, and one scene features a most ingenious gimmick: Marjorie and Lou run head on into each other, but being ghosts they both pass through without a collision: the only result is that their clothes are switched. The film also has fine contributions from wise cracking Binnie Barnes, and Gale Sondergaard as the housekeeper. Unfortunately, the film has never received its due because people who dislike Abbott and Costello are unwilling to give it a chance.

From experimentation in THE TIME OF THEIR LIVES, the team went into a tried and true formula which resulted in one of their funniest outings in years, BUCK PRIVATES COME HOME. The 1947 release brought BUCK PRIVATES up to date by having the soldiers returning home after World War Two with a little war orphan named Evie, and getting involved in a get-rich-quick scheme with racing-car mechanic Tom Brown. Nat Pendleton repeated his role from the 1941 film as the sergeant who is also the cop on their beat, forever frustrated in his attempts to get even with Bud and Lou. The film's climax is a masterfully arranged sequence with Lou driving the boys' souped-up racing car, which goes off the track, in and out of houses and buildings, and through an airport.

Count Dracula (Bela Lugosi) has Lou under his spell in ABBOTT AND COSTELLO MEET FRANKENSTEIN.

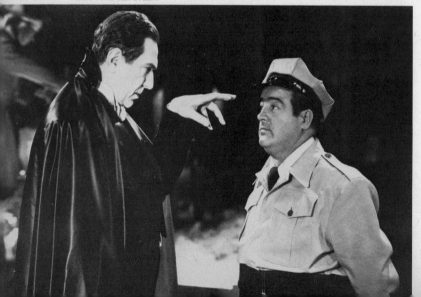

Lou drives through a billboard, which breaks over his head and forms wings for the car; before he knows what's going on, the car takes to the sky and flies over the city streets. The special effects are convincing enough to make the sequence one of the funniest the team ever did. Their next film opens with this subtitle: "MONTANA—In the Days when Men were Men—with Two Exceptions." The two exceptions are Abbott and Costello, and the film is THE WISTFUL WIDOW OF WAGON GAP. The two heroes are traveling salesmen who get in the middle of a shoot-out in the town of Wagon Gap. Lou is accused of killing one of the town's ornery outlaws, and by law he is given the responsibility of supporting the dead man's wife and children. The widow turns out to be raucous Marjorie Main, and her children comprise quite a brood. Through a series of circumstances Lou becomes sheriff, and in the film's funniest segment, he walks around town unafraid, because everyone knows that killing him will mean having to support his widow and family. Lou takes on new courage with this fact backing him up (he has a photo of the family in his pocket in case anyone needs reminding) and all goes well until he and Bud get involved in a stagecoach holdup engineered by the local bigshot (Gordon Jones—later Mike the Cop on their TV series). The film has its slow moments, but generally it is quite amusing, with Miss Main adding some fine moments.

THE NOOSE HANGS HIGH, made independently at Eagle-Lion studios in 1948, was pretty undistinguished, except for Lou's delightful byplay with veteran comic Leon Errol. But following this venture, the team returned to Universal for a film that propelled them back into the highest ranks of box-office popularity, and gave them the impetus to continue making films for Universal for the next seven years: ABBOTT AND COSTELLO MEET FRANKENSTEIN. Combining horror and comedy was nothing new in 1948; the team had tried it seven years earlier in HOLD THAT GHOST. Most other screen comics got tangled up with mad doctors or monsters at one point in their adventures. But working for Universal, Abbott and Costello had the rights to use the studio's copyrighted screen monsters, Frankenstein, Dracula and the Wolfman. In addition, Universal was able to secure the services of Bela Lugosi to play Count Dracula, Lon Chaney, Jr., to play the Wolfman, and Glenn Strange to do service as the Frankenstein monster, as he had done twice before in HOUSE OF FRANKENSTEIN and HOUSE OF DRACULA. The result was Abbott and Costello's best film, certainly the best horror-comedy ever made, and in many ways one of the best horror films ever produced at Universal. The studio had pioneered the talking horror-film with such greats as FRANKENSTEIN and DRACULA. While both were classic films, they suffered from some of the awkwardness still evident in talkies of the early 1930's. FRANKENSTEIN in particular cried for a musical score. Later films in the series had more studio polish in their favor, but with few exceptions they lacked the strong story lines and direction that had made the early films great. ABBOTT AND COSTELLO MEET FRANKENSTEIN, however, created a truly eerie atmosphere, especially in Count Dracula's castle, and the scenes with the Count and the Monster coming to life were as exciting as any in the "legitimate" horror films. For all of Abbott and Costello's clowning, the monsters played their roles straight; contrasted to the madcap antics around them, they were that much more terrifying. The special effects were superb, with Lugosi's transformation from a bat into the human form of Dracula (done via animation) standing out. The film was a tremendous success in 1948, and it remains a first-rate film today.

Unfortunately, neither of the team's next two films was a worthy successor. MEXICAN HAYRIDE (minus its Broadway score by Cole Porter) was strictly ordinary. AFRICA SCREAMS, a jungle-picture spoof, was no bull's-eye, but had some very

Boris Karloff is in command in ABBOTT AND COSTELLO MEET THE KILLER, BORIS KARLOFF.

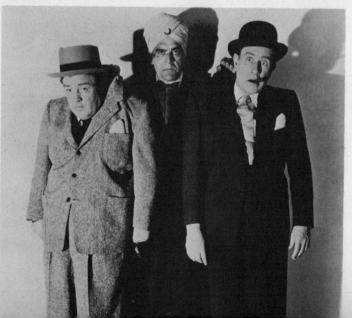

funny moments, with a fine comic supporting cast including
Shemp Howard, Joe Besser, and Hillary Brooke. Universal
then decided to cash in on FRANKENSTEIN's success by nam-
ing the team's next picture ABBOTT AND COSTELLO MEET THE
KILLER, BORIS KARLOFF. Few marquees could accommodate
all that, and Karloff's name was frequently omitted from the
film's title. Why it was included in the first place proved
quite a mystery, for his role in the film was clearly a supporting one, and his scenes with the team were few and far
between. The film is an amusing comedy-whodunit, with a
series of murders occurring in the hotel where Lou works as
a bellboy and Bud is house detective. Karloff is a phony
swami who turns out to be a red herring only indirectly
involved in the murders. His key scene has him trying to
hypnotize Lou into committing suicide. "You'll kill yourself
if it's the last thing you do," he declares. Some of the humor
involving dead bodies is rather strained, but the film moves
briskly to an unexpectedly exciting climax in a maze-like
cavern near the hotel. The mysterious murderer, wearing a
hood, traps Lou into meeting him there, and then delights in
watching him slip and slide on the narrow ledges above the
seemingly bottomless pits and craggy rocks below. The special effects are excellent in this scene, and unusually elaborate for what is essentially a medium budget picture.

No, that's not Bud Abbott. It's a mirage from ABBOTT AND COSTELLO IN THE
FOREIGN LEGION.

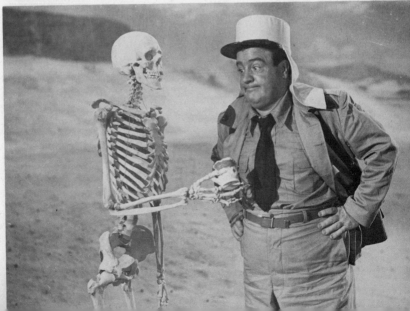

ABBOTT AND COSTELLO IN THE FOREIGN LEGION is not quite so elaborate, nor as good. It moves, which is more than one can say for some films, but the belly-laugh scenes never come. The closest the film comes is one sequence where Lou inadvertently engages in a slave auction—he's only waving to one of the girls, but his gestures are interpreted as bidding signals; the other key scene has Bud and Lou lost in the desert, and envisioning a series of mirages. AB-BOTT AND COSTELLO MEET THE INVISIBLE MAN continued their "horror" cycle, and turned out to be the best of all the sequels they made to A & C MEET FRANKENSTEIN. This one has them recently graduated from a detective school (Bud had to pay the dean $20 to give Lou his diploma) and getting involved with a young fighter (Arthur Franz) who's been framed for murder by racketeer Sheldon Leonard. Franz's doctor friend has been experimenting with an invisibility formula passed on to him by its inventor (Claude Rains' picture is on the wall), but he refuses to let the young doctor try it, for fear of his sanity. When the doctor isn't looking, however, Franz injects himself and remains invisible for the rest of the film. He hits upon a scheme to get the goods on Leonard by making Lou look like a great fighter. They all go down to work at the local gym, and with invisible Franz

Lou and Bud graduate from detective school; but Bud had to bribe Walter F. Appler $20 to give Lou a diploma. From ABBOTT AND COSTELLO MEET THE INVISIBLE MAN.

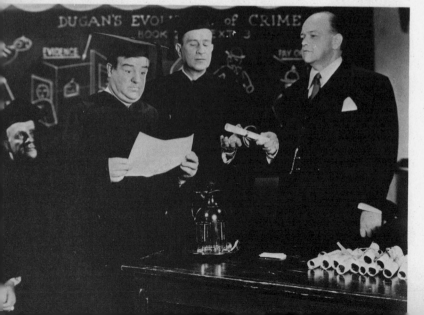

doing all the work, Lou effortlessly beats the daylights out of a punching bag. As they had expected, Lou quickly becomes the leading contender for the next championship, and at the same time, becomes the target of more of Leonard's corruption. The climactic fight scene has Lou astounding observers by knocking out his opponent seemingly without hitting him! In the dressing room afterward, there is a shootout, and Franz is hit, but Leonard is caught and arrested by the police. Meanwhile, at the hospital, Costello gives Franz a blood transfusion and saves his life. Due to some back up, Lou also becomes invisible momentarily, reappearing only to find his feet facing the wrong way. INVISIBLE MAN is one of the team's funniest outings, and the special effects are just about the best ever devised for this kind of film. Scenes like the one where Franz unwraps his bandages, revealing nothing but air, are eye-popping.

Unfortunately, ABBOTT AND COSTELLO MEET THE INVISIBLE MAN was the duo's last really good film; several of their subsequent efforts were amusing, but none came up to the level of hilarity reached during the 1940's, and revived in this 1951 release. Amid some halfhearted Universal films, the team journeyed to Warner Brothers for the first time, under the aegis of producer Alex Gottlieb, who had worked on many of their films at the home studio. Their first for Warners was JACK AND THE BEANSTALK, which started in black and white and switched to color (à la WIZARD OF OZ), but never generated many laughs. Bud and Lou are baby sitters, and as Lou reads the famous fairy tale to a bratty

Lou is Jack, Buddy Baer is the Giant in JACK AND THE BEANSTALK.

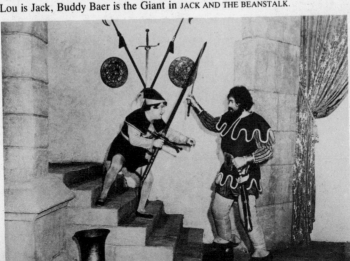

youngster, he dreams that he is Jack, and the story begins. The production itself is nicely mounted, and Buddy Baer makes a convincing giant, but there is very little Abbott and Costello in the film. It comes off better as a children's fantasy than as a comedy. Their second Warners film, also in color, was ABBOTT AND COSTELLO MEET CAPTAIN KIDD, with Charles Laughton playing foil for the team's usual antics. The film was not inspired, however, and a potentially good idea was wasted, with Laughton only coming to life in the final scenes, and the team's material remaining average throughout.

In 1951 Abbott and Costello made their TV debut on NBC's popular *Colgate Comedy Hour*. The one-hour show was a typical variety hodgepodge, with A & C doing a handful of old routines—from "Who's on First?" to the perennial "Crazy House," with Lon Chaney, Jr. adding some equally time-worn "scare comedy." Critics berated them for hauling out this old material, but the vaudeville-like setting of a TV variety show at that time was a perfect setting for Bud and Lou—and the perfect showcase for their kind of comedy. Audiences ate it up, and the team was integrated into the series' pattern of rotating hosts for the next three years. In 1952 they decided to produce their own show, on

Charles Laughton isn't amused by the antics of Bud and Lou in ABBOTT AND COSTELLO MEET CAPTAIN KIDD.

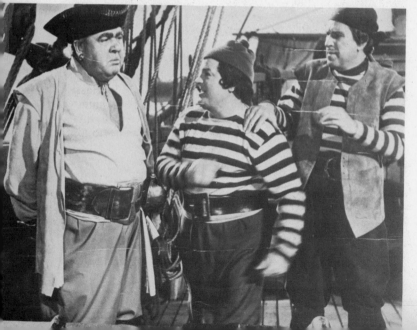

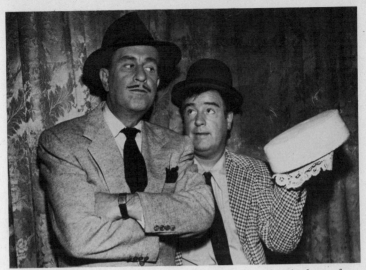

Bud and Lou as they appeared in their filmed TV series, in front of a proscenium curtain.

film, and two seasons of *The Abbott and Costello Show* resulted. The show is still in syndication today. Fifty-two episodes were filmed, with Pat Costello (Lou's brother) acting as executive producer and Jean Yarbrough (who worked on some of their films) functioning as producer-director. These half-hour shows are a strange blend of disjointed burlesque and vaudeville routines, material borrowed from old A & C movies, and the type of two-reel comedy material most studios did during the 1930's and 40's. The resemblance in all cases is more than coincidental. Sidney Fields, who played their landlord in the series, wrote many of the scripts. He was an ex-burlesque comic himself, steeped in the classic skits and blackouts familiar in that field of entertainment, and he didn't hesitate to lift old routines and place them verbatim into the A & C shows. Clyde Bruckman, who also contributed many scripts, started as Buster Keaton's head writer in the 1920's and later wrote and directed for Laurel and Hardy, the Three Stooges and many other film comics. In Bruckman's scripts, one can see gags and often entire situations lifted from many of his earlier films. One episode, for example, uses the classic gag from Keaton's THE NAVI-GATOR where an oil-painting portrait hangs outside a window, and gives the illusion of a man peeking inside. Other shows used material that had first appeared in A & C movies like HOLD THAT GHOST, NAUGHTY NINETIES, and MEXICAN HAYRIDE—including "Who's on First," which popped up in at least two different episodes. Another similarity to the two-reel comedies was seen in the casts of the TV series: one program had Walter Catlett as a fanatical bird lover; comedy heroine Dorothy Granger (for years Leon Errol's wife in his two-reelers) was in three different shows; and still another featured Laurel and Hardy's perennial nemesis Charlie Hall as a man working on a roof. Such familiar character actors as Allen Jenkins, Thurston Hall, Lucien Littlefield and James Flavin were frequently seen in the cast, along with some fading starlets of the 1940's (Mary Beth Hughes) and some upcoming ones of the 1950's (Joan Shawlee). The show's regulars were Sidney Fields, as the landlord, Gordon

Shades of burlesque: Abbott and Costello do "the lemon bit" on TV's *Colgate Comedy Hour.*

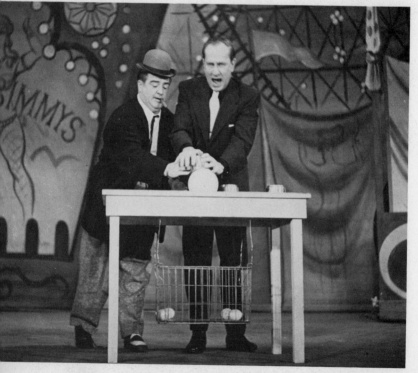

Jones, as Mike the Cop, Hillary Brooke, as a lovely neighbor, Joe Besser, as Stinky, the obnoxious brat, and Joe Kirk,
as Mr. Bacciagalupe. The shows were filmed on an assembly
line basis, with an audience laughtrack (often quite shrill)
added later. The show is strained and silly, often outland-
ishly incoherent, but it does contain some hilarious routines—
and some amusing ad-libs from Lou. It also serves as a
filmed record of virtually every classic burlesque routine
ever performed.

Reviewing ABBOTT AND COSTELLO GO TO MARS on its TV
page in recent years, *The New York Times* remarked, "And
about time." The joke was unfair to Bud and Lou, but not
to that particular film, which was one of their dreariest. And
for some reason, the planet on which the film took place was
not Mars at all, but Venus. Their next film, ABBOTT AND
COSTELLO MEET DR. JEKYLL AND MR. HYDE, was one of their
most disappointing efforts. It has good special effects, with
transformation scenes of man-into-monster that rival any of
Universal's earlier horror films, but the laughs are few and
the "straight" plot involving mad doctor Boris Karloff is

Even Mack Sennett himself couldn't liven up ABBOTT AND COSTELLO MEET THE
KEYSTONE KOPS.

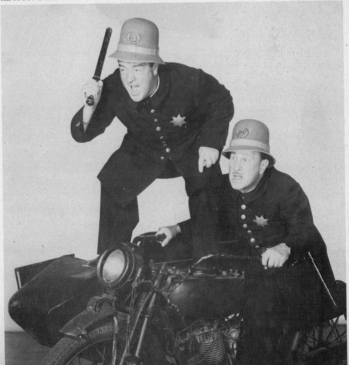

rather limp. The film's best scene comes when Lou, inside a horror museum, inadvertently sets off a live wire which brings a Frankenstein statue to life. In 1954, Bud and Lou were set to appear in a comedy with bandleader Spike Jones and his City Slickers called FIREMAN SAVE MY CHILD. Stunt sequences were filmed with doubles for A & C—but then the team bowed out. Stories conflict as to why (Costello's illness, a producer's change of heart, Costello's refusal to participate in the film)—but Universal salvaged its footage by casting physical look-alikes Hugh O'Brian and Buddy Hackett in the film!

Abbott and Costello were off the screen until 1955 when Universal made ABBOTT AND COSTELLO MEET THE KEYSTONE KOPS. Here, it seemed, was a "natural" for the team, a subject that would allow for silent-movie spoofs and plenty of slapstick. What resulted was another big disappointment, with a token appearance by Mack Sennett in one scene, and very little of the verve and action of silent comedy. Fred Clark, playing a conniving movie producer, was easily the film's greatest asset. Oddly enough, the team's last film for the studio, ABBOTT AND COSTELLO MEET THE MUMMY, was quite good, the best film they had done since INVISIBLE MAN. Co-star Marie Windsor recently recalled that the two stars delighted in confounding their assistant director, answering other players' dialogue with "What?" during rehearsals, and just enjoying themselves as much as possible. One wishes the film could have had that same carefree spirit; it sticks to a straight plot for the most part, but Bud and Lou's scenes are good and they receive above-average support from a good cast: Marie Windsor, Richard Deacon, Michael Ansara and Dan Seymour, among others. One of the film's best scenes is a throwback to the team's earliest work, a play on words along the lines of "Who's on First." Somehow, these verbal exchanges had disappeared from their films of the 1950's, even though John Grant, who wrote most of their best material, was still working on the scripts. A & C MEET THE MUMMY made up for the loss when the two were told to dig a ditch. Lou has a bunch of tools and tells Abbott to take his pick. Bud grabs a shovel and gets to work. "Wait a minute," says Lou. "I told you to take your pick." "That's what I did," Bud replies. "The shovel is my pick." Lou can't grasp this, and he asks them to start all over again. He takes back the tool, and tells Bud to take his pick. Again Abbott grabs a shovel, explaining, "The shovels is my pick; my pick is the shovel." "How can a shovel be a pick?" Lou wants to know. Finally, with Bud's help, he recites, "The shovel is your pick and your pick is the shovel and the pick is my pick." "Now you've got it," says Bud encouragingly. "I don't even know what I'm talking about!" protests Lou in a whiny voice reminiscent of their best radio sketches of the 1930's and 40's.

After MUMMY, Universal dropped Abbott and Costello. The 1950's were strange times in Hollywood, and it was surprising that the team had stayed with their original studio as long as they did. Every other studio in town was tearing up contracts, and stars were moving into television or branching out into independent feature films. Nothing turned up for Abbott and Costello until late the following year, 1956. An independent producer, Bob Goldstein, hired them for a picture to be released through United Artists. The film was DANCE WITH ME, HENRY, and while it was pleasant, it was far from being hilarious. Bud and Lou are amusement-park owners who are also taking care of two youngsters. Gangsters and stolen money enter into the scene and create havoc for the duo, climaxing in a wild chase through the amusement park one night. To Goldstein's credit, he hired a director who had worked with the team many times, Charles Barton, but his scenarists did not include their right-hand

Abbott and Costello, older but not wiser, in DANCE WITH ME, HENRY, their last film.

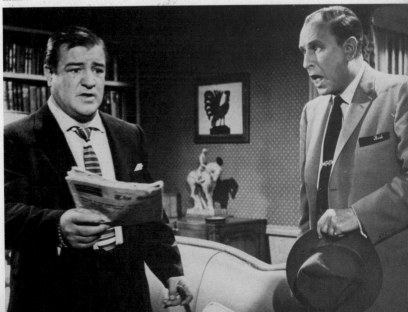

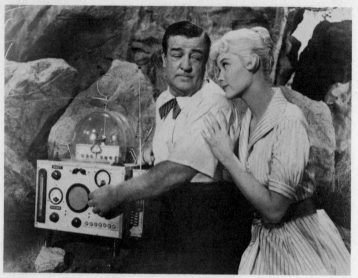

Lou Costello in his only film without Bud Abbott, THE 30 FOOT BRIDE OF CANDY ROCK. Dorothy Provine has the title role.

man, John Grant, and the script simply lacked the old-time energy.

In 1957, Lou Costello started making solo appearances on the Steve Allen TV show, but not until an Associated Press reporter cornered him in July did any official announcement come: Abbott and Costello had split up. It happened after a final engagement in Las Vegas.

Bud Abbott had no immediate prospects for work, but Lou Costello kept busy for the next two years, playing Las Vegas (including a Minsky's burlesque show that brought his career full circle) and making guest appearances on TV, including a pair of dramatic performances, on *G.E. Theater* and *Wagon Train*. His fondest wish was to make a film about the life of New York City's colorful mayor Fiorello LaGuardia, and it's too bad this never came about. He had great simpatico for the subject and even looked a bit like the famed "little flower." This might have been the perfect opportunity for Lou to stretch his talent—and try giving a realistic portrayal. Instead, he starred in a low-budget comedy feature for Columbia called THE THIRTY-FOOT BRIDE OF CANDY ROCK, as a meek handyman whose girlfriend, through strange circumstances, is inflated to gargantuan proportions. Though looking much older than the "bad boy" of his Hollywood heyday, Costello gave an enjoyable performance as a Casper Milquetoast character and was surrounded by fine comedy players. The humor in the film was aimed at younger viewers, who responded appropriately when the film was released. Unfortunately, it was released after Lou Costello's death, on March 3, 1959. Years of illness and strain on a weakened heart finally took their toll.

Bud Abbott lived until 1978, beset by tax problems and failing health. There was barely any work during those twenty years. He made his solo acting debut on *G.E. Theater*, playing an agent, and briefly returned to nightclubs doing the old A & C routines with comedy veteran Candy Candido. But demand for Abbott without Costello was virtually nil. Bud's last real spurt of activity came when he provided his own voice for an Abbott and Costello cartoon series produced by Hanna-Barbara (Stan Irwin did the voice of Lou).

Much has been written in recent years about the off-screen lives of Bud and Lou, revealing the depth of rivalry that existed between the two and discussing the various demons that haunted both men. What is astonishing is how these long-time partners were able to suppress their feelings and camouflage their problems whenever they stepped before an audience. They were troupers in the best sense of the word—and in the performance of such classic routines as "Who's on First?" they demonstrated that there was more to their success than the mere memorization of dialogue. Bud Abbott had us convinced that he really believed every word he was saying—and Lou Costello was equally credible in his portrayal of utter confusion and gullibility.

The sharpster and the patsy may not have been the most subtle characters in all of show business, but Abbott and Costello played them to absolute perfection.

The Films of Abbott and Costello

(Director's name follows year.)

1. **One Night in the Tropics**—Universal 1940—A. Edward Sutherland—Allan Jones, Nancy Kelly, Robert Cummings, Leo Carrillo, Mary Boland, Peggy Moran, Barnett Parker, William Frawley, Nina Orla, Richard Carle, Don Alvarado, Kathleen Howard, The Theodores, Viv-

ian Fay, Francis McDonald, Eddie Acuff, Edgar Dearing, Tyler Brooke, Eddie Dunn, Sally Payne, Charles Hall, Cyril Ring, Barry Norton. 82 minutes.

2. **Buck Privates**—Universal 1941—Arthur Lubin—Lee Bowman, Alan Curtis, The Andrews Sisters, Jane Frazee, Nat Pendleton, Samuel S. Hinds, Harry Strang, Nella Walker, Leonard Elliott, Shemp Howard, Mike Frankovich, Jeanne Kelly (Jean Brooks), Nina Orla, Dora Clement, Elaine Morey, Kay Leslie, Dorothy Darrell, Douglas Wood, Charles Coleman, Selmer Jackson, James Flavin, Tom Tyler, Harold Goodwin, Jack Mulhall, William Gould, Stanley Blystone, Carleton Young, Bob Cason, Stanley Smith, William Hall, Kenne Duncan. 84 minutes.

3. **In the Navy**—Universal 1941—Arthur Lubin—Dick Powell, The Andrews Sisters, Claire Dodd, Dick Foran, Butch and Buddy, Shemp Howard, Sunnie O'Dea, Don Terry, William B. Davidson, Thurston Hall, Robert Emmett Keane, Edward Fielding, Douglas Wood, Eddie Dunn, Ralph Dunn, Dick Alexander, Richard Crane, Hooper Atchley, Jack Mulhall, Claire Whitney, Lyle Latell, Patsy O'Byrne. 85 minutes.

4. **Meet the Stars**—Republic 1941—Harriet Parsons—A & C appeared with Judy Garland, Mickey Rooney, Milton Berle and other stars in this episode entitled "Los Angeles Herald Examiner Benefit." One reel.

5. **Screen Snapshots**—Columbia 1941—Ralph Staub—A & C, Rita Hayworth, and Burns and Allen are among the stars shown entertaining at U.S. Army bases. One reel.

6. **Picture People**—RKO 1941—Another behind-the-scenes short featuring footage of A & C, Rita Hayworth, and Ray Bolger. One reel.

7. **Hold that Ghost**—Universal 1941—Arthur Lubin— Richard Carlson, Joan Davis, Mischa Auer, Evelyn Ankers, Marc Lawrence, Shemp Howard, Russell Hicks, William B. Davidson, Don Terry, Edward Pawley, Nestor Paiva, Edgar Dearing, Frank Penny, Thurston Hall, Janet Shaw, William Ruhl, Frank Richards, Bobby Barber, Kay, Kay, and Katya, Howard Hickman, Harry Hayden, William Forrest. 86 minutes.

8. **Keep 'Em Flying**—Universal 1941—Arthur Lubin— Carol Bruce, Martha Raye, William Gargan, Dick Foran, Charles Lang, William B. Davidson, Doris Lloyd, Frank Penny, Stanley Smith, James Horne, Jr., James Seay, William Forrest, Earle Hodgins, Carleton Young, Richard Crane, Princess Luana. 86 minutes.

9. **Ride 'Em Cowboy**—Universal 1942—Arthur Lubin—Dick Foran, Anne Gwynne, Johnny Mack Brown, The Merry Macs, Ella Fitzgerald, Samuel S. Hinds, Douglass Dumbrille, Morris Ankrum, The High Hatters, The Buckaroo Band, The Ranger Chorus, Charles Lane, Russell Hicks, Wade Boteler, James Flavin, Isabel Randolph, Eddie Dunn, James Seay, Harry Cording, Ralph Peters, Linda Brent, Chief Yowlachie, Bob Baker. 86 minutes.

10. **Rio Rita**—MGM 1942—S. Sylvan Simon—Kathryn Grayson, John Carroll, Patricia Dane, Tom Conway, Peter Whitney, Barry Nelson, Eros Valusia, Arthur Space, Dick Rich, Joan Valerie, Inez Cooper, Mitchell Lewis, Julian Rivero, Frank Penny, David Oliver. 91 minutes.

11. **Pardon My Sarong**—Universal 1942—Erle C. Kenton—Virginia Bruce, Robert Paige, Lionel Atwill, Leif Erickson, Nan Wynn, Samuel S. Hinds, Four Ink Spots, Tip, Tap and Toe, Katherine Dunham Dancers, Charley the seal, Marie McDonald, Irving Bacon, Susan Levine, Jack LaRue, Joe Kirk, Hans Schumm, Frank Penny, Jennifer Holt, Charles Lane, Chester Clute, Tom Fadden, George Chandler, Eddie Acuff, Sig Arno, Herb Vigran, Teddy Infuhr, Florine McKinney, Jayne Hazard, Audrey Long, Lona Andre. 84 minutes.

12. **Who Done It?**—Universal 1942—Erle C. Kenton—Patric Knowles, Louise Allbritton, Don Porter, Mary Wickes, William Gargan, William Bendix, Jerome Cowan, Thomas Gomez, Ludwig Stossel, Walter Tetley, Joe Kirk, Crane Whitley, Paul Dubov, The Pinas, Milton Parsons, Edward Keane, Alice Fleming, Gladys Blake, Frank Penny, Bobby Barber, Harry Strang, Duke York, Jerry Frank. 74 minutes.

13. **It Ain't Hay**—Universal 1943—Erle C. Kenton—Patsy O'Connor, Grace McDonald, Leighton Noble, Cecil Kellaway, Eugene Pallette, Eddie Quillan, Shemp Howard, Dave Hacker, Samuel S. Hinds, Richard Lane, Wade Boteler, Selmer Jackson, Andrew Tombes, Pierre Watkin, William Forrest, Ralph Peters, Bobby Watson, Charles Coleman, James Flavin, Jack Norton, George Humbert, Robert Homans, Matt Willis, Harry Harvey, Herb Vigran, Harry Strang, Mike Mazurki, Herbert Heyes, Paul Dubov, Kate Drain Lawson, Janet Ann Gallow, Frank Penny, Kit Guard, Spec O'Donnell. 80 minutes.

14. **Hit the Ice**—Universal 1943—Charles Lamont—Ginny Simms, Patric Knowles, Elyse Knox, Sheldon Leonard,

Marc Lawrence, Joe Sawyer, Johnny Long and Orchestra (with Helen Young, Gene Williams, The Four Teens), Mantan Moreland, Minerva Urecal, Virginia Sale, Wade Boteler, Joseph Crehan, Pat Flaherty, Ed Gargan, Eddie Dunn, Dorothy Vaughan, Ken Christy, Harry Strang, Rebel Randall, Billy Wayne, Eddie Parker, Bobby Barber, Cordelia Campbell. 82 minutes.

15. **In Society**—Universal 1944—Jean Yarbrough—Marion Hutton, Kirby Grant, Anne Gillis, Arthur Treacher, Thomas Gomez, George Dolenz, Steven Geray, Margaret Irving, Murray Leonard, Thurston Hall, Nella Walker, William B. Davidson, Will Osborne Orchestra, Three Sisters, Luis Alberni, Don Barclay, Edgar Dearing, Cyril Ring, Ian Wolfe, Charles Coleman, Alice Fleming, Gladys Blake, Mabel Todd, Tom Dugan, Dorothy Granger, Ralph Dunn, Tom Fadden, Charles Hall, Roxanne Hilton. 75 minutes.

16. **Lost in a Harem**—MGM 1944—Charles Riesner—Marilyn Maxwell, John Conte, Douglass Dumbrille, Lottie Harrison, J. Lockard Martin, Murray Leonard, Adia Kuznetzoff, Milton Parsons, Ralph Sanford, Jimmy Dorsey Orchestra, Harry Cording, Frank Penny, Tor Johnson, Jody Gilbert, Paul Newland, Mitchell Lewis, Eddie Dunn, Sondra Rodgers, Elinor Vandivere, Dick Alexander, Feodor Chaliapin, John Lipson, Heinie Conklin, Bill Wolfe, Jimmy Conlin, John Indrisano, Al Hill, Frank Hagney, Bud Jamison, Frances Ramsden. 89 minutes.

17. **The Naughty Nineties**—Universal 1945—Jean Yarbrough—Alan Curtis, Rita Johnson, Henry Travers, Lois Collier, Joe Sawyer, Joe Kirk, Barbara Pepper, Jack Norton, The Rainbow Four, Ben Johnson, Sam McDaniel, John Indrisano, Lillian Yarbo, Emmett Vogan, John Hamilton, Ed Gargan, Donald Kerr, Ruth Lee, Cyril Ring, Gladys Blake, Jack Rice, Jack Overman, Arthur Loft, Carol Hughes, Tom Fadden, Milt Bronson, Rex Lease, Sarah Selby, Sidney Fields, William Desmond. 76 minutes.

18. **Abbott and Costello in Hollywood**—MGM 1945—S. Sylvan Simon—Frances Rafferty, Robert Stanton, Jean Porter, Warner Anderson, Carleton Young, "Rags" Ragland, Donald McBride, Mike Mazurki, Dean Stockwell, Sharon McManus, Marion Martin, Arthur Space, William "Bill" Phillips, Chester Clute, Marie Blake, Harry Tyler, William Tannen, Garry Owen, Dick Alexander, Hank Worden, King Baggott, Betty Blythe, Broderick O'Far-

rell, Frank Penny, Sarah Edwards, Anne O'Neal, Bert Roach, Frank Hagney, Clancy Cooper, Nicodemus (Nick Stewart), Milton Kibbee, Joe Devlin, Dell Henderson, Chester Conklin, Gerald Perreau (Richard Miles), The Lyttle Sisters; guest stars Lucille Ball, Preston Foster, Butch Jenkins, Robert Z. Leonard. 83 minutes.

19. **Here Come the Co-eds**—Universal 1945—Jean Yarbrough—Peggy Ryan, Martha O'Driscoll, June Vincent, Lon Chaney, Donald Cook, Charles Dingle, Richard Lane, Joe Kirk, Bill Stern, Phil Spitalny Orchestra, Anthony Warde, Dorothy Ford, Ruth Lee, Don Costello, Donald Kerr, Rebel Randall, Jayne Hazard, Jean Carlin, Maxine Gates, Dorothy Granger, Eddie Dunn, Gene Roth, Pierre Watkin, Baby Marie Osborne. 87 minutes.

20. **Little Giant**—Universal 1946—William A. Seiter— Brenda Joyce, Jacqueline De Wit, George Cleveland, Elena Verdugo, Mary Gordon, Pierre Watkin, Donald MacBride, Victor Kilian, Margaret Dumont, George Chandler, Beatrice Gray, Lane Chandler, Chester Conklin, Ed Gargan, Ralph Peters, Florence Lake, Bert Roach, Mary Field, Eddy Waller, Ralph Dunn, Dorothy Christy, Anne O'Neal, William "Red" Donahue and mule Euhanod, Joe Kirk, Ethelreda Leopold, Donald Kerr, Milton Bronson, Pat Costello (Lou's brother), Sebastian Cristillo (Lou's father). 91 minutes.

21. **The Time of Their Lives**—Universal 1946—Charles Barton— Marjorie Reynolds, Binnie Barnes, John Shelton, Gale Sondergaard, Jess Barker, Robert H. Barrat, Donald MacBride, Anne Gillis, Lynne Baggett, William Hall, Rex Lease, Harry Woolman, Selmer Jackson, Walter Baldwin, Boyd Irwin, Marjorie Eaton, Kirk Alyn, Myron Healey, John Crawford. 82 minutes.

22. **Buck Privates Come Home**—Universal-International 1947—Charles T. Barton—Tom Brown, Joan Fulton (Joan Shawlee), Nat Pendleton, Beverly Simmons, Don Beddoe, Don Porter, Donald MacBride, Lane Beban, Jr., Lennie Dremen, Al Murphy, Bob Wilke, William Haade, Janne DeLoos, Buddy Roosevelt, Chuck Hamilton, Joe Kirk, Patricia Alphin (Audrey Young), Charles Trowbridge, Jimmy Dodd, Russell Hicks, Ralph Dunn, Cliff Clark, Lyle Latell, Eddie Acuff, Milton Kibbee, Ottola Nesmith, Eddie Dunn, Billy Curtis, Myron Healey, Rex Lease, Frank Mayo, Lee Shumway, Ernie Adams, Donald Kerr, Knox Manning, Milburn Stone. 77 minutes.

23. **The Wistful Widow of Wagon Gap**—Universal-International 1947—Charles T. Barton—Marjorie Main, George Cleveland, Gordon Jones, William Ching, Peter Thompson, Olin Howlin, Bill Clauson, Bill O'Leary, Pamela Wells, Jimmie Bates, Paul Dunn, Diana Florentine, Rex Lease, Glenn Strange, Edmund Cobb, Wade Crosby, Murray Leonard, Iris Adrian, Charles King, Dave Sharpe, Dewey Robinson, Emmett Lynn, Billy Engle, Lee Lasses White, George Lewis, Jack Shutta, Frank Hagney, Ed Piel. 78 minutes.

24. **10,000 Kids and a Cop**—Nassour 1947—Charles Barton—James Stewart, William Bendix, Truman Bradley. Bud and Lou appeared briefly in this film extolling the virtues of the Lou Costello Jr. Youth Foundation in Los Angeles. Two reels.

25. **The Noose Hangs High**—Eagle-Lion 1948—Charles Barton—Joseph Calleia, Leon Errol, Cathy Downs, Mike Mazurki, Fritz Feld, Russell Hicks, Benny Rubin, Bess Flowers, Joe Kirk, Matt Willis, Ben Welden, Jimmy Dodd, Ellen Corby, Isabel Randolph, Pat Flaherty, Murray Leonard, Sandra Spence, Elvia Allman, Alvin Hammer, Herb Vigran, James Flavin, Lyle Latell, Paul Maxey, Fred Kelsey, Minerva Urecal, Lois Austin. 77 minutes.

26. **Abbott and Costello Meet Frankenstein**—Universal-International 1948—Charles T. Barton—Lon Chaney, Bela Lugosi, Glenn Strange, Lenore Aubert, Jane Randolph, Frank Ferguson, Charles Bradstreet, Howard Negley, Joe Kirk, Helen Spring, Paul Stader, the voice of Vincent Price. 92 minutes.

27. **Mexican Hayride**—Universal-International 1948—Charles T. Barton—Virginia Grey, Luba Malina, John Hubbard, Pedro de Cordoba, Fritz Feld, Tom Powers, Pat Costello, Frank Fenton, Chris-Pin Martin, Sidney Fields, Fiores Brothers Trio, Mary Castle, Reed Howes, Argentina Brunetti, Eddie Kane, Pedro Regas, Joe Kirk, Julian Rivero, Kippee Valez, Charles Miller. 77 minutes.

28. **Abbott and Costello Meet the Killer, Boris Karloff**—Universal-International 1949—Charles T. Barton—Boris Karloff, Lenore Aubert, Gar Moore, Donna Martell, Alan Mowbray, James Flavin, Roland Winters, Nicholas Joy, Mikel Conrad, Morgan Farley, Victoria Horne, Percy Helton, Claire DuBrey, Harry Hayden, Vincent Renno, Patricia Hall, Murray Alper, Marjorie Bennett, Gail Bonney, Frankie Van, Billy Gray. 94 minutes.

29. **Abbott and Costello in the Foreign Legion**—Universal-International 1950—Charles Lamont—Patricia Medina, Walter Slezak, Douglass Dumbrille, Fred Nurney, Wee Willie Davis, Leon Belasco, Jack Raymond, Henry Corden, Chuck Hamilton, Jack Shutta, Dan Seymour, Alberto Morin, Ted Hecht, John Cliff, Buddy Roosevelt, David Gorcey, Charmienne Harker. 79 minutes.

30. **Abbott and Costello Meet the Invisible Man**—Universal International 1951—Charles Lamont—Nancy Guild, Arthur Franz, Adele Jergens, Sheldon Leonard, William Frawley, Gavin Muir, Sam Balter, John Day, George J. Lewis, Frankie Van, Bobby Barber, Paul Maxey, Ed Gargan, Herb Vigran, Ralph Dunn, Harold Goodwin, Rory Mallinson, Jack Shutta, Milt Bronson, Donald Kerr, Kit Guard. 82 minutes.

31. **Comin' Round the Mountain**—Universal-International 1951—Charles Lamont—Dorothy Shaye, Kirby Grant, Joe Sawyer, Glenn Strange, Ida Moore, Shay Cogan, Guy Wilkerson, Bob Easton, Swats Taylor, Morg Hamilton, Russell Simpson, Hank Wordern, Jack Kruschen, O. Z. Whitehead, Norman Leavitt, Peter Mamakos, Stanley Waxman, Dean White, Joe Kirk, William Fawcett, Harold Goodwin, Jane Lee. 77 minutes.

32. **Jack and the Beanstalk**—Warner Brothers 1952—Jean Yarbrough—Buddy Baer, Dorothy Ford, Barbara Brown, David Stollery, William Farnum, Shaye Cogan, James Alexander. Color—87 minutes.

33. **Lost in Alaska**—Universal-International 1952—Jean Yarbrough—Mitzi Green, Tom Ewell, Bruce Cabot, Minerva Urecal, Emory Parnell, Michael Ross, Howard Negley, Harry Tyler, Maudie Prickett, Billy Wayne, Paul Newlan, Iron Eyes Cody, William Gould, Donald Kerr, Bobby Barber, Sherry Moreland. 76 minutes.

34. **Abbott and Costello Meet Captain Kidd**—Warner Brothers 1952—Charles Lamont—Charles Laughton, Hillary Brooke, Fran Warren, Bill Shirley, Leif Erickson, Rex Lease, Sid Saylor, Frank Yaconelli. Color—70 minutes.

35. **News of the Day**—MGM 1952—A & C made an appearance with Charles Laughton in this newsreel to promote U.S. Bonds.

36. **Abbott and Costello Go to Mars**—Universal 1953—Charles Lamont—Robert Paige, Mari Blanchard, Martha Hyer, Horace McMahon, Jack Tebler, Hal Forrest, Harold Goodwin, Joe Kirk, Jack Kruschen, Jean Willes, Anita Ekberg, Jackie Loughery, James Flavin, Russ

Conway, Sid Saylor, Paul Newlan, Grace Lenard, William Newell, Stanley Waxman, Milton Bronson, Rex Lease, Dale Van Sickel, Gloria Paul, Jack Shutta, Stanley Blystone, Bobby Barber, Rickey Van Dusen, Cora Shannon, and the Miss Universe Contest winners. 76 minutes.

37. **Abbott and Costello Meet Dr. Jekyll and Mr. Hyde**—Universal 1953—Charles Lamont—Boris Karloff, Craig Stevens, Helen Westcott, John Dierkes, Reginald Denny, Carmen De Lavallade, Henry Corden, Marjorie Bennett, Harry Cording, James Fairfax, Arthur Gould-Porter, John Rogers, Clyde Cook, Hilda Plowright, Jimmy Aubrey, Donald Kerr. 76 minutes.

38. **Hollywood Grows Up**—Columbia 1954—Ralph Staub —A Screen Snapshots reel, with Staub and Larry Simms (from the BLONDIE series) reviewing World War II footage of Burns and Allen and Abbott and Costello routines. 10 minutes.

39. **Abbott and Costello Meet the Keystone Kops**—Universal 1955—Charles Lamont—Fred Clark, Lynn Bari, Frank Wilcox, Maxie Rosenbloom, Henry Kulky, Sam Flint, Mack Sennett, Heinie Conklin, Hank Mann, Roscoe Ates, Harold Goodwin, Paul Dubov, Joe Besser, Harry Tyler, Joe Devlin, William Haade, Byron Keith, Murray Leonard, Colin Campbell, Marjorie Bennett, Donald Kerr, Frank Hagney, Carole Costello. 79 minutes.

40. **Abbott and Costello Meet the Mummy**—Universal 1955—Charles Lamont—Marie Windsor, Michael Ansara, Dan Seymour, Kurt Katch, Richard Karlan, Richard Deacon, Eddie Parker, Mel Welles, George Khoury, Peggy King, Mazzonne-Abbott Dancers, Chandra-Kaly Dancers, Veola Vonn, Jan Arvan, Kem Dibbs, Ted Hecht, Michael Vallon, Mitchell Kowal, Robin Morse, Hank Mann, Paul Marion, Donald Kerr, Carole Costello. 79 minutes.

41. **Dance with Me, Henry**—United Artists 1956—Charles Barton—Gigi Perreau, Rusty Hamer, Mary Wickes, Ted de Corsia, Ron Hargrave, Sherry Abarrone, Frank Wilcox, Richard Reeves, Paul Sorenson, Robert Shayne, John Cliff. 79 minutes.

42. **The World of Abbott and Costello**—Universal 1965— Produced by Max J. Rosenberg and Milton Subotsky; narration written by Gene Wood; narrated by Jack E. Leonard—a compilation including scenes from BUCK PRIVATES, IN THE NAVY, RIDE 'EM COWBOY, WHO DONE IT?,

HIT THE ICE, IN SOCIETY, THE NAUGHTY NINETIES, LITTLE
GIANT, BUCK PRIVATES COME HOME, THE WISTFUL WIDOW
OF WAGON GAP, A & C MEET FRANKENSTEIN, MEXICAN
HAYRIDE, A & C IN THE FOREIGN LEGION, COMIN' ROUND
THE MOUNTAIN, LOST IN ALASKA, A & C GO TO MARS, A &
C MEET THE KEYSTONE KOPS, A & C MEET THE MUMMY. 75
minutes.

Lou Costello made the following solo appearance:

The 30-Foot Bride of Candy Rock—Columbia 1959—
Sidney Miller—Dorothy Provine, Gale Gordon, Jimmy
Conlin, Charles Lane, Robert Burton, Will Wright, Lenny
Kent, Ruth Perrott, Peter Leeds, Robert Nichols, Veola
Vonn, Jack Straw, Russell Trent, Arthur Walsh, Joey
Faye, Joe Greene, Bobby Barber, Doodles Weaver,
Jack Rice. 75 minutes.

MARTIN and LEWIS

Few acts in the history of show business have exploded onto the scene with as much force as Martin and Lewis. Their loud, raucous shenanigans convulsed TV, nightclub and movie audiences for ten years. Their greatest success came in the 1950's, and with it, other comedy teams like Abbott and Costello were pushed out of the spotlight. The fresh zaniness and incomparable energy of Martin and Lewis put them in a class by themselves, and by the early 50's they were the hottest entertainers in the country. An explosive team on and off stage, they eventually split in 1956 and went their separate ways. Today both men are stars on their own, and the days of Martin and Lewis seem part of the distant past.

In the beginning . . . Dean Martin and Jerry Lewis as they appeared in their first film, MY FRIEND IRMA.

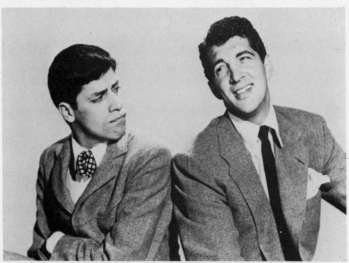

People have always marveled at Dean Martin's easygoing style of performing. He never makes it seem like work—which is quite a feat for someone who had to work very hard to make something of himself. Nowadays, Dino feels he's entitled to take it easy. Born in Steubenville, Ohio, in 1917, Dino Crocetti struggled through school until the eleventh grade, when he quit and sought work around town. He delivered bootleg liquor during prohibition, worked as a gas station attendant, and then turned to boxing. By the time he was twenty he was featured locally as a welterweight. Crocetti was quick and agile, and reportedly won 24 out of his first 30 bouts. One opponent injured Dino's nose, causing him to seek plastic surgery. Perhaps because of this experience, he quit the fight game and moved into another lively field: gambling. Maurice Condon, writing in *TV Guide*, found that most natives of Steubenville remembered Dino best from this period, when he gained quite a reputation as a dealer and croupier in the local back rooms. He also loved to sing, and when several of his gambling friends offered to back him in a show-business career, he went along with the idea. Dino was able to find work with several local bands, and stayed with Sammy Watkins' Ohio-based band for three years. In the early 1940's, he left Watkins for more lucrative work in nightclubs, and started to make a name for himself.

Jerry Lewis (born Joseph Levitch) came from a show-business family, and, unlike Martin, knew what he wanted to do from a very early age. Born in 1926 in Newark, New Jersey, he was forced to live with relatives while his performing parents were on the road. Every summer, however, Rea and Danny Lewis were entertainers-in-residence at a Catskills resort in New York State. Their son spent his summers with them, and got his first taste of show business. He would beg his father to let him perform for the Catskills crowds, and although Danny Lewis didn't relish the idea of his son becoming an entertainer, there was little he could do to suppress the boy's enthusiasm. After suffering through the first year of high school, the youngster quit and sought a job ushering at the Paramount Theater in New York. There, at the scene of many later Martin and Lewis successes, he whetted his appetite for the life of an entertainer, and decided to set out on his own with a "record act," mimicking various people whose records would be played off stage. His father convinced agent Abby Greshler to catch his son's act one night, and Greshler agreed to take him on as a client. Jerry Lewis, as he then called himself, was 18, without experience, and extremely nervous. For several years he moved from one flea-bag hotel and nightclub to another.

One day in 1946, Martin and Lewis were introduced, so the story goes, on a street corner in New York City. They were casual acquaintances, but coincidentally they appeared on the same bills at local nightclubs during the next few months. At the 500 Club in Atlantic City, the two young performers appeared together on stage for the first time with an impromptu act. As Martin sang, Lewis would cavort with the orchestra and generally break up his routine. This was essentially what Martin and Lewis did for ten years in personal appearances, with new pieces of material added every once in a while, and occasional breaks for an uninterrupted song or two from Martin, with Lewis trying out his terpsichorean talent. As Maurice Zolotow put it in a magazine article on the team, "Martin and Lewis were not witty or sophisticated or sharp, but they made you laugh even if you felt guilty about it."

Guilt complexes notwithstanding, Martin and Lewis scored a hit, and quickly built up steam. They worked at the Latin Casino in Cherry Hill, New Jersey; the Riviera in Fort Lee, New Jersey; the Chez Paree in New York; Slapsie Maxie's in Hollywood, and finally, New York's Copacabana. By the late 1940's, Martin and Lewis were cabaret headliners, packing in wild, enthusiastic crowds wherever they went. In 1949, producer Hal Wallis brought them to Hollywood for their

Marie Wilson is Irma; Diana Lynn, Dean and Jerry are her pals in MY FRIEND IRMA.

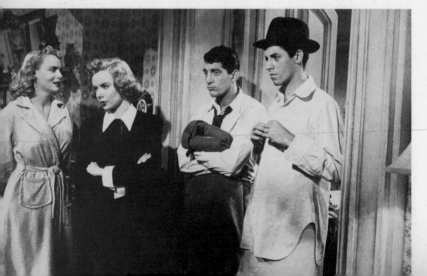

first film. Dean Martin and Jerry Lewis were billed fifth and sixth in the cast listing of MY FRIEND IRMA, but there was no doubt as to whose film it was. *Irma* was a popular radio show at the time, and Wallis thought a film version would be a sure-fire hit. It was, but not just because of the radio series. *The New York Times'* Bosley Crowther found the film worthless, but added "Let us amend that ever so slightly. We could go along with the laughs which were fetched by a new mad comedian, Jerry Lewis by name. This freakishly built and acting young man, who has been seen in nightclubs hereabouts with a collar-ad partner, Dean Martin, has a genuine comic quality. The swift eccentricity of his movements, the harrowing features of his face and the squeak of his vocal protestations, which are many and frequent, have flair. His idiocy constitutes burlesque of an idiot, which is something else again. As a hanger-on in the wake of Irma, he's the funniest thing in this film." Crowther was unimpressed by Martin, but not as much as Howard Barnes in the *Herald-Tribune*, who dismissed the comedy team as "incredibly boring."

In retrospect, IRMA proved a good springboard for Martin and Lewis. It gave them good exposure in a film with built-in box-office appeal, and introduced them to many people who had not seen them in nightclubs. In addition, they were able to work without much responsibility to the plot, since their roles were incidental in the film's story line. When the film opened at New York's Paramount Theater, Martin and Lewis headlined the stage show accompanying the film, and at-

Dean and Jerry in "their" medium—television. Here they clown with guest star Jack Webb.

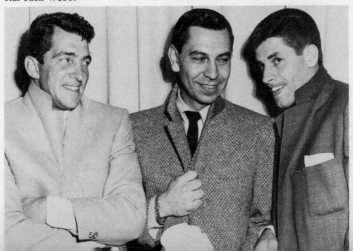

tracted a huge crowd, comprised mostly of youngsters who
were becoming Martin and Lewis fans. The reception at the
Paramount was enthusiastic, but a mere foreshadowing of
what was to come over the next few years. When MY FRIEND
IRMA GOES WEST opened a half-year later at the Paramount,
Bosley Crowther had to admit that he couldn't hear much of
the film's dialogue over the din created by screaming, laughing fans who filled the theater to capacity on opening day.
The film was no better than MY FRIEND IRMA, but once again
it gave Martin and Lewis some good scenes, which cemented
the duo as movie comedians of the first rank.

Around this time, Dean and Jerry tried their hand at
radio. It was the only medium they never conquered. One
critic concluded that they had to be seen to be believed. His
thought was echoed many times over by people who ran to
the nearest theater when the team was playing, but passed
them by when they were featured on Bob Hope's radio
show. Martin and Lewis were much more successful on
television, which they invaded in 1950 as frequent stars of
the *Colgate Comedy Hour*. The Colgate show had rotating
stars (Abbott and Costello, Fred Allen, etc.) who show-
cased their talent on this popular show. Martin and Lewis
made their debut on the program with an hour of frenzied
comedy and music that was just an extension of their nightclub act. They clowned through every act in the show, breaking each other up and winning tremendous weekly audiences.
Martin and Lewis were the first star team of the television
age.

In December of that same year, Paramount released the
team's first starring comedy, AT WAR WITH THE ARMY. The
director was Hal Walker, a Paramount contractee who specialized in brisk, fast-moving comedies like the Bob Hope-
Bing Crosby ROAD series. AT WAR WITH THE ARMY starts
with Jerry, a private on perpetual KP duty, singing "The
Navy gets the Gravy but the Army Gets the Beans." The
rest of the film follows a pattern that the team used for many
years: Dean is in a more secure position than Jerry (he's a
sergeant here), and his chief concern is going after a pretty
girl and serenading her with songs written by Mack David and
Jerry Livingston. Jerry is a hapless, helpless private who
seems to do everything wrong, and gets into the wildest
situations (finding himself the victim of a Coke machine that
doesn't stop delivering bottles, dressing as a woman to en-
tice officer Mike Kellin, etc.). AT WAR WITH THE ARMY
shapes up as a lively, entertaining comedy that shows Martin

and Lewis at their best, following a formula that worked for several years.

Their next film, THAT'S MY BOY, is the story of "Jarring Jack" Jackson, whose disappointment in his son (Jerry) is profound, because Junior will never be a football star. Dean, on the other hand, is an athletic ace whose college tuition is paid by Jarring Jack on the condition that he work with Junior to build up his abilities as a footballer. Junior redeems himself at the last minute by going into the last game of the season and winning singlehandedly in the final seconds. The odd part about THAT'S MY BOY is that while audiences and reviewers found it hilarious in 1951, it seems more melancholy than anything else when seen today. Both pigheaded father (played by Eddie Mayehoff) and fumbling Junior are such pathetic figures that it's difficult to laugh at them; their phobias are portrayed too realistically. Mayehoff had better opportunities when he starred in a broader, funnier TV series, also called THAT'S MY BOY, some years later. The team's next film, SAILOR BEWARE (originally titled AT SEA WITH THE NAVY) was back on-target, largely because of the people connected with it. The adaptation was by Elwood Ullman, a long-time writer of Columbia's comedy shorts, and additional dialogue was contributed by John Grant, who provided Abbott and Costello with their best material for fifteen years. SAILOR BEWARE has virtually no plot. Dean and Jerry are in the Navy, battling with their superior officer

A military misunderstanding from JUMPING JACKS, with Don DeFore, Jerry, Dean, Danny Arnold and Robert Strauss.

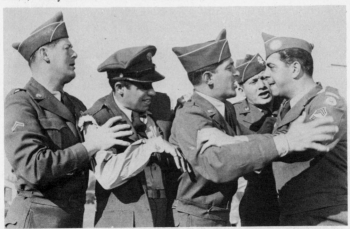

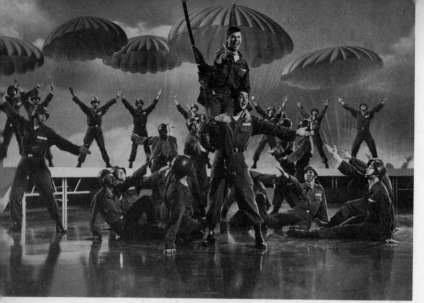

One of JUMPING JACKS' silly production numbers.

(Robert Strauss) and falling for two lovelies, Corinne Calvet
and Marion Marshall. With overtones of Abbott and Costello's
BUCK PRIVATES, they go through induction (the doctor can't
find any blood pressure in Jerry's body), appear on a local
TV show where Jerry conducts a straight-faced chorus as
Dean tries to sing (a routine Lewis uses to this day), and
wind up in the boxing ring with Jerry pretending to be a
cauliflower champion. Trying to act professional, he talks to
Dean about his career. "What are you, a boxer?" Dean
asks. "What do I look like, a cocker spaniel?" Jerry snaps,
continuing, "I was fighting Gene Tierney once, and . . ."
"You mean Gene Tunney," Dean interrupts. "You fight
who you want, I'll fight who I want," Jerry replies. The fight
scene itself is the funniest boxing spoof ever devised since
Chaplin went through his paces in CITY LIGHTS. SAILOR
BEWARE is one of the team's all-time best films, hysterically
funny at times.

For unknown reasons, after this film, Martin and Lewis
appeared in THE STOOGE, a very offbeat film that departed
radically from their usual formula. Paramount, worried about
the response to this film, shelved THE STOOGE and put their
comedy stars into another military vehicle, JUMPING JACKS,
which they felt would be safer. It *was* safe material, and
even had Robert Strauss repeating his role as their superior
from SAILOR BEWARE. But JUMPING JACKS is only medium
Martin and Lewis, the sign of a good idea wearing thin. THE
STOOGE was finally released in early 1953, and while it did

good business (the team never had a box-office dud) it confirmed the studio's original reaction. Dean Martin plays a conceited vaudeville star who works with a stooge, Jerry Lewis. Dean treats his foil with contempt, but Jerry is too naive and good natured to quit. Finally, Martin's ego becomes too overpowering, and he and Lewis split. Then Dean realizes that he is nothing without his partner, and humbly goes to him for forgiveness. If the film sounds mawkish and old-hat, that's because it is. THE STOOGE was an experiment with different material, but in 1953 neither critics nor fans wanted to see an acting Dean Martin or a serious Jerry Lewis going for pathos. Significantly, Jerry Lewis names this as his favorite Martin and Lewis picture.

SAILOR BEWARE was a loose remake of two earlier Paramount films: LADY BE CAREFUL (1936) and THE FLEET'S IN (1942). After THE STOOGE, Paramount began combing its files to see what other properties might be reworked for its star team. The first one that seemed a likely prospect was Bob Hope's mystery-comedy GHOST BREAKERS, originally filmed in 1940 with Hope and Paulette Goddard. The writers got to work and came up with SCARED STIFF, Martin and Lewis' next starring vehicle. The material was contrived when Bob Hope had done it, however, and in 1953 it seemed even more so. The film's only bright moments are those that have nothing to do with the original story: Jerry imitating Humphrey Bogart in order to fool a gang of thugs, dancing

Jerry coaches Dean at an important golf tournament in THE CADDY, as Donna Reed stands by.

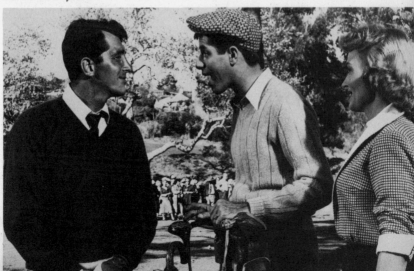

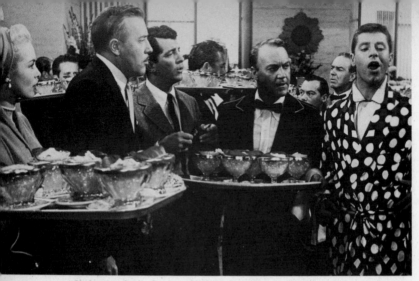

"Shrimp cocktails for everybody," cries Jerry in this scene from LIVING IT UP, as Janet Leigh, Fred Clark, Dean and Ralph Montgomery try to curb his enthusiasm.

and mimicking Carmen Miranda, and a guest appearance by Bing Crosby and Bob Hope (Dean and Jerry had appeared in their film ROAD TO BALI the year before). Their next film, THE CADDY, was one of their weakest, with good moments here and there and the only hit song to come from a Martin and Lewis film: "That's Amore." The most interesting aspect of this film is the opening sequence where Dean and Jerry play, in effect, themselves, with actual footage of mobbing fans waiting to see them outside the Paramount Theater in New York. Dean's father (Joseph Calleia) stands backstage as the boys go into their act, and tells their life story to a reporter. The rest of the film is a flashback about Jerry, whose father was a great golfer, coaching Martin to become a prize-winning pro. There simply isn't enough comedy, and the heart-tugging plot about success going to Martin's head is all too familiar.

MONEY FROM HOME covered familiar ground again. In it, Dean is heavily in debt to gangster Sheldon Leonard, and is forced to become one of his hirelings. Sent to make sure a certain horse doesn't run in a steeplechase race, he encounters Jerry, his cousin and a would-be veterinarian who loves animals. The film runs smoothly but predictably to the slapstick race finale, with Jerry as jockey! This, and the fact that the film was shot and released in 3-D, are the chief distinctions of MONEY FROM HOME. The next film was a remake of David O. Selznick's 1937 film NOTHING SACRED, which was later musicalized on Broadway as *Hazel Flagg*. The 1937

film is considered a comedy classic, but LIVING IT UP holds
its own quite nicely, with Jerry in the part originated by
Carole Lombard, Dean replacing Charles Winninger, Janet
Leigh taking Fredric March's place, Fred Clark instead of
Walter Connolly, and Sig Ruman repeating his hilarious role
as a Viennese doctor. The story has Jerry believing that he is
dying of radiation poisoning in a small Midwestern town.
Reporter Janet Leigh hears of this and envisions a human-
interest story of unlimited potential. She convinces her edi-
tor (Clark) that she should bring the dying Lewis to New
York for one last fling—with appropriate press coverage, of
course. As she arrives in the small town where the victim
lives, doctor Martin tells Jerry that he doesn't have radiation
poisoning at all—just a bad sinus condition—but convinces
him that the New York trip is too good a deal to pass up.
The rest of the film follows Jerry's escapades in the big city,
including one hilarious scene where he is given the honor of
tossing out the first ball at Yankee Stadium, with unexpected results. LIVING IT UP is probably Martin and Lewis'
best film, but in many ways it marks a change from their
earlier efforts. Dean and Jerry are essentially the same, but
they are not as frenetic as they were in their earlier films.
LIVING IT UP presents a more restrained, yet very funny,
Jerry Lewis, and the effect is salutary. Reviewing their next
film, THREE RING CIRCUS, Howard Thompson in *The New
York Times* noted that the duo seemed more relaxed, and

Jerry gets to throw out the first ball at Yankee Stadium in LIVING IT UP, with
unexpected results.

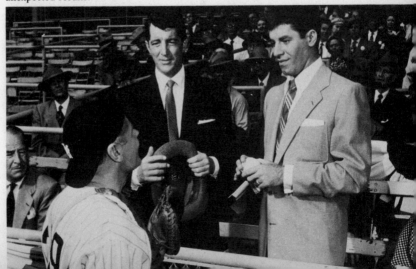

expressed his hope that this trend would be continued; it seemed to the critic to be a great improvement over their former brand of humor. THREE RING CIRCUS is a far cry from the unabashed zaniness of AT WAR WITH THE ARMY, but it rates as a very pleasant film, with a few inspired moments as the boys go to work for Joanne Dru's circus, and encounter such characters as the bearded lady, played by Elsa Lanchester. CIRCUS also has a well-done sequence with Jerry trying to make a crippled child laugh. It has elements of pathos, but it is kept well under control. It was only in later years that Jerry Lewis, working on his own, went overboard in this department.

Martin and Lewis' contract now called for two pictures a year at Paramount. They were the industry's biggest money-making act in the 1950's, and between films they continued to work on NBC television shows, make records, and appear around the country in personal-appearance extravaganzas. In 1952, *Variety* headlined, "IF BIGTIME VAUDE IS REALLY DEAD, HOW COME M & L KILL 'EM IN TEX.?" Movie-fan magazines had a field day with the comedy team, for their film sets were not far removed from lunatic asylums, with directors, writers, cameramen, grips and electricians armed with water pistols and clowning vigorously with the two stars. Norman Taurog, a director since the 1920's, told Maurice Zolotow, "I find that I get the best results when I treat them like little boys. It reminds me of the days when I was directing Jackie Cooper in the SKIPPY comedies."

Dean and Jerry, playing themselves on stage at the Paramount Theatre in New York, in THE CADDY.

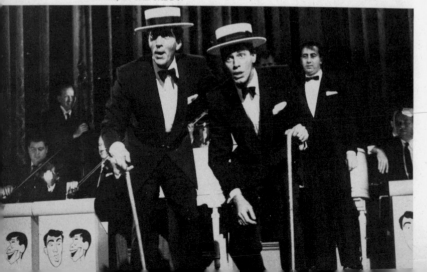

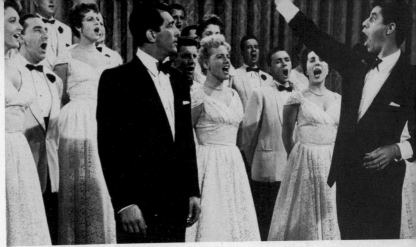

One of Martin and Lewis' best routines, with Jerry giving frantic instructions to a dead-pan chorus. From YOU'RE NEVER TOO YOUNG.

Like little boys, however, both Martin and Lewis had explosive tempers which were liable to be set off at a moment's notice. In 1954, after one flare-up, there were serious rumors that the two were going to break up. Shortly thereafter, the disagreement was smoothed over and the team was back together again. Lewis, nine years younger than Martin, always considered his partner something of a big brother; Martin's affection for Lewis was also strong. But being together constantly, working night after night at one-night stands, days on end in movie studios, tended to keep the partners on edge. Andrew Sarris has written, "Martin and Lewis, at their best—and that means not in any of their movies—had a marvelous tension between them . . ." The tension did account for some of the team's most memorable

A climactic chase scene from YOU'RE NEVER TOO YOUNG.

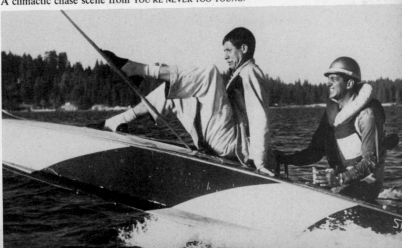

appearances, and it is true that Martin and Lewis were seen to their best advantage performing live. They did, however, adapt themselves to movies quite well, and recorded some of their best moments together on film.

Dusting off another oldie, Paramount revamped THE MA-JOR AND THE MINOR for Martin and Lewis, retitling it YOU'RE NEVER TOO YOUNG. Once again Jerry played a male version of an original female role (played by Ginger Rogers in the 1942 film), and Diana Lynn took the role played by Ray Milland in the earlier film. With some new plot twists involving some stolen gems, and a memorable "heavy" in the person of Raymond Burr, YOU'RE NEVER TOO YOUNG turned out quite well, although a notch below the team's best efforts. ARTISTS AND MODELS, their next film, was the team's first encounter with director Frank Tashlin, a former cartoonist and comedy writer who started directing films in 1949. Tashlin was noted for his vivid imagination in the field of visual comedy, and he brought to ARTISTS AND MODELS some of the most enjoyable, far-out ideas Martin and Lewis ever worked with. The story has comic-book publisher Eddie Mayehoff in trouble because his comics don't have enough blood and gore to remain best sellers. He hires artist Dean Martin to spice up his product, but Dean can't come up with the necessary material until he meets comic-book devotee Jerry, who dreams in comic-book style. Martin gets him to relate all of his dreams, which makes him a hit in the comic field, and allows him to go off in pursuit of female artist Dorothy Malone. The film also serves as an excuse to display the obvious talents of Shirley MacLaine, Anita Ekberg

Jerry faces some formidable foes: Jeff Morrow, Lon Chaney and Bob Steele (back to camera) in PARDNERS.

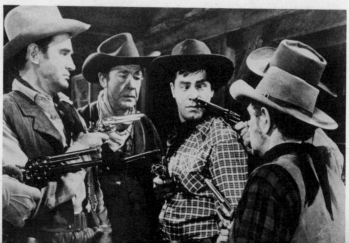

and Eva Gabor, all of whom were seen to best advantage in Technicolor and VistaVision. One of the film's comic highlights comes when Jerry appears on a TV panel show as an example of moral decay brought about by reading too many comic books.

By the time PARDNERS was being filmed in 1956, rumors were rampant about the biggest feud yet between Martin and Lewis. The filming went smoothly, however, and the remake of Bing Crosby's 1936 RHYTHM ON THE RANGE turned out to be one of the comedy duo's better endeavors, with some truly funny scenes of the pardners Out West, encountering such adversaries as Jeff Morrow, Lon Chaney and Bob Steele. After finishing PARDNERS, Martin and Lewis came to New York for an extended engagement at the Copacabana nightclub. It was a tremendous success, and it proved that whatever their feelings off stage, on stage they were still a hit. The columns and fan magazines were running wild with stories of the team splitting up, and their reports appeared to be accurate when Dean Martin complained about his role in the team's upcoming film, HOLLYWOOD OR BUST. The film was made, however, and completed in late 1956. It turned out to be the last film starring Dean Martin and Jerry Lewis, and the story that the Copacabana stint was a farewell appearance turned out to be true.

HOLLYWOOD OR BUST was directed by Frank Tashlin, who again brought his inventive mind to a usual Martin and Lewis plot about a movie-mad kid (Jerry) doing everything imaginable to get himself to the movie capital and a face-to-face meeting with his idol, Anita Ekberg. But Dean Martin's complaint was justified. Here, in the team's seventeenth film, he was still being used as a singing prop, a "necessary evil" to offset the madcap comedy of his popular partner. This was particularly frustrating to Martin because he was possessed of fine comic talent himself, and a natural wit which has finally emerged in recent years. Martin also accused Lewis of taking himself too seriously, considering himself to be another Chaplin. Many show-business friends tried to reconcile the two partners, to no avail. There was no official statement of a split, but the situation became obvious when Jerry Lewis starred on his own in THE DELICATE DELINQUENT for Paramount Pictures, with Darren McGavin in the role originally intended for Dean Martin. Likewise, Martin starred in a film for MGM called TEN THOUSAND BEDROOMS. Both films were released in early 1957, and in April of that year Martin sold out his interest in York

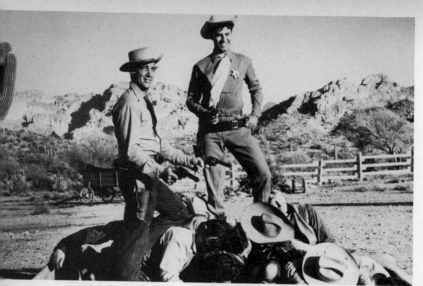
How the West was won. Dean and Jerry triumph in PARDNERS.

Pictures Corporation, the Martin and Lewis production company that controlled their films. When that announcement was made, the die was cast: Martin and Lewis were finished as a team.

Jerry Lewis' first film on his own, DELICATE DELINQUENT, turned out to be one of his best, and determined that the comedian could function quite well on his own. Dean Martin, however, did not fare quite as well. TEN THOUSAND BEDROOMS was a bomb. Lewis continued his happy association with Paramount Pictures, doing two films a year, every one of which made money. Dean Martin had an uphill struggle, and it wasn't until he landed good roles in dramatic films like SOME CAME RUNNING and CAREER that people sat up and took notice. His records were always popular, and his association with Frank Sinatra in "the Clan" helped build his image of an easygoing, fun-loving boozer. Both men had their anxious moments in the years following their split: Lewis in trying to promote himself as a serious singer, and Martin in trying to erase the "Jerry Lewis' partner" image. On September 30, 1958, they had a memorable encounter in front of millions of television viewers. Lewis was a guest on Eddie Fisher's TV show, and told his host that he wanted to sing a tune. Suddenly, from the wings came Dean Martin and Bing Crosby, who did their best to break up the show. "Don't sing!" cried Martin as he walked on stage. He and his former partner proceeded to chase each other around the stage, as Crosby heckled and Fisher doubled up with laughter. The appearance was completely spontaneous and made headlines the next day as columnists around the country speculated about a reteaming. Nothing ever came of it.

In the years since the breakup of Martin and Lewis, both men have enjoyed great individual success. Martin alternated dramatic film roles with lighter comedy vehicles before settling into a nine-year run on TV with a weekly variety show that was unrivaled for casual atmosphere (and which required Dino to work just one day a week). In recent years he's worked mainly in Las Vegas. Jerry Lewis's movie career took a nose dive in the 1970s, and a prime-time variety show lasted just two years; for a while his most prominent showcase was an annual telethon for the Muscular Dystrophy Association (where, in 1976, Dean Martin made a surprise appearance). He's enjoyed something of a renaissance in the 1980s, however, with new film projects including a widely praised dramatic performance opposite Robert DeNiro in *The King of Comedy*.

When Martin and Lewis were both working at NBC in Hollywood on their respective shows, there was talk of the possibility of exchanging guest shots. Jerry Lewis denied it, and explained, "You don't live and work with a guy as long as I did without the divorce being painful. How do you tell your audience you loved the guy? To kid what was and still is painful, because it might be saleable today, would be beneath my dignity. I'm still too sensitive about it. Dean can do it because the character he plays lets him do it. I can't."

So it is that Dean Martin and Jerry Lewis are now separate entities, both stars in their own right whose names are seldom mentioned in the same breath. It's hard to believe that not so long ago they were, together, the hottest act in show business and—for a time—the most successful comedy team in America.

The Films of Dean Martin and Jerry Lewis

(Director's name follows year.)

1. **My Friend Irma**—Paramount 1949—George Marshall—John Lund, Diana Lynn, Don DeFore, Marie Wilson, Hans Conried, Kathryn Givney, Percy Helton, Erno Verebes, Gloria Gordon, Margaret Field, Charles Cole-

man, Douglas Spencer, Ken Niles, Francis Pierlot, Dewey Robinson, Chief Yowlachie, Jack Mulhall, Nick Cravat, Jimmy Dundee, Felix Bressart. 103 minutes.

2. **My Friend Irma Goes West**—Paramount 1950—Hal Walker—John Lund, Marie Wilson, Diana Lynn, Co-rinne Calvet, Lloyd Corrigan, Donald Porter, Harold Huber, Joseph Vitale, Charles Evans, Kenneth Tobey, James Flavin, Wendell Niles, George Humbert, Roy Gordon, Gregg Palmer, Chief Yowlachie, Jody Gilbert, Jimmy Dundee. 91 minutes.

3. **At War with the Army**—Paramount 1950—Hal Walker—Mike Kellin, Jimmy Dundee, Dick Stabile, Tommy Far-rell, Frank Hyers, Danny Dayton, William Mendrek, Kenneth Forbes, Paul Livermore, Ty Perry, Jean Ruth, Angela Greene, Polly Bergen, Douglas Evans, Steven Roberts, Al Negbo, Dewey Robinson, Lee Bennett. 93 minutes.

4. **That's My Boy**—Paramount 1951—Hal Walker—Ruth Hussey, Eddie Mayehoff, Marion Marshall, Polly Bergen, Hugh Sanders, John McIntyre, Tom Harmon, Francis Pierlot, Lillian Randolph, Selmer Jackson, Torben Myer, Leon Tyler, Greg Palmer, Mickey Kuhn, Bob Board, Don Haggerty, Hazel (Sonny) Boyne. 98 minutes.

5. **Sailor Beware**—Paramount 1951—Hal Walker—Corinne Calvet, Marion Marshall, Robert Strauss, Leif Erickson, Don Wilson, Vince Edwards, Skip Homeier, Dan Bar-ton, Mike Mahoney, Mary Treen, Donald MacBride, Louis Jean Heydt, Elaine Stewart, James Flavin, Don Haggerty, Mary Murphy, Dick Stabile, The Mayo Broth-ers, Marshall Reed, Jimmy Dundee, Duke Mitchell, James Dean, The Marimba Merry Makers, The Freddie Troupe, guest star Betty Hutton. 108 minutes.

6. **Jumping Jacks**—Paramount 1952—Norman Taurog—Mona Freeman, Don DeFore, Robert Strauss, Richard Erdman, Ray Teal, Marcy McGuire, Danny Arnold, Charles Evans, James Flavin, Alex Gerry, Jody Gilbert. 96 minutes.

7. **Hollywood Fun Festival**—Columbia 1952—Ralph Staub—A Screen Snapshots reel; Staub and Dick Haynes narrate footage of Martin and Lewis at the Photoplay Awards banquet, and later at Barney's Beanery, where the an-nual "Mickey" awards are given. 10 minutes.

8. **Road to Bali**—Paramount 1952—Hal Walker—Bob Hope, Bing Crosby, Dorothy Lamour, Murvyn Vye, Peter Coe, Ralph Moody, Leon Askin, guest stars: Jane

Russell, Bob Crosby, (Humphrey Bogart in a scene from THE AFRICAN QUEEN), Bunny Lewbel, Michael Ansara, Harry Cording, Carolyn Jones, Allan Nixon. Martin and Lewis were guest stars in their first color feature. Color—91 minutes.

9. **The Stooge**—Paramount 1953—Norman Taurog—Completed March, 1951; released 1953—Polly Bergen, Marion Marshall, Eddie Mayehoff, Richard Erdman, Frances Bavier, Percy Helton, Mary Treen, Donald Mac-Bride, Charles Evans, Don Haggerty, Tommy Farrell, Oliver Blake. 100 minutes.

10. **Scared Stiff**—Paramount—1953—George Marshall—Lizabeth Scott, Carmen Miranda, George Dolenz, Dorothy Malone, William Ching, Paul Marion, Jack Lambert, Tom Powers, Tony Barr, Leonard Strong, Henry Brandon, Hugh Sanders, Frank Fontaine, Nolan Leary, Chester Clute, Percy Helton, Billy Daniel, Dick Stabile, guest stars Bing Crosby and Bob Hope. 108 minutes.

11. **The Caddy**—Paramount 1953—Norman Taurog—Donna Reed, Barbara Bates, Joseph Calleia, Fred Clark, Clinton Sundberg, Howard Smith, Marshall Thompson, Marjorie Gateson, Frank Puglia, Lewis Martin, Romo Vincent, Argentina Brunetti, Houseley Stevenson, Jr., John Gallaudet, William Edmunds, Charles Irwin, Freeman Lusk, Keith McConnell, Henry Brandon, Maurice Marsac, Donald Randolph, Stephen Chase, Tommy Harmon, Ben Hogan, Sammy Snead, Byron Nelson, Julius Boros, Jimmy Thompson, "Lighthorse" Harry Cooper, Wendell Niles, Mary Treen, Mary Newton, Mike Mahoney, Hank Mann, Dick Stabile, King Donovan, Ned Glass, Torben Meyer, Dick Wessel, Frank Richards, Elaine Riley, Nancy Kulp, Mario Siletti, Johnny Downs. 95 minutes.

12. **Money from Home**—Paramount 1953—George Marshall—Marjie Millar, Pat Crowley, Richard Haydn, Richard Strauss, Gerald Mohr, Sheldon Leonard, Romo Vincent, Jack Kruschen, Lou Lubin, Joe McTurk, Frank Mitchell, Sam (Society Kid) Hogan, Phil Arnold, Louis Nicoletti, Charles Horvath, Dick Reeves, Frank Richards, Harry Hayden, Henry McLemore, Mortie Dutra, Wendell Niles, Ed Clark, Grace Hayle, Bobby Barber, Al Hill, Drew Cahill, Buck Young, Jack Roberts, Ben Astar, Arthur Gould Porter, Robin Hughes, Elizabeth Slifer, Gertrude Astor, Maidie Norman, Rex Lease, Mara Corday, Mike Mahoney. Color—100 minutes.

13. **Living It Up**—Paramount 1954—Norman Taurog—Janet Leigh, Edward Arnold, Fred Clark, Sheree North, Sammy White, Sid Tomack, Sig Ruman, Richard Loo, Raymond Greenleaf, Walter Baldwin, Marla English, Kathryn Grandstaff (Grant), Emmett Lynn, Dabbs Greer, Clancy Cooper, John Alderson, Booth Colman, Stanley Blystone, Fritz Feld, Torben Meyer, Art Baker, Grady Sutton, Lane Chandler, Mike Mahoney, Gino Corrado, Bobby Barber, Al Hill, Hank Mann, Frankie Darro. Color—95 minutes.

14. **Three Ring Circus**—Paramount 1954—Joseph Pevney—Joanne Dru, Zsa Zsa Gabor, Elsa Lanchester, Wallace Ford, Sig Ruman, Gene Sheldon, Nick Cravat, Douglas Fowley, Sue Casey, Mary L. Orosco, Frederick E. Wolfe, Phil Van Zandt, Ralph Peters, Chick Chandler, Kathleen Freeman, Robert McKibbon, Neil Levitt, Al Hill, Robert LeRoy Diamond, George E. Stone, Lester Dorr, Donald Kerr, James Davies, Louis Lettieri, Sandy Descher, Billy Curtis, Harry Monty, Milton A. Dickinson, Bobby Kay, Sonnie Vallie, Robert Locke Lorraine, John Minshull, Joe Evans, George Boyce, Mike Mahoney, Drew Cahill, Buck Young, Mike Ross, Mark Hanna. Color—103 minutes.

15. **You're Never Too Young**—Paramount 1955—Norman Taurog—Diana Lynn, Nina Foch, Raymond Burr, Mitzi McCall, Veda Ann Borg, Margery Maude, Romo Vincent, Nancy Kulp, Tommy Ivo, Milton Frome, Hans Conried, Donna Percy, Emory Parnell, James Burke, Whitey Haupt, Mickey Finn, Peggy Moffitt, Johnstone White, Dick Simmons, Louise Lorimer, Isabel Randolph, Robert Carson, Dick Cutting, Mary Newton, Paul Newlan, Stanley Blystone, Bobby Barber, Bob Morgan. Color—102 minutes.

16. **Artists and Models**—Paramount 1955-Frank Tashlin—Shirley MacLaine, Dorothy Malone, Eddie Mayehoff, Eva Gabor, Anita Ekberg, George "Foghorn" Winslow, Jack Elam, Herbert Rudley, Richard Shannon, Richard Webb, Alan Lee, Otto Waldis, Kathleen Freeman, Art Baker, Emory Parnell, Carleton Young, Nick Castle, Jr., Margaret Barstow, Martha Wentworth, Sara Berner, Steven Geray, Ralph Dumke, Clancy Cooper, Charles Evans, Mortimer Dutra, Frank Jenks, Mike Ross, Ann McCrea, Patti Ross, Glen Walters, Larri Thomas, Sharon Baird, Eve Meyer, Dale Hartleben, Mickey Little, Patricia Morrow, Sue Carlton, Tommy Summers, Max

Power, Frances Lansing, Don Corey, Frank Carter, Dorothy Gordon, Rudy Makoul, Jeannette Miller. Color—106 minutes.

17. **Pardners**—Paramount 1956—Norman Taurog—Lori Nelson, Jeff Morrow, Jackie Laughery, John Baragrey, Agnes Moorehead, Lon Chaney, Jr., Milton Frome, Richard Aherne, Lee Van Cleef, Stuart Randall, Scott Douglas, Jack Elam, Bob Steele, Mickey Finn, Douglas Spencer, Philip Tonge, Valerie Allen, Emory Parnell, James Parnell, Gavin Gordon, Johnstone White, William Forrest, Elaine Riley, Ann McCrea, Mary Newton, Stanley Blystone, Charlie Stevens, Matt Moore, Hank Mann, Bobby Barber. Color—82 minutes.

18. **Hollywood or Bust**—Paramount 1956—Frank Tashlin—Anita Ekberg, Pat Crowley, Maxie Rosenbloom, Willard Waterman, Jack McElroy, Mike Ross, Wendell Niles, Frank Wilcox, Kathryn Card, Richard Karlan, Tracey Roberts, Ben Welden, Ross Westlake, Gretchen Houser, Sandra White, Adele August, Drew Cahill, Torben Meyer, Chief Yowlachie, Minta Durfee, Dick Alexander, Valerie Allen, Dean's daughters Claudia, Gail, and Dena Martin. Color—95 minutes.

OTHER TEAMS

Moran and Mack

It is doubtful that the comedians who were known as "The Two Black Crows" are in for a revival today, but no one will dispute their great popularity in the 1920's and early 1930's. To understand their success, one must appreciate the fact

Moran and Mack in one of their dismal two-reelers, TWO BLACK CROWS IN AFRICA.

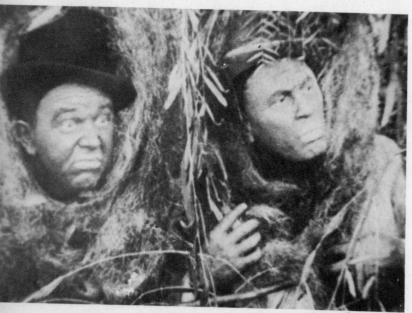

that ethnic humor was at its height in the 1920's, in vaudeville, burlesque and even in movies. Jewish comedians, Irish comedians, Dutch comedians, Italian comedians, all displaying the most outlandish stereotypes of their groups, were very much in vogue. Into this world came two ex-minstrels who caught on with the public by doing a first-rate dialogue act in blackface: Moran and Mack.

Charles E. Mack (real name: Sellers) was born in 1887 in White Cloud, Kansas. His partner, George Moran (real name: Searcy) was born not far away, in Elwood, Kansas. Both men had similar backgrounds, working at a variety of odd jobs before drifting into show business. They both spent their early years in minstrel shows, which gave them the background for their later act. When he reached New York, Mack teamed with another ex-minstrel man, John Swor, for a blackface act that appeared in *The Passing Show of 1916*. The act was well-received, and Mack went on to appear in other Broadway revues like *Maid in America*. In *Over the Top* he shared comedy honors with a young man he had met on the vaudeville circuit some years before, George Mack. The two men had been acquaintances before, but now they became close friends, and decided to try their luck together in vaudeville. Moran served as the fast-talking straight man of the act, and Mack, with an air of perpetual worry and frustration, delivered the punchlines. Their patter was fresh and funny, with a limitless series of puns that made audiences howl.

After two years on the vaudeville circuit, Moran and Mack returned to Broadway as featured players in *The Passing Show of 1921*, which established them as star comics and assured their success for the rest of the decade. They appeared in *Earl Carroll's Vanities, Ziegfeld Follies, George White's Scandals, The Greenwich Village Follies*, and other top shows. In 1928 the comedy team appeared on a weekly radio show, and around the same time made a series of comedy records that amazed everyone by selling a reported seven million copies. In 1929, Paramount Pictures signed the Two Black Crows (as they were known to most fans) for feature films, and mounted an impressive production for their film debut. Evelyn Brent co-starred, George Abbott directed, and the story was taken from Octavus Roy Cohen, a popular writer whose stories of Negro life were filmed as a series of Paramount shorts. The resulting features was an odd blend of music, comedy and maudlin drama called WHY BRING THAT UP? (the title being a Moran and Mack catch line).

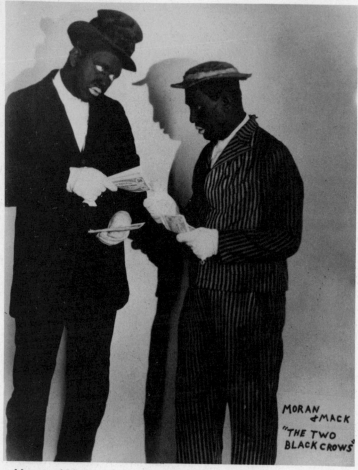

Moran and Mack exchange some money in a publicity still.

After the release of WHY BRING THAT UP? the blackface team was riding high professionally, but off stage there was disharmony. In December 1929, George Moran left the act, charging that Mack had been paying him $200 a week, with occasional bonuses, while the "team" was making $5000 a week in vaudeville engagements and film work. A Los Angeles judge ruled that since Mack was the official owner of the act, and originator of the team, he had the right to adjust Moran's salary, and furthermore, had the exclusive use of the team name. George Moran walked out, and was replaced by Mack's old partner Bert Swor (who had played a supporting role in WHY BRING THAT UP?). Continuing as "Moran and Mack" as if nothing had happened, the team appeared in another Paramount feature, ANYBODY'S WAR, which was not successful. Paramount dropped the comedy team from its roster without fanfare.

Charlie Mack recruited various men to work with him in the "Two Black Crows" act before he and the original George Moran were reconciled. By this time, however, the popularity of the team was being eclipsed by a pair of radio comedians known as Amos 'n' Andy. Moran and Mack found it harder to secure first-rate bookings in the early 1930's, but seemed to be back on the road to success when they headlined a bill at the Palace in May of 1932. They were then approached by the former King of Comedy, Mack Sennett, to return to Hollywood for another feature film. Sennett was on the downgrade by this time, forced to work with Sono Art-World Wide Pictures, a fly-by-night company of the early 1930's, but he saw a chance for a comeback with Moran and Mack. He directed the team in a feature-length musical comdey, HYPNOTIZED. Its quality was indicated by Richard Watts, Jr., in his review in the New York *Herald-Tribune*: "There is a certain academic interest to be found in HYPNOTIZED, for if you haven't seen it you cannot realize how bad a motion picture can be."

Moran and Mack followed this triumph with a series of two-reel comedies for Educational Pictures, which specialized in cheap products using once-famous comedy stars. The Moran and Mack shorts hit rock bottom, with tiresome gags and none of the snappy dialogue that had made the team famous. In 1933 they were guests on Fred Waring's radio show, but write-ups in the press indicated how far the team had fallen. Most of them used the past tense, and had to remind readers of the comedy team "remembered as The Two Black Crows." On January 11, 1934, Myrtle Mack,

Charlie's wife, was driving her husband, daughter, George Moran, and Mack Sennett through Arizona on their way to Hollywood, when a rear tire was punctured and the car went out of control. It skidded off the road and toppled over several times, killing Charlie Mack instantly, and injuring the others.

George Moran tried to continue the act with new partners, with minimal success, and did a USO tour during World War II with the old vaudeville material. In 1949 he suffered a stroke, and died August 1. In Moran's obituary, *Variety* noted: "Earthy comedy of the team, which projected Moran as the wise-cracking straight man for the slow-and-easy Mack, was rated the top blackface comedy act of the era. Although their deliveries were in caricature vein, it never brought criticism and they presumably had as many Negro fans as white. Their material and comedy were tops— and that's all that mattered."

Smith and Dale

When Smith and Dale made their first movie in 1929, they were already show-business veterans. Theirs was one of the longest partnerships in comedy history, spanning some seventy years and relying on material that never failed to get laughs . . . even when it started showing its age. At a 1962 tribute given them by The Lambs, an actors' club in New York City, a *New York Times* reporter tried to ask the comic duo how they came together. "We met in 1898," said Joe Smith. "Don't remind me," interrupted Charlie Dale.

The fact remains that it *was* 1898 when (according to the oft-told story) young Joe Seltzer was riding a bicycle north on Eldridge Street while Charlie Marks was riding east on Delancey Street, in New York. This explosive meeting led to a fast friendship between the two young men who agreed to become partners in show business. Show business for the two neophytes was restricted to saloons, beer halls, and other rowdy establishments in such colorful sections of New York as the Bowery, Chinatown and the Lower East Side. At this time, Seltzer and Marks did a dance routine that met with mixed response from the rough patrons of these establishments. Several years later, the story goes, when they

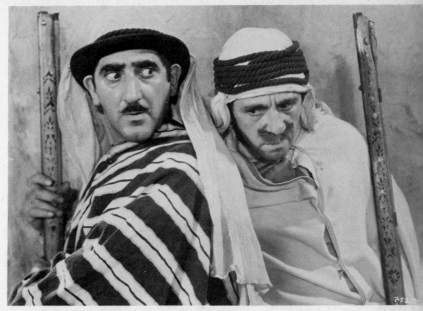

Joe Smith and Charlie Dale in the Paramount short THE ARABIAN SHRIEKS.

were booked into a vaudeville house, a local signmaker was selling a surplus of signs advertising a defunct team named Smith and Dale. The price seemed right to Seltzer and Marks, so they bought the signs and changed the name of their act.

At the turn of the century, the two performers became part of an act called the Avon Comedy Four that experienced modest success for two decades doing a variety of well timed sketches including one that introduced a character named "Dr. Kronkheit." The Avon Four made its Broadway debut in 1916 in *Why Worry?*, which featured a comedienne and singer named Fanny Brice. In 1919 the act broke up, and Smith and Dale found success on their own in a host of Broadway revues, in vaudeville houses around the country and even in burlesque. Reportedly, the team even made some silent comedy shorts, although the appeal of these films must have been limited, for by this time Smith and Dale were known for their marvelous timing and delivery of verbal gags. Many of their sketches became vaudeville staples, such as "S.S. Malaria" and "La Schnapps, Inc.," but the routine with which Smith and Dale became indelibly identified was "Dr. Kronkheit and his Only Living Patient."

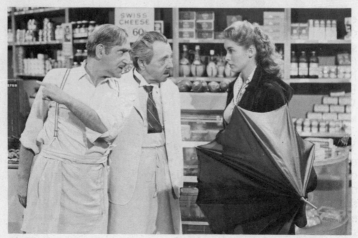

Smith and Dale offer some sage advice to Janet Leigh in TWO TICKETS TO
BROADWAY.

This uproarious routine has been printed verbatim by
Bennett Cerf in his *Encyclopedia of Modern American Humor*, labeled an American vaudeville classic, and that it is.
Charlie Dale comes to see Dr. Kronkheit, and is told by a
nurse to take a chair. "Wrap it, I'll take it on my way out,"
he replies. When he finally gets to see the doctor he begins
by saying "Doctor, I'm dubious." "Pleased to meet you, Mr.
Dubious," Joe Smith replies, in one of the all-time great
comedy exchanges. The skit builds in hilarity to a perfect
finish. "You owe me $10," Dr. Kronkheit announces. "For
what?" "$10 for my advice," he explains. "Here's $2," says
Mr. Dubious, "Take it, Doctor—that's *my* advice."

In 1929, Smith and Dale were among the scores of vaudevillians drafted into service by the movies. They filmed a
number of their skits and also appeared in some specially
written short subjects, both at Warner Bros.' Vitaphone
studio in Brooklyn and at Paramount's studio in Astoria,
New York. Titles included THE FALSE ALARM FIRE CO.,
KNIGHTS IN VENICE, ANYTHING BUT HAM, and WHERE EAST
MEETS VEST. Their Jewish-stereotype characters did not appeal to everyone in the movie audience, nor did their humor
(one trade magazine referred to them as "Hebrew comedians" and complained about their "stale gags"—this in 1930!).
But they always scored on stage, and it was there that they
enjoyed their greatest success yet in a show called *Mendel,
Inc.* Warner Bros. then decided to film the play, retaining its

ethnic quality but giving it a more general title, THE HEART OF NEW YORK. George Sidney, from the *Cohens and Kellys* series, played opposite Smith (as Sam Shtrudel) and Dale (as Bernard Schnaps) in this entertaining bit of hokum set in New York's Lower East Side. It was to become Smith and Dale's most sustained piece of work on film. (While at Warner Bros. they appeared in another, much inferior film, MANHATTAN PARADE.)

From that time on, Smith and Dale made their home in New York, with only occasional forays into the world of movie-making, with short subjects for Universal and Columbia and occasional trips to Hollywood. In 1939 they starred in a pair of slapstick two-reelers for Columbia that were directed by the talented Charley Chase, but neither A NAG IN THE BAG nor MUTINY ON THE BODY were particularly well suited to the style of Smith and Dale. In 1945 they were signed by 20th Century–Fox to appear in the musical feature NOB HILL, but all their footage was left on the cutting-room floor.

Then in 1951 they had one last fling in films—with very pleasing results. Joe and Charlie were cast as delicatessen owners who aspire to be in show business in Howard Hughes' RKO production TWO TICKETS TO BROADWAY, starring Tony Martin, Janet Leigh, Gloria DeHaven, and Eddie Bracken. The script allowed them to perform some of their best patter routines, which were definitely the highlights of an otherwise standard musical. John Rosenfeld wrote in the *Dallas News,* "There are some of the best looking legs and things in TWO TICKETS TO BROADWAY, but maybe we are getting old. We only had eyes for Joe Smith and Charlie Dale, a pair of stage-struck delicatessen owners, who virtually give us their 'Dr. Kronkheit' routine." The sentiment was echoed by many fans.

When New York's legendary Palace Theatre experimented with a return to two-a-day vaudeville in 1951, Smith and Dale were on hand to head the bill. Several years later, when Judy Garland made history with her dazzling engagement at the Palace, she hired Smith and Dale to fill out the bill—telling the press that she'd always enjoyed the team when she was in vaudeville herself and was happy to have them working on the same stage with her.

Smith and Dale continued to work for years to come, recording comedy albums, appearing in off-Broadway revues, and making guest appearances on television, repeatedly on *The Ed Sullivan Show.* Their timing was as sharp as ever when they celebrated their seventieth anniversary as a team.

Charlie Dale died in 1971 at the age of ninety, but Joe Smith continued to be active even while living at the Actors Fund Home in Englewood, New Jersey. He took delight in visiting local schools and talking about vaudeville. A teacher, Terry McGrath, became his latter-day partner in demonstrating classic Smith and Dale routines for children who'd never seen this kind of humor before. In recognition of his volunteer work, Hackensack, New Jersey High School presented Joe Smith with something he'd always wanted—a diploma—on the eve of his eighty-seventh birthday.

Joe Smith died on February 22, 1981, having just celebrated his ninety-seventh birthday. He lived a full and rich life, and died with the knowledge that Smith and Dale had carved a special niche in show-business history, and (fortunately for us) preserved some of their brightest moments on film.

The Wiere Brothers

The Wiere Brothers were a popular act in America for more than thirty years, but it always seemed to this observer that they were taken for granted. Not enough people stopped to realize that in this act were three of the most versatile performers in show business. They could sing, dance, do acrobatics, play various instruments—and do all of this to perfection—in addition to being naturally funny men. In the late 1960s, Joey Bishop had them as guests on his late-night television show. After doing their act, they sat and talked with him for several minutes. "Do you mind if I ask how long you've been together?" Bishop asked innocently. "Yes," replied Sylvester with a smile. "Do you ever have arguments?" Bishop persisted. "Only when we talk," answered Herbert.

The Wiere Brothers come from an impressive show-business family. Their grandmother sang in the Prussian State Opera, and their grandfather, for variety, did an acrobatic act. Their grandmother arranged for them to study dancing with the company ballet, and they appeared with the troupe in *Aida* and *The Poet and the Peasant* during the Elverside Music Festival in Germany. Their father was a comedian, and their sister a singer and dancer; consequently the family was al-

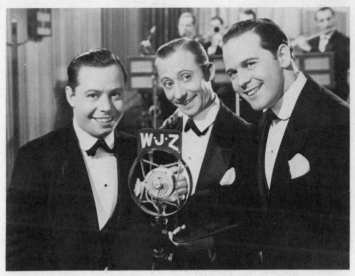

The Wiere Brothers pose during a mock radio show in THE GREAT AMERICAN BROADCAST.

ways on the road, and the three brothers were born in different countries. Harry was born in Berlin in 1908, Herbert in Vienna in 1909, and Sylvester in Prague in 1910. In 1922, when Sylvester, the youngest, was 12, the family troupe was staying in Dresden, Germany, with an ailing father and a working sister. The three brothers decided to form an act for themselves, and the local theater manager put them to work immediately. Reportedly, it is (with minor changes) the same act they have done ever since.

In 1935 the brothers made their first trip to America, and played at the French Casino in Chicago. They returned to the Continent, but came back to the U.S. each of the next two years. In 1937 they decided to stay, and opened at Ben Marden's Riviera Club in New Jersey, billed as "the Continental Comedy Trio, the Wiere Brothers." They tried their luck in Hollywood, and were featured briefly—and unmemorably—in a sequence of Walter Wanger's *Vogues of 1938*. The following year they were awarded a plaque by the National Humor Foundation citing them as "the comedy find of the year," and in December 1938, they opened Kurt Robitschek's *Vaudeville Marches On*, an attempt to revive

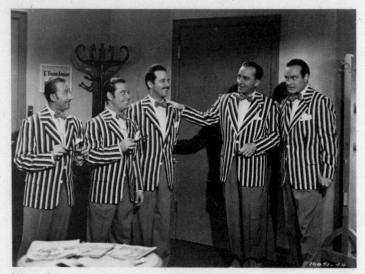

Harry, Sylvester and Herbert act as American jazz musicians to help Bing Crosby and Bob Hope out of a jam in THE ROAD TO RIO.

the three-a-day show policy at Broadway's Majestic Theater. Wrote Brooks Atkinson, "After a dull and talentless beginning the show that opened at the Majestic last evening catches up with the Wiere Brothers, 'Europe's foremost comedians,' as the bill ballyhoo puts it. Without traveling all over Europe it is easy to recognize them as perfect vaudevillians—fast, expert, and vastly amusing. They are brothers three, diminutive and perfectly matched, and for rapid nonsense it would be hard to improve on their sleight-of-hand routine. Give them three derby hats and they can exorcize the ghost of the lamented variety show in a couple of gags and a few pieces of absurd business. Night clubs and radio have developed techniques that lack the pungency and precision of vaudeville and are a horse of several different colors. But the Wiere Brothers still work in that crisp and demented style of comedy. Let them take as many bows as time permits."

The Wieres have been taking bows ever since, in nightclubs, on such stages as New York's Radio City Music Hall, Roxy, and Paramount theaters, and on television. But Hollywood never quite knew what to do with the Wiere boys. In 1941 they were hired by 20th Century-Fox, along with several other "specialty acts," to appear in THE GREAT AMERICAN BROADCAST, a heavily fictionalized account of the birth and development of commercial radio. They only had two scenes, but both showed them to best advantage, and the second segment allowed them to do virtually their entire vaudeville act for the camera. The great blessing is that this routine is preserved on film. But, after BROADCAST, Fox had no further use for the Wiere Brothers, and did not sign them to a contract. Throughout the 1940's, they were featured in occasional films like SWING SHIFT MAISIE for MGM and HANDS ACROSS THE BORDER for Republic.

In 1947 they were given another chance to shine, with Bing Crosby and Bob Hope in THE ROAD TO RIO, where they played three Brazilian musicians who are hired by Hope and Crosby to impersonate jive-talking members of their American band. Since the brothers (in the film) speak no English, they are taught several expressions by rote, which they fire *too* readily at anyone within earshot. All Herbert can remember to say is "You solid, Jackson!" and his brothers mimic similar slangish greetings which eventually give Hope and Crosby away as imposters.

In the 1950's, the Wieres toured with such shows as *Roberta* and *Rosalinda*. *Roberta* allowed them to do some musical routines kidding the classics, in which Herbert would introduce "Beethoven's Fit Thymphony." The orchestra would play four bars, then he would explain, "It goes on and on like that." In *Rosalinda*, presented on NBC-TV's *Producer's Showcase* series, they were interpolated into the script of this old operetta chestnut as Frosh, Frish and Frush, roles they were to repeat twelve years later during an engagement of the same show at the Los Angeles Music Center. In the late 1950's and early 1960's, the Wiere Brothers enjoyed tremendous popularity on TV as frequent guest stars on every major variety program. One of their classic gags would have one brother stand in the middle of the screen, singing. On each chorus, his brothers would move in on each side of the screen and put their hands on the middle brother's shoulders while singing their lines. When they would move back out of camera range, their hands would remain on his shoulders!

In 1960, producer-director Jules White created a half-hour pilot film for CBS called OH, THOSE BELLS! starring the Wiere Brothers. White had just completed 25 years as head of Columbia Pictures' short-subjects department, producing and directing two-reelers with Buster Keaton, Andy Clyde and the Three Stooges, among others. OH, THOSE BELLS! was his idea to perpetuate the slapstick comedy genre that seemed

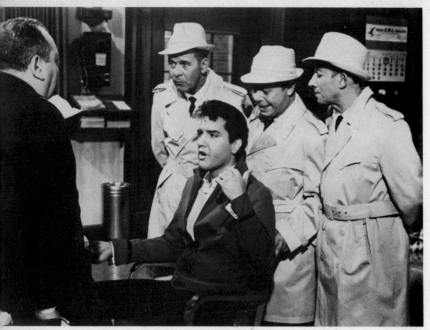

Leon Askin delivers orders to his three ace detectives, the Wiere Brothers, who have been trailing Elvis Presley in DOUBLE TROUBLE.

to be dying, and CBS liked the idea. White, however, concluded, "At CBS there were all chiefs, no Indians. The film was so bad, I quit—who needs such a rat race?" Nevertheless, CBS liked the show, and commissioned 13 segments. Then, at the last minute, they canceled the show and put the 13 episodes on the shelf, where they remained until May 1962, when a summer replacement was needed for an unsuccessful situation-comedy starring Bob Cummings. OH, THOSE BELLS! was finally aired, and reaction was mixed. *The New York Times'* Jack Gould thought the show was a sleeper, but *Show* magazine provided the best analysis:

"For [the Wiere Brothers'] club act, they originate all their own routines, which have a certain endearing zaniness. 'Slapstick suggests a lack of subtlety,' says brother Harry Wiere. 'You think of people throwing pies and hitting each other over the head. We are not roughnecks by nature. We are gentle people. Our style is more European. Everything we do is gentle. Our personalities carry the comedy.' But slapstick they have become. In theory, the brothers were supposed to go over each script and give it the whimsical Wiere touch by adding comedy business where they saw fit. However, CBS' eager writers tended to provide scripts that were already a full twenty-four minutes long—the maximum script length for a half-hour show—leaving little time for insertions without cutting into the story line. Being gentle people, Herby, Harry and Sylvester, with their ideas about subtlety, were at an understandable disadvantage against a fevered television task force. But the brothers' silent-film brand of humor conquers occasionally, and lifts them above the predictable situations of small-screen, assembly-line comedy."

In 1967 the Wieres made their first movie in twenty years, DOUBLE TROUBLE, with Elvis Presley. Although their contribution to the film was minor, it was still fun to see them cavorting as three bumbling detectives on Elvis' trail.

Through the 1960's, the Wiere Brothers continued to convulse audiences in top nightclubs and stages around the country, doing essentially the same act that made them popular thirty years ago. A recent addition had the trio playing violin, guitar and bass fiddle. Herbert, trying to do a serious piece on his violin, would be frustrated by his brothers' hillbilly antics, and with a shrug would stop playing and instead, balance the violin on his chin. Harry, noticing his brothers' accomplishment, would take the guitar and do the same. This would leave Sylvester, smiling blandly at the audience, plucking his bass fiddle. When he saw his two brothers balancing their instruments on their chins, he did a long take, turning from them to his huge fiddle and back. Finally he would lift the bass into the air, and miraculously, manage to balance it on his chin for the finale to their delightful act.

On talk and variety shows, on TV's popular *Laugh-In*, and on tour, the Wieres were as funny in 1970 as they ever were. Then, in July, Sylvester, the lovable moon-faced member of the trio, suffered a heart attack in his home and died at the age of sixty. Understandably, the brothers suffered a tremendous blow, but Herbert and Harry have done their best to carry on an act—and a tradition—that has delighted audiences around the world for so many, many years.

Mitchell and Durant

In the days of silent comedy, most slapstick comics were comedians first, and acrobats second. Mitchell and Durant, who never made a silent film, started as acrobats, and carried their gymnastic skills over into a comedy act that relied on hitting, kicking, slapping, tripping and falling more than anything else. Jack Durant started at the age of nine in an acrobatic act. He met Frank Mitchell at a gym where they both went to work out. The two became friends, and broke into vaudeville together with a roughhouse act, during which Durant always seemed to get the worst of the situation. Somehow or other they were considered worthy of a featured spot in the 1929 edition of *George White's Scandals* on Broadway, and continued to appear in such shows as *Earl Carroll's Vanities* and *Hit the Deck*. In 1934 the call came from Hollywood, and the comedy team reported to Fox

Jack Durant, Ray Walker, Alice Faye and Frank Mitchell pose during MUSIC IS MAGIC.

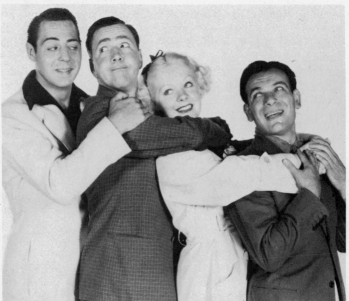

Studios, where they appeared in a rapid succession of brisk comedies and Alice Faye musicals, injecting their own material into the scripts wherever possible.

The New York Times wrote, in a review of SHE LEARNED ABOUT SAILORS, ". . . the knockabout team of Mitchell and Durant are present almost continually in the picture. Having the interests of their audience at heart, they will kill themselves with a little encouragement. They bite, kick, scratch, punch, and gouge each other with such a cheerful disregard for their personal safety that it is impossible not to be impressed and ungrateful not to be amused. But it happens that the law of diminishing returns cannot be suspended even for Mitchell and Durant. If a spectator could forget how much he laughed while the clowns were pummeling each other during the first thirty minutes of the film, he would be in the happy position of being able to enjoy them all over again in the last thirty minutes."

In 1938 the team split, Mitchell to continue in films as a supporting player, and Durant to go on to a very successful solo career on the stage (replacing Gene Kelly in *Pal Joey* on Broadway), in films (notably Orson Welles' JOURNEY INTO FEAR), and especially in nightclubs, where he became a popular stand-up comic. Today, the antics of Mitchell and Durant, in their surviving films, are hard to stomach, and it is difficult to see what made them so popular. If any team deserves to be obscured in the annals of film history, it is they, but as long as there are Alice Faye fans, people will have to endure Mitchell and Durant in such 1930's musicals as SHE LEARNED ABOUT SAILORS, 365 NIGHTS IN HOLLYWOOD, and MUSIC IS MAGIC.

Fibber McGee and Molly

Fibber McGee and Molly were hardly movie comedians, but they were one of show-business' most enduring teams, and like most radio stars, they were often drafted to go through their paces in Hollywood. Marian Driscoll was born in 1898, Jim Jordan in 1897, in Peoria, Illinois. The two met when they became members of the same local choir. They were teen-agers at the time, but Jim fell in love with Marian, and courted her for the next few years. Jim held down a

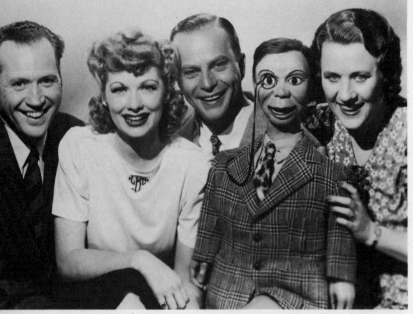

LOOK WHO'S LAUGHING with Jim Jordan (Fibber McGee), Lucille Ball, Edgar Bergen, Charlie McCarthy, and Marian Jordan (Molly).

variety of odd jobs in Peoria, but he longed to be a professional singer, and made several attempts to break into show business. Marian earned her living by giving piano lessons in Peoria, and once went out as Jim's partner when he thought he had a chance in vaudeville. Three times out, and three times back, the two were battered down in defeat and always ended up where they started, in Peoria. In 1918 they were married, and supplemented their nine-to-five income by entertaining at local affairs.

Time and time again Jim Jordan went out on the road, only to return to Peoria and his wife, who by this time had a baby to raise and couldn't travel with him. One day when they were visiting relatives in Chicago, they heard commercial radio for the first time, and decided that it was worth a try. They were hired as singers on station WENR, which didn't pay much but gave them a start. The turning point came in 1931 then they met an ambitious young man named Don Quinn, who wanted to make radio writing his profession. Over the next few years the threesome collaborated on several false start endeavors, culminating in 1935 with the birth of *Fibber McGee and Molly*.

The original *McGee* show, broadcast locally in Chicago, raised few eyebrows. It was considered a lackadaisical, uninspired domestic comedy by the critics. But the warmth and sincerity of Marian and Jim Jordan was communicated to the show's audience, and in a very short time the program was a tremendous success on the NBC radio network. By 1938 Paramount Pictures was beckoning the radio team to Hollywood, where they made their movie debut in THIS WAY, PLEASE, with Betty Grable and Jackie Coogan. Fibber and Molly returned to Hollywood several years later with a contract to do one film a year with RKO Radio Pictures. These films can best be described as lightweight, and while Marian and Jim Jordan come across very nicely on the screen, it is safe to say that had their success depended on these films, they never would have enjoyed the longevity they possessed. LOOK WHO'S LAUGHING and HERE WE GO AGAIN teamed Fibber and Molly with Edgar Bergen and Charlie McCarthy, among others, for short-running hodge-podges of music and comedy that are best forgotten. HEAVENLY DAYS (1944) attempts to give the radio characters a real story to work with, but gets tangled up in wartime morale boosting and a sticky

Raymond Walburn isn't pleased with Fibber and Molly in this scene from HEAVENLY DAYS.

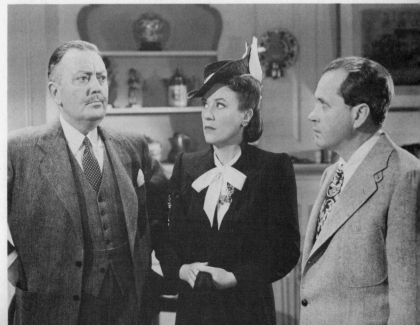

subplot involving some refugee children. The film's best scene has Jim Jordan harmonizing with the Kings' Men quartet, playing soldiers traveling with them on an East-bound train.

Whatever the quality of these films, Fibber McGee and Molly were radio stars of the top magnitude, and continued their weekly program through 1956. Like most radio stars, they attempted to transfer their format to television in the early 1950's, with disastrous results. The blame was given to their writers, who had not worked with the team on radio and did not understand their basic appeal. After the demise of their weekly show, Fibber and Molly continued to do five-minute spots for the NBC radio network *Monitor* show on weekends, until Marian Jordan fell ill in the late 1950's. In 1959 NBC unveiled a new TV version of *Fibber McGee and Molly*—"new" because it did not star the Jordans, but instead Bob Sweeney as Fibber and Cathy Lewis as Molly. With or without the Jordans, the show was not successful and also not very good.

The Jordans lived in happy retirement in Encino, California, where Marian Jordan died in her sleep in April 1961, bringing an end to one of the best-loved American couples of all time.

Brown and Carney

Success or failure in show business depends largely on being in the right place at the right time. In the mid-1940's, two vaudevillians were under contract to RKO Radio Pictures, playing supporting roles in sundry "A" and "B" pictures, when somebody got the bright idea of creating a comedy team to rival Abbott and Costello. The result was the energetic but short-lived comedy team of Wally Brown and Alan Carney. Brown, then in his 40's, had done fairly well in vaudeville as a low-key comedian, but yearned for greener pastures and accepted an RKO contract in 1942. Alan Carney was also a successful comic on the vaudeville circuits, with a rubber face, and an equally flexible voice that enabled him to do impressions and dialect jokes. His first film break came in RKO's MR. LUCKY (1943) with Cary Grant.

In 1944 RKO started building up Brown and Carney as the studio's answer to Abbott and Costello. Brown was the Abbott prototype, the fast-talking straight man, more or less, with Carney the Costello figure, the butt of most of the jokes. They made their debut together in ADVENTURES OF A ROOKIE, a film reminiscent of BUCK PRIVATES in more ways than one. RKO assigned the film, and its sequel (ROOKIES IN BURMA) to producer Bert Gilroy and director Leslie Goodwins of their short-subjects department, and stocked the casts with other RKO contract players. No one was particularly impressed, but the Brown and Carney movies were more than adequate time fillers for the lower berths in RKO double features around the country, and the team continued for the next three years. In 1944, RKO sent their comedy duo out for a vaudeville tour together, in which theater patrons saw Brown and Carney at their best, not confined by contrived scripts or low budgets, but doing their old tried-and-true routines.

Good supporting roles in STEP LIVELY (1944), with Frank

Alan Carney has had an accident; among the witnesses, Wally Brown, Anne Jeffreys, Lionel Atwill and Bela Lugosi.

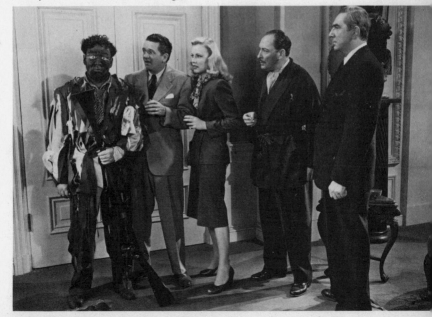

Sinatra, and more vehicles like RADIO STARS ON PARADE, THE GIRL RUSH, SEVEN DAYS ASHORE, and ZOMBIES ON BROADWAY followed. ZOMBIES attracted more attention than most of the others, because it treaded familiar and sure-fire ground—combining horror and comedy—and employed the services of Bela Lugosi. Unfortunately, Lugosi was going from one grade-Z film to another at this point, and he could not muster much enthusiasm for the low-grade roles he was given. His next film with the comedy team was even sadder; GENIUS AT WORK cast Lugosi as Lionel Atwill's butler, with little dialogue and just as little action. Brown and Carney fared well with the material, playing opposite lively young starlet Anne Jeffreys for the second time, but Atwill's villainy was very standard, and Lugosi's unfortunate casting was rather sad.

After GENIUS AT WORK in 1946, some genius at RKO decided that Brown and Carney were no longer useful to the studio, and dropped their contracts. Just as the team was created by the studio, so were they dissolved. Wally Brown

Wally Brown, George Murphy, Alan Carney, Frank Sinatra, and Gloria DeHaven in STEP LIVELY, a remake of the Marx Brothers' ROOM SERVICE.

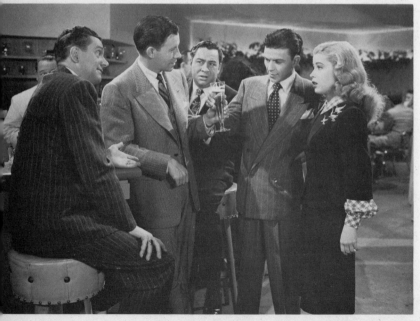

continued to work in many films and dozens of TV shows like *I Married Joan, Wagon Train, My Three Sons* and others, until his death in 1961. Alan Carney likewise found steady work in feature films, and continued to appear in many Walt Disney films, among others. He was given a good cameo role, along with scores of other veterans, in Stanley Kramer's IT'S A MAD, MAD, MAD, MAD WORLD (1964). He died of a heart attack in 1973.

In retrospect, Brown and Carney weren't all that bad, but their teaming was a contrivance—based on someone else's formula for success. Had they met in vaudeville and teamed up at that time, they might have created their own style and enjoyed a more lasting partnership as a result.

Noonan and Marshall

In the wake of Martin and Lewis, several comedy teams tried to establish themselves, including one duo (Duke Mitchell and Sammy Petrillo) who impersonated Dean and Jerry to the nth degree. Around 1950 an actor-comedian named Tommy Noonan teamed with a handsome singer-straightman named Peter Marshall, planning to take the country by storm. Noonan and Marshall enjoyed modest success, but they never really hit it big as a team. Both men fared better on their own.

Tommy Noonan had made his acting debut with his brother, John Ireland, in 1934, when Ireland enlisted in the ranks of New York's experimental-theater movement. Between 1934 and 1938 Noonan appeared in some sixty plays, gaining invaluable experience. He started his own repertory theater in Delaware, and after Navy service in World War II made his broadway debut in a flop called *Men to the Sea*. He came to Hollywood after this endeavor, and was placed under contract by RKO. Noonan made his movie debut in *George White's Scandals*, and for the next few years was kept busy in scores of RKO two-reelers, "B" pictures, and occasional "A" movies. He met Pete Marshall when Marshall's sister, Joanne Dru, married John Ireland. The two hit it off and decided to team up. They managed to land a job in Warner Brothers' all-star film STARLIFT in 1951, which gave them little to do but at least got them going.

The duo split and reteamed several times during the 1950's, when Noonan began to land good film roles: Judy Garland's musician friend in A STAR IS BORN, Marilyn Monroe's boyfriend in GENTLEMEN PREFER BLONDES, the floorwalker in BUNDLE OF JOY, and so on. When he reteamed with Pete Marshall in the late 1950's, it was with the intention of supervising a series of movies for the team. The first film under this arrangement was THE ROOKIE, one of the most abominable movies ever made, produced and coscripted by Noonan on a shoestring budget. A second film, SWINGIN' ALONG, was somewhat better, but failed to ignite the team, and Noonan and Marshall flickered out.

Noonan went on to fame and notoriety as the producer-director-writer-co-star of PROMISES PROMISES, a nudie film starring Jayne Mansfield, and THREE NUTS IN SEARCH OF A BOLT, with Mamie Van Doren. In April 1968 he entered a hospital with a brain tumor, and died on April 24 at the age of forty-six. Peter Marshall's career took a turn upward with his landing the job of emcee on a successful daytime television show, which lasted fourteen years, and made him a house-

Stunning Julie Newmar was the only thing that made THE ROOKIE worth watching; Noonan and Marshall were the nominal stars.

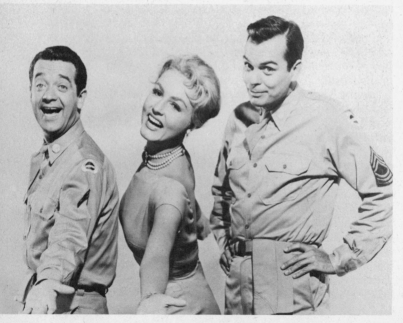

hold name. This in turn gave him the ability to pursue more personal projects—recording, playing Las Vegas, and touring the country as an actor and singer. He also worked for a time with a partner, Dick Gautier, and revealed once again the pleasant personality and sense of humor that made him an ideal straight man.

Rowan and Martin

The first comedy team to enjoy any lasting popularity after Martin and Lewis was Rowan and Martin, who scored their greatest success on television with *Rowan and Martin's Laugh-In* in the late 1960s and early 70s. This "overnight" stardom was the culmination of many years' steady work in nightclubs and TV, however. As to the team's movie career,

Veteran character actor James Gleason with movie newcomers Dick Martin and Dan Rowan in ONCE UPON A HORSE.

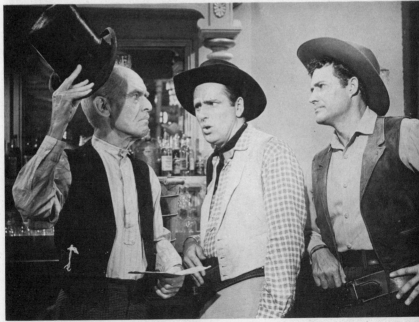

it was nipped in the bud on two different occasions—some twelve years apart!

Dan Rowan was born in 1922 in Beggs, Oklahoma, where his parents, both performers, were stopping on a cross-country tour. They appeared in a carnival-type revue, and their starry-eyed son joined them on stage as soon as he could learn the rudiments of singing and dancing. His parents died when he was eleven, and the rest of his childhood was spent in an orphanage. He later was adopted, and when he reached the age of nineteen he set out on his own, hitchhiking to Los Angeles. Rowan had held down several jobs, but in school he developed a liking for writing. When he arrived in California he set out to become a writer, and was hired by Paramount Pictures in an apprentice-like position. After World War II, he married and settled down in a more secure field, selling automobiles.

Dick Martin, also born in 1922, was a native of Battle Creek, Michigan. Always possessed of a keenly comic mind, he became a staff writer for the *Duffy's Tavern* radio show at the age of twenty-two. He wanted very much to be a

Dick Martin makes love to Doris Day in THE GLASS BOTTOM BOAT, his only film without partner Dan Rowan.

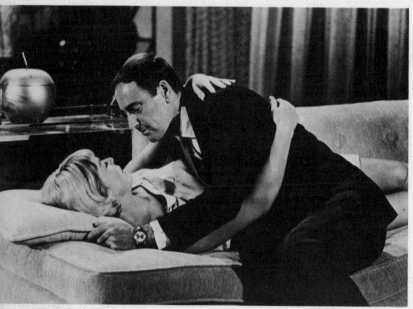

popular comedian, but his determined efforts never led to success. In 1946 he and another aspiring newcomer, Artie Lewis, billed themselves as the real Martin and Lewis, to no avail. He subsequently launched several acts with other partners, but none of them caught on. He remained a comedy writer during the day, and tended bar at night to supplement his income.

In the early 1950's, Dan Rowan got bored with the car business and decided to try his luck as an actor. He put himself into training and hired an agent. But it was a close friend, comedian-actor Tommy Noonan, who saw Rowan's comic possibilities and introduced him to Dick Martin. Dan and Dick liked each other, and decided to try working as a team, writing their own material. At first, Rowan was the comic and Martin was the straight man in the act, but in Rowan's words, "Dick's one of the worst straight-men in the world. He couldn't remember any line unless it was funny . . ." The two switched roles and found steady, if not presti-

Dan Rowan doesn't know that Julie Newmar is really a werewolf in THE MALTESE BIPPY.

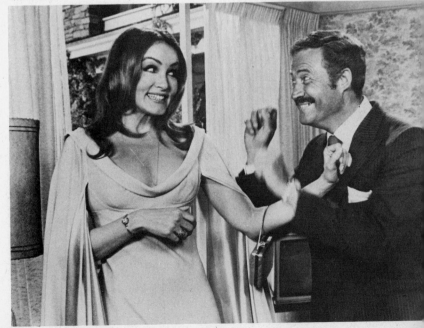

gious work. They played in dingy nightclubs, crowded bars, noisy burlesque houses, and other such establishments.

Even though his popularity had diminished since the 1930's, when he was the king of the columnists, Walter Winchell still wielded great power in the 1950's, and when he saw Rowan and Martin work in Miami Beach, he started to "plug" the team as much as possible. Their bookings improved, and they were featured in top niteries like the Copacabana and the Coconut Grove. In the mid-1950's they got their first television offers, and for years they appeared on the top variety shows. But really big-time success eluded them, even though they never lacked jobs and their salaries were more than adequate.

In 1957 they were signed to star in a comedy feature for Universal called ONCE UPON A HORSE. Produced, directed, and written by comedy pro Hal Kanter, this Western spoof could—and should—have been a turning point for Rowan and Martin. But the film was treated as a B-picture and never made much of an impression on audiences or critics—a shame, since it has some very clever touches and an offbeat sense of humor.

By the 1960s Rowan and Martin were a polished, very funny duo who never seemed to be doing rote material but simply interacted: Dick in a funny, funky, non-sequitur stream of consciousness, and Dan in a calm and slightly incredulous manner, reacting to Dick's off-the-wall remarks. "There was a lot of Burns and Allen in us," Martin later explained, and the comparison was apt. "We didn't sing, didn't dance, didn't do impressions. We just developed this wonderful ability to read each other's minds. We never had anything written down."

They always seemed to have work, but their career really picked up steam in 1966 when they headlined in Las Vegas and were chosen to host Dean Martin's summer replacement series on NBC-TV. This led to other offers, and in 1967 they starred in a special for NBC called *Rowan and Martin's Laugh-In,* produced by George Schlatter. The format was frenetic and freewheeling, with a large cast of young comics delivering one-liners, doing blackouts, and participating in wild sight gags. The special was a great success, and in the midst of the next TV season, NBC commissioned a weekly series, which became a national sensation. With such catch phrases as "Sock it to me," "Ver-r-y interesting," and "Look it up in your Funk and Wagnall's," and a talented cast including Goldie Hawn, Arte Johnson, Ruth Buzzi, Jo Anne

Worley, and later Lily Tomlin, the show took off like a skyrocket. And so did Rowan and Martin.

MGM signed them to star in a comedy feature (which most publicity claimed was their first, conveniently ignoring ONCE UPON A HORSE). Playing on one of the buzzwords of the TV show, it was titled THE MALTESE BIPPY. Dan and Dick were surrounded by fine actors and had an experienced comedy director, Norman Panama. But the script (about a werewolf) was only intermittently funny, and the film fizzled at the box office. Plans for a second feature, titled THE MONEY GAME, were quietly dropped.

Laugh-In ran for six years on NBC, after which time Rowan and Martin went their separate ways, Dan to retire and enjoy the good life, Dick to pursue a successful comedy-directing career in television. There was a brief reunion in 1982 for a gimmicky TV show called *Ultraquiz*, but there was no return to movies.

Rowan and Martin were together for some thirty years, then split up without rancor, career disintegration or bankruptcy lurking in the wings. And that, in the annals of comedy teams, may be unique.

Cheech and Chong

Cheech and Chong couldn't have existed before the 1960s. They wouldn't have stood a chance to get on screen before the 1970s. But their sweeping success—in several media—has taken them into the 1980s as the daring duo of counterculture humor.

Cheech and Chong are the most radically different comedy team of all time. Other comedians have been irreverent, but in their films, Cheech and Chong are positively oblivious of society and its mores. And yet the roots of their humor are not really so different from those of their famous predecessors.

Drugs and the street life are the fuel for their humor. They make jokes about all manner of body functions and seem to revel in the sheer tastelessness of it all. It's not attractive, but it certainly appeals to an enormous number of people. Cheech and Chong's record albums have sold an estimated ten million copies. Their first film, predicted to be little more than a cult item, grossed $47.5 million in 1978. It cost just $2 million to make.

Their movies are blissfully incoherent. Some of them are crudely made. Hollywood has never presented such spaced-out stars before, and the sheer novelty of watching two total screw-ups stumble through life seems to please millions of fans.

Cheech and Chong's success is nothing short of a phenomenon. And the most interesting thing about it is that the two men who play these dopes so convincingly are so very different in real life. Richard "Cheech" Marin (nicknamed in childhood after the Chicano food dish cheecharone—or cracklings) is the son of a Los Angeles police officer. He was a straight-A student in school, though he earned a reputation early on as a class clown. He worked his way through college, earning a B.A. degree in English, though his strongest interests were rock music and pottery. He fled to Canada to dodge the draft in 1968, and it was there that he met Thomas Chong.

Thomas Chong's mother was Scotch-Irish, and his father was Chinese. He grew up outside of Calgary, Alberta, and developed a youthful interest in music. He quit school in the tenth grade and supported himself in a variety of jobs, but worked hardest at making it in the music business. While playing with a group called The Vancouvers, he cowrote a hit song for the group called "Does Your Mama Know About Me."

But Chong's interests soon spread from music to comedy, and he spent several years developing his skills by doing improvisation. Eventually he formed an improv group called City Works at his brother's nightclub in Vancouver, and one night a young man named Cheech Marin showed up looking for work.

They performed together for two years in the cast of City Works and then hit the nightclub trail as Cheech and Chong. A Los Angeles gig led to their first record album and an astonishing string of successes—including a prestigious Grammy Award.

Their record producer, Lou Adler, took director's reins for the team's first movie, UP IN SMOKE, and the results took a great many people by surprise. C & C's fans lapped up the free-wheeling comedy about two fuzz-brained fellows who will go anywhere and do anything to get some "good grass." But the movie's utter amiability proved disarming even to nonfans, and even viewers who had no great love for the drug culture found themselves surrendering to laughter.

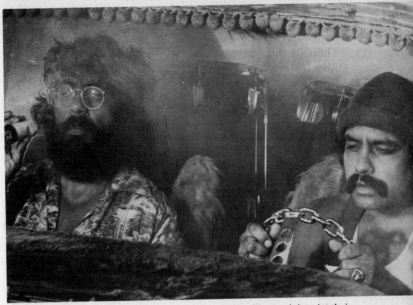

Thomas Chong and Cheech Marin with the world's biggest joint, in their debut movie UP IN SMOKE.

The fact is, none of C & C's subsequent films have maintained that same air of friendly abandon. Or perhaps it *is* just a one-joke idea being stretched too thin with scatological jokes.

But such criticism didn't keep CHEECH & CHONG'S NEXT MOVIE from being a hit. Or CHEECH & CHONG'S NICE DREAMS. Or even THINGS ARE TOUGH ALL OVER, which broke new ground by actually getting C & C involved in a story (and casting them in dual roles, as themselves and as a pair of Arabs who hire them to drive a car full of hidden cash from Chicago to Las Vegas). Thomas Chong has even taken over the directing chores on a number of these films, surrounding the team with compatible, street-wise improv performers. What is the secret of Cheech & Chong's screen success? "We've managed to incorporate the basic humor of poverty into our appeal, which makes it universal—the underdogs against the world," Chong explained in a *Playboy* magazine interview. "We give people hope."

Cheech Marin added, "We represent the frustrations of modern man. Guys who fantasize themselves in great situations they'll never have. To us—I dunno—it's funnier if you

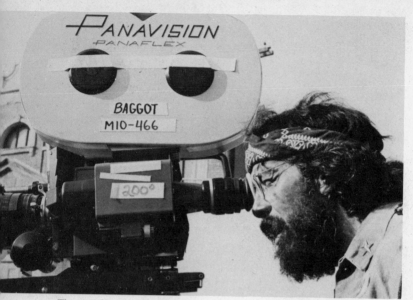

Thomas Chong goes behind the camera to direct CHEECH & CHONG'S NEXT
MOVIE.

don't get laid. It's existentially perfect, somehow. Like
Zen . . ."

The team made token appearances in a compilation film,
IT CAME FROM HOLLYWOOD, and an all-star comedy disaster
called YELLOWBEARD. Then, after the flop of a particularly
poor—and poorly made—vehicle called STILL SMOKIN', which
incorporated live concert footage with some thin plot tissue,
the team decided to try something completely different.
"God came to us in the form of a marijuana joint and said,
'No more dope films,' " joked Chong as the team embarked
ON CHEECH & CHONG'S THE CORSICAN BROTHERS. This costume comedy didn't hit the mark but did prove that C & C
could retain their basic style of humor in a different kind of
setting—here, the era of King Louis XIV in a send-up of
Alexander Dumas' famous story of twins who share each
other's physical sensations. It was widely lambasted by critics—
and audiences—but it was hard to completely dislike a film
that used stale French bread as a weapon and boasted in its
credits that it was filmed entirely on location "somewhere in
France."

Cheech and Chong may not know everything about the art

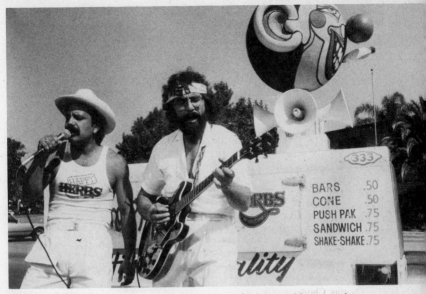

Cheech and Chong play ice-cream vendors with a little something extra in
CHEECH & CHONG'S NICE DREAMS.

of film, but they seem to have mastered the art of living
well: their wives and children are involved with their films
(spouses Rikki Marin and Shelby Fiddis Chong have served
as actresses and associate producers on C & C projects).

And if, at this writing, they've suffered some setbacks in a
fantastic movie career, they're certainly resilient and resourceful enough to bounce back—to the delight of some
and the mystification of others. They're not to everyone's
taste, goodness knows, but Cheech and Chong speak to
their audiences as persuasively, and successfully, as any of
the great comedy teams of the past.

Index

Abbott and Costello team, 87, 242, 268, 270, 275–311, 312, 316, 318, 351; in vaudeville and burlesque, 275, 277; in Broadway revue, 275, 277; film making by, 278–296, 299, 300; on radio, 277; in nightclubs, 279; "Who's on First" routine of, 287, 298; on TV, 296; split-up of team, 302; list of films of, 303–311

Abbott, George, 268, 333

Abbott, William (Bud), *see* Abbott and Costello team

Academy Award, 27, 190

Adler, Lou, 360

Agee, James, 1; on Marx Brothers, 128

Albertson, Frank, 123

Allen, Fred, 316

Allen, Gracie, *see* Burns and Allen team

Allen, Irwin, 131

Allen, Steve, 282, 302

Ameche, Don, 236, 251

Anderson, "Bronco Billy," 4

Andrews Sisters trio, 241, 280, 281

Anita Louise, 87

Ankers, Evelyn, 281

Ansara, Michael, 300

Appleby, Dorothy, 194

Arlen, Harold, 125

Arlen, Richard, 170

Arno, Peter, 71

Arnold, Danny, 317

Askin, Leon, 344

Astaire, Fred, 72, 90, 171, 172, 173–174

Astor, Gertrude, 256

Atkinson, Brooks: on Clark and McCullough, 67, 71; on Olsen and Johnson, 263; on Abbott and Costello, 277; on the Wiere Brothers, 342

Atwill, Lionel, 238, 283, 351, 352

Auer, Mischa, 257, 261

Avalon Four, 158

Baer, Buddy, 296

Baggett, Lynne, 288

Bailey, Bob, 45

Baker, Kenny, 125

Ball, Lucille, 124, 131, 160, 195

Barclay, Don, 151

Barnes, Binnie, 238, 288, 290

Barnes, Howard, on Martin and Lewis, 315

Barr, Charles, 13

Barrat, Robert, 127

Barton, Charles, 301

Barty, Jack, 153

Beddoe, Don, 192

Bedini, Jean, 67, 77

Beebe, Marjorie, 68

Beery, Noah, 90, 92, 93

Beery, Noah, Jr., 269

Beery, Wallace, 33

Benadaret, Bea, 177

Bendix, William, 283, 284

Benedict, Richard, 269

Bennett, Bruce, 195

Benny, Jack, 166, 170, 180, 250

Bergen, Edgar, 348

Berle, Milton, 93, 233

Berlin, Irving, 67, 235, 250

Bernds, Edwards, 193, 206

Bernie, Ben, 250

Besser, Joe, 196, 202, 203–206, 208, 263, 299

Best, Willie, 93

Related Reading from PLUME